Handbook
of Psoriasis

This book is dedicated to my wife Kathryn
and children Amanda, Charles Jr., and Kristen

Handbook of Psoriasis

SECOND EDITION

Charles Camisa, MD

Senior Staff Dermatologist
Cleveland Clinic Foundation
Naples, Florida

Affiliate Associate Professor
Department of Dermatology
University of South Florida
Tampa, Florida

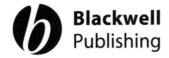
Blackwell
Publishing

© 1998, 2004 by Blackwell Publishing Ltd
Blackwell Publishing, Inc., 350 Main
Street, Malden, Massachusetts
02148-5020, USA
Blackwell Publishing Ltd, 9600 Garsington
Road, Oxford OX4 2DQ, UK
Blackwell Publishing Asia Pty Ltd, 550
Swanston Street, Carlton, Victoria
3053, Australia

First published 1998
Second edition 2004

Library of Congress Cataloging-in-
Publication Data

Camisa, Charles.
 Handbook of psoriasis / Charles Camisa.
 —2nd ed.
     p.   ;   cm.
 Includes bibliographical references and
index.
    ISBN 1-4051-0927-0
 1. Psoriasis—Handbooks, manuals, etc.
 [DNLM: 1. Psoriasis—Handbooks.
 WR 39 C183h 2003] I. Title.
 RL321.C257 2003
 616.5′26—dc22
                        2003017766

ISBN 1-4051-0927-0

A catalogue record for this title is available
from the British Library

Set in 9.5/12.5pt Photina by Graphicraft
Limited, Hong Kong
Printed and bound in the United States
by Sheridan Books, Inc.

Commissioning Editor: Stuart Taylor
Editorial Assistant: Katrina Chandler
Production Editor: Karen Moore
Production Controller: Kate Charman

For further information on Blackwell
Publishing, visit our website:
http://www.blackwellpublishing.com

Contents

A colour plate faces p. 34

Contributors

Kenneth Gordon
Loyola University Medical Center, Maywood, Illinois

Thomas N. Helm
Buffalo Medical Group, Williamsville, New York

Allison Holm
30 North Union Street Suite 105, Rochester, New York

Thomas Osborn
Division of Rheumatology, Mayo Clinic Foundation, Rochester, Minnesota

William S. Wilke
Department of Rheumatic and Immunologic Disease, Cleveland Clinic Foundation, Cleveland, Ohio

Preface

The *Handbook of Psoriasis*, second edition, is intended to be a convenient complete reference work on the diagnosis and treatment of psoriasis. The format is designed to be used by the busy practitioner, primary care and specialist alike; each chapter stands on its own, but cross-reference to other chapters may be necessary to fill in details. This book may also be employed as a brief textbook on psoriasis to be read from cover-to-cover by novices in dermatologic therapy: medical students, house officers, physician's assistants, and nurse practitioners.

The first edition of the *Handbook of Psoriasis* was an abbreviated companion to the complete hard-cover text *Psoriasis* (Blackwell Science 1994). This second edition is an up-to-date stand-alone text that emphasizes how to employ standard treatment protocols such as ultraviolet light, methotrexate, retinoids, and cyclosporine as well as newer combinations of topical corticosteroids and calcipotriene or tazarotene, which have been lately approved or studied.

Every chapter has been extensively updated or rewritten when necessary. The chapter "Childhood psoriasis" was coauthored by a new contributor, Dr Allison Holm, a pediatric dermatologist, and Dr Thomas Helm. Because most of the clinical research in psoriasis since 1998 has involved the novel designer drugs, a new chapter on "Biologic immunotherapy of psoriasis" was written by Dr Kenneth Gordon, a renowned investigator in the field. The advent of biologic agents has also drastically changed the paradigms of pathogenesis and therapy for psoriatic arthritis. Therefore, my Cleveland Clinic rheumatology colleagues, Drs Thomas Osborn and William Wilke, have masterfully rewritten and updated their chapter.

For ease of reading, only selected literature and reviews published since 1998 and important earlier articles are cited at the end of each chapter; however, the number of references has increased. I have also incorporated the appendices containing lists of ultraviolet light therapy equipment and accessories as well as formulae for evaluating psoriasis into the appropriate chapter with websites when applicable. As always, it is assumed that the reader will select the combination of treatments that works best for each individual patient.

Foreword

Why another book on psoriasis? Even though psoriasis affects only 1–3% of the world's population, it has clearly staked an important position among dermatologic diseases. Because of the chronic nature of psoriasis, its severity, which can range from very mild to life-threatening, and the many different forms in which it presents, it remains one of our most challenging diseases. Over the past three decades, more treatments have been developed for psoriasis than perhaps for any other dermatologic disorder. It should therefore be no surprise that the National Psoriasis Foundation is dermatology's largest patient support group. It is the equivalent of the American Diabetes Association for endocrinologists, the Arthritis Foundation for rheumatologists, or the American Heart Association for cardiologists.

Over the past few years, Camisa's first edition of *Handbook of Psoriasis* has proved to be an invaluable tool, one which I have regularly used as a reference in the day-to-day management of my patients. This second edition is equally valuable. There are individual chapters on hard-to-treat body sites such as the nails, scalp, and joints, and new chapters on childhood psoriasis and biologics. But this handbook's most useful features lie in the numerous therapy tables scattered throughout the book. Those tables range from the most up-to-date listing of topical corticosteroid potency rankings to a listing of vendors and models of home phototherapy units. Useful pearls of information are sprinkled throughout the text and tables. For example, how many of us know the amount of ointment required to treat the face and neck twice daily for one week? The answer, 17.5 g, lies in Table 11.5. Detailed instructions on how to use anthralin, how to set up a day care center, how to administer UVB phototherapy, and how to perform minimal erythema dose testing, are only a few of the many subjects covered. Perhaps the most useful chapters are those containing tables outlining the monitoring requirements for drugs such as methotrexate, cyclosporine, and even drugs that are less commonly used, such as hydroxyurea. By virtue of those tables, this book is useful not only for physicians caring for psoriasis patients, but for dermatologists using the aforementioned drugs for any dermatologic disorders.

We are entering an exciting time in dermatology with the development of biologic agents that can target specific steps in the pathogenesis of cutaneous diseases. It is my expectation that we will need a third edition of Camisa's *Handbook of Psoriasis* as we develop new drugs for this disease.

Mark Lebwohl, M.D.

Acknowledgments

This book was made possible by the encouragement and sacrifices of my family, the expert typing by Ms Lisa Meadows, the superb clinical photography of Ms Flora Williams, and the professional editing by the Blackwell staff.

Special thanks are extended to Thomas N. Helm for his contributions to Chapters 8, 10, and 14 and for photomicrography; to Carl Allen for photomicrography; to Ms Williams and Craig Eichler for helpful advice regarding Figure 1.1; to Steven Feldman and Alan Fleischer for permission to use the SAPASI questionnaire; and to Peter Farr for permission to use Figure 13.1. However, I alone accept responsibility for any unintentional factual inaccuracies or errors of omission.

Note: The indications and dosages of all drugs in this book have been recommended in the medical literature and conform to the practices of the general medical community. The medications described do not necessarily have specific approval by the U.S. Food and Drug Administration for use in the diseases and dosages for which they are recommended. The package insert for each drug should be consulted for use and dosage as approved by the FDA. Because standards for usage change, it is advisable to keep abreast of revised recommendations, particularly those concerning new drugs.

1   Overview of psoriasis

Charles Camisa

Psoriasis is at once both a common and complex disease. The prevalence of psoriasis in the population of the U.S. and U.K. is estimated to be about 2%. Severity ranges from a single fingernail pit to skin lesions on a fraction of the skin's surface area to a total-body skin involvement that is associated with disabling arthritis. Psoriasis usually does not take lives, but it does ruin them. The negative effect of psoriasis on a patient's quality of life does not necessarily correspond to the extent of body surface area involved. Patients with psoriasis perceive a reduction in mental and physical functioning comparable to those with cancer, diabetes, and depression.

The cause of this vexing condition is still not known although it is agreed that the clinical lesions represent the end-result of hyperproliferation and abnormal differentiation of the epidermis. Many hypotheses of the pathogenesis of psoriasis have been advanced. Some have been disproved outright or have just fallen out of favor due to lack of evidence. Other hypotheses remain viable candidates to explain the primary pathophysiologic alterations or else they have been validated only as epiphenomena.

Before the advent of modern technology with its sophisticated instrumentation for identifying and quantitating molecules in skin, dermatologists relied on clinical and histopathologic morphology for correlating cause and cure to a skin disease (Table 1.1).

Referring to psoriasis, Goeckerman said, "The comparative frequency with which psoriasis occurs demands that not only the specialist but the general practitioner should be familiar with effective therapeutic measures directed against it." Many different treatments exist for psoriasis; they are individually and in combination frequently effective, and nearly completely so for some subsets of psoriatic patients. Psoriasis is the third most common reason for office visits to dermatologists (behind acne and warts). It has been

1

Table 1.1 Clinicopathological correlations and psoriasis therapy.

Clinical morphology	Histopathological morphology	Treatment
Scales	Hyperkeratosis/parakeratosis	Keratolytics, emollients
Thickness	Acanthosis ("psoriasiform hyperplasia")	Coal tar, anthralin, retinoids, vitamin D analogues, phototherapy
Redness	Dilated and tortuous capillaries	Corticosteroids
	Lymphocytes in dermis	Cyclosporine, tacrolimus, phototherapy, biologic immunotherapies
Pustules	Neutrophils in epidermis	Retinoids, methotrexate

estimated that there are 1.5 million visits per year to hospital or office-based practitioners for psoriasis; 80% are to dermatologists and 20% to physicians of other specialties. Another 1.5 million visits are for outpatient UVB or PUVA. Approximately 58% of new cases of psoriasis are first encountered by primary care physicians, which emphasizes the importance of recognizing psoriasis in practice and treating it competently. A study designed to compare the ability of primary care physicians to diagnose common skin diseases from color slides showed that psoriasis was recognized correctly 85% of the time (compared to 100% for dermatologists).

Managed care created new responsibilities for general practitioners (GPs) and dermatologists. Both groups learned how to practice in a cost-conscious manner without compromising the optimal outcome for the patient with psoriasis. Collaboration between the dermatologist and GP is essential: the dermatologist should educate the GP in differential diagnosis and the fundamentals of topical treatment. The two parties must come to terms as to what constitutes "primary care of the skin." Based on interest and available time, the GP may pursue more advanced dermatologic training via reading, attending continuing medical education courses, or spending time seeing patients with the dermatologist.

Given all of the advances made in anti-psoriasis therapy since 1925 (Fig. 1.1), it is surprising that topical steroids are still prescribed at 70% of visits to dermatologists for psoriasis. The more complex systemic therapies (PUVA, methotrexate, retinoids, etc.) for the more severe forms of psoriasis are prescribed at about 10% of visits to dermatologists. No wonder that 32% of patients with

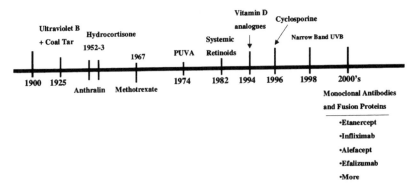

Figure 1.1 Timeline of breakthroughs in psoriasis therapy.

severe psoriasis reported that the treatment they are receiving is not "aggressive" enough in a telephone survey conducted by the National Psoriasis Foundation.

For the purpose of this book, "psoriasis" is considered a single disease entity with several morphologic variants, and a full range of severity and expression based on:

1 Heredity (certain HLA types and psoriasis susceptibility genes).

2 Environmental factors (such as trauma and climate).

3 Associated diseases (particularly infections and emotional stress).

4 Concomitant medications.

5 Immunologic status of the host.

The first four factors mentioned have been studied by direct observation, simple laboratory techniques, and statistical analysis, but the fifth had to await the development of in vitro assays of cellular function and the accurate identification and measurement of nanomolar quantities of chemokines elaborated by cells in blood and skin. Historically, polymorphonuclear leukocytes and mononuclear phagocytes were examined first because they were readily retrieved and purified in large quantities from circulating blood. The roles of lymphocytes and Langerhans' cells were subsequently explored by in situ monoclonal antibody labeling techniques. It was soon recognized that differences in the microenvironment of skin could be influenced by soluble mediators secreted by all of the cell types involved, including the keratinocyte itself. A "new" skin cell with antigen-processing capability, the dermal dendrocyte, has been proposed as the pivotal cell type in the autoimmune pathogenesis of psoriasis. The immunosuppressive drugs used in organ transplantation, cyclosporine and tacrolimus, block inter-leukin-2 production and the cascade of cytokines and receptors before slowing hyperproliferation and blunting the concomitant inflammatory responses in the skin. This finding suggests that some aberration in the regulation of interleukins, growth factors, or adhesion molecules is the primary pathologic process in psoriasis. Taking the lead from these clues, further advances in molecular biologic techniques have allowed the synthesis of novel fusion proteins, recombinant human interleukins, and monoclonal antibodies that target specific cell types, block T-cell activation and migration into skin, skew the cytokine response of psoriasis from predominantly type 1 towards type 2, and inhibit the action of proinflammatory cytokines that induce or maintain psoriatic changes.

Where then does arthritis fit into this picture? Although less common than the skin disease, occurring in about 10% of cases of psoriasis, psoriatic arthritis, by its nature, can be more physically disabling. A joint space is about as far removed anatomically and functionally from hyperproliferative epidermis as one can get. Mucous membranes and the eye are more closely related to skin embryologically than synovium is but are infrequently affected by psoriasis. Is psoriasis therefore a systemic inflammatory autoimmune disease like lupus erythematosus? Other than the skin and the articular involvement in a minority of cases, other organ systems such as the liver, gut, and kidney are rarely affected by psoriasis. The hypothesis of aberrant immunoregulatory control, combined with genetic and environmental factors, may help to explain the accumulation of inflammatory cells in such disparate sites and influence fibroblasts in the dermis and synovium to induce proliferation of keratinocytes or synoviocytes, respectively. T-lymphocytes with the same restricted T-cell receptor have been found in skin lesions and synovial fluid of patients, suggesting that one super-antigen may have activated the cells that play a role in the initiation and maintenance of psoriasis and psoriatic arthritis. Some systemic treatments, e.g. sulfasalazine, methotrexate, cyclosporine, and etanercept, ameliorate both the skin and joint disease.

The total annual expenditure for cutaneous psoriasis treatment in the U.S. was estimated to be between $1.6 billion and $3.2 billion (Sander *et al.*) even before the use of biologic immunotherapy, currently the most expensive systemic treatment available. When tailoring therapy to the individual patient, physicians should base selections on efficacy, toxicity, accessibility, and cost. Sander *et al.*

Table 1.2 Psoriasis treatments listed in descending order of estimated annual cost.

Treatment	Results
Infliximab	Excellent
Alefacept	Good–Excellent
Etanercept	Good–Excellent
Cyclosporine	Excellent
Day Goeckerman	Excellent
PUVA	Good–Excellent
Narrowband UVB	Good–Excellent
Acitretin	Good
Methotrexate	Excellent
Hydroxyurea	Fair
Tazarotene (topical)	Fair–Good
Calcipotriene (topical)	Good
Potent topical corticosteroids	Fair
Commercial tanning bed	Poor–Fair

in 1993 determined that excellent results can be achieved at high cost with the Goeckerman regimen in a psoriasis day treatment center (although less expensive than hospitalization) and that methotrexate was the most cost-effective systemic treatment at the time. The new biologic immunotherapies will have to be compared to methotrexate in this regard. The cost of using a single treatment includes the cost of the drug as well as office visits and laboratory tests for efficacy and safety monitoring, respectively. It does not include time lost from employment or time spent receiving or applying the treatments. Moreover, in actual practice, two or more treatments are routinely employed simultaneously for additive or synergistic effects. While a cure for psoriasis remains elusive in the twenty-first century, the treatments listed in Table 1.2, as well as some of the investigational and less popular ones discussed later in this book, offer incalculable advantages compared to those of less than a century ago.

Selected references

Feldman S. R., Clark A. R. (1998) Psoriasis. *Med Clin N Am* **85**, 1135–1144.
Goeckerman W. H. (1925) The treatment of psoriasis. *Northwest Med* **24**, 229–231.
Kirsner R. S., Federman D. G. (1995) Managed care: the dermatologist as a primary care provider. *J Am Acad Dermatol* **33**, 535–537.

Krueger G., Koo J., Lebwohl M. *et al.* (2001) The impact of psoriasis on quality of life. Results of a 1998 National Psoriasis Foundation Patient-Membership Survey. *Arch Dermatol* **137**, 280–284.

Lebwohl M. G., Feldman S. R., Koo J. Y. M., Menter M. A. (2002) *Psoriasis Treatment Options and Patient Management.* National Psoriasis Foundation Portland, OR.

Ramsay D. L., Fox A. B. (1981) The ability of primary care physicians to recognize the common dermatoses. *Arch Dermatol* **117**, 620–622.

Sander H. M., Morris L. F., Phillips C. M. *et al.* (1993) The annual cost of psoriasis. *J Am Acad Dermatol* **28**, 422–425.

Stern R. S. (1996) Utilization of outpatient care for psoriasis. *J Am Acad Dermatol* **35**, 543–545.

2 The clinical variants of psoriasis

Charles Camisa

Introduction

The prevalence of psoriasis in the U.S. and U.K. populations is about 2%. The prevalence of psoriasis is much lower in Native Americans, African-Americans, and Asians. Most African-Americans trace their ancestry to West Africa where the prevalence of psoriasis is 0.7%. There are between 150,000 and 260,000 new cases of psoriasis per year in the U.S. The sex incidence is equal. The mean age of onset is about 30 years, with the range being from birth to 100 years. Females may be affected earlier in life than males.

The cause of psoriasis remains an enigma.

The most common pattern of psoriasis is that of a symmetric inflammatory papulosquamous disease (see Plate 1, facing p. 34). Recognition of the classic morphology of the skin lesions by an experienced clinician is usually sufficient for confirmation of the diagnosis, but simple diagnostic maneuvers, such as examination of scales for hyphal elements using potassium hydroxide (KOH), serologic testing for syphilis, and skin biopsy, may be necessary to rule out other considerations.

Koebner phenomenon

One of the hallmarks of psoriasis is the Koebner phenomenon, or isomorphic response, which occurs in some patients with unstable or flaring psoriasis. Physical trauma results in linear or figurate patterns of psoriasis that conform to the localization of injury from a scratch, burn, surgical incision (Fig. 2.1), or skin graft donor site. Apparently, injury to the epidermis alone can induce the Koebner phenomenon, as shown by cellophane "tape stripping," a technique commonly employed by investigators that removes the entire stratum

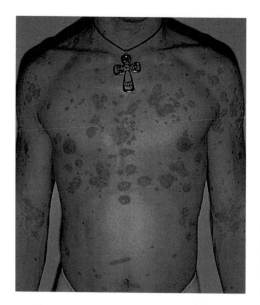

Figure 2.1 Generalized plaque psoriasis with linear lesion above umbilicus secondary to laceration (Koebner phenomenon).

corneum but leaves the granular layer and stratum spinosum intact. Needle scarification is an alternate method. The isomorphic response is not unique to psoriasis: it can occur with lichen planus, lichen nitidus, vitiligo, and other skin diseases. Routine daily trauma may be partly responsible for the prominent involvement of the scalp, elbows, knees, hands, fingernails, sacrum, and genitalia. Because the scales of about 50% of psoriatic plaques are colonized by pathogenic staphylococci, it is important to clear psoriasis as much as possible prior to elective surgery, particularly orthopedic surgery, in order to reduce the risks of postoperative infection and psoriasis developing in the healing incision.

Certain drugs have been associated with a kind of "endogenous Koebner phenomenon," notably, lithium, antimalarials, beta-adrenergic-blocking agents, and interferons, which can induce psoriasis or aggravate preexisting disease in some patients. Flare-ups of psoriasis may be triggered by streptococcal tonsillitis or pharyngitis and upper respiratory viral infections. Acute guttate psoriasis is frequently the initial episode of chronic psoriasis.

Genetics

There is no doubt that heredity plays a role in the development of psoriasis. Earlier onset of psoriasis tends to be associated with familial aggregation and more severe disease. For example, 40% of patients with an early age of onset had immediate family members who were also affected. Farber and Nall found that, of psoriatics indicating familial aggregation, 73% had onset before the age of 30 years. But when a patient developed psoriasis after the age of 20 years and no parent had psoriasis, only 3% of siblings had psoriasis. In cases when psoriasis developed before the age of 15 years and one parent had psoriasis, 50% of siblings developed psoriasis by the age of 60 years. Patients with severe psoriasis with onset at the age of 15 years or earlier were three times more likely to have siblings with psoriasis than were patients with onset after the age of 30. Twin studies showed 67% concordance for monozygotic twins compared to 18% for dizygotic twins. The lack of complete concordance in monozygotic twin pairs suggests that environmental factors are also important and supports the theory of multifactorial inheritance of psoriasis.

Christophers and Henseler have distinguished two types of non-pustular psoriasis on the basis of family history, HLA associations, and age of onset. They designated as type I those patients with a positive family history, onset during the second decade, and a close association between HLA-Cw6, -B13, and-Bw57 (a subtype of B17). Type II psoriasis manifests during the fifth decade, does not involve parents and siblings, and is associated with HLA-Cw2 and -B27, with relative risks of developing psoriasis of 6.1 and 3.1, respectively. Swanbeck *et al.* analyzed age of onset for 11,366 psoriasis patients and found a definite peak around puberty and maxima at about 30 and 50 years with a great deal of overlap.

Farber and Nall disputed the bimodal age incidence. Their peak age of incidence is in the second and third decades. They posited that the bimodal or trimodal curves reported may be an artifact of an excess number of HLA-B13- and -B17-positive individuals who tended to have disease at an earlier onset.

A study of 12 Canadian families with 15 sibling pairs with psoriasis was analyzed for haplotype sharing. The results suggest that either more than one gene contributes to psoriasis susceptibility or that there is a gene–dosage effect. All sib pairs shared at least one haplotype, and 13 of the 15 pairs were HLA identical compared to an expected frequency of four. The extended haplotype CW6-B57-DRB1*0701-DQA1*0201-DQB1*0303 was found in 35% of type I psoriatics and 2% of controls. (DRB1*0701 is a subtype of DR7; DQB1*0303 encodes the DQ9 molecule.) A new haplotype was detected at a significantly higher frequency in Croatian type I patients. It differed from the Canadian psoriatics only by the substitution of DQB1*0201.

The development of psoriasis is related to the effects of one or more genes located near the HLA region that are able to influence autoreactivity. However, no differences in the patterns of T-cell receptor variable regions could be detected in lesional biopsy specimens from patients with type I and type II nonpustular psoriasis.

The Cw6 antigen is probably not the causative gene for psoriasis but rather a marker for the gene determining susceptibility to psoriasis. The putative gene, dubbed PSORS1, is located on the short arm of chromosome 6 within the major histocompatibility locus and is mapped just beyond HLA-C toward HLA-A. Positional candidate genes include corneodesmin and alpha-helix coiled-coilrod homologs as well as HLA-C. Specific alleles of the three candidate genes within the PSORI region are associated with guttate psoriasis and psoriasis vulgaris but *not* palmoplantar pustulosis. Overall, the relative risk for developing psoriasis in patients with Cw6 is 13.3. The risk is doubled if Cw6 is associated with HLA-B57 (but not -B13). In ethnic groups with very low frequencies of HLA-B57, such as Native Americans and Eskimos, psoriasis is rare. A mutation replacing alanine at position 73 on many HLA-C alleles has been found in some ethnic groups with psoriasis, but its significance is uncertain. Psoriasis is the only disease showing HLA-C as a predominant marker, but the class II antigens, DR4 and DR7, also show significantly increased association with psoriasis. Patients with type I psoriasis are more likely to express Cw6 (85%) and DR7 alleles (70%) than type II patients (14 and 30%, respectively).

Among 369 Icelandic Caucasians with familial psoriasis who were typed for HLA-C, significant clinical differences were found between the positive and negative groups. For example, Cw6-positive patients had an earlier age of onset of psoriasis, more guttate-type onset, more extensive disease, and a higher incidence of the Koebner phenomenon. Cw6-negative patients were more likely to demonstrate psoriatic nail changes and psoriatic arthritis. In a separate study of 29 consecutive Caucasians with guttate psoriasis associated with a history of a sore throat, 100% carried the Cw*0602 allele.

Genome-wide linkage scans of multiply affected families has uncovered psoriasis susceptibility genes on chromosomes 1q, 3, 4q, 6q, 10, 16q, 17q, 19, and 20p. Not all loci have been independently confirmed by more than one research group; new ones will probably be discovered. Only 10% of carriers of PSORS1 on chromosome 6q (discussed above) develop psoriasis, supporting the polygenic theory of inheritance of the disease. Genes regulating epidermal differentiation are located on chromosome 1q. The susceptibility locus at chromosome 17q does not require HLA-Cw6 positivity. Elder *et al.* have proposed the existence of "severity genes" which contribute to the susceptibility to other autoimmune diseases. For example, there is a gene implicated in Crohn's disease that is located in the same region as PSORS 8 in chromosome 16.

Plaque-type psoriasis

Plaque-type psoriasis is the most common morphologic variant encountered in practice and is called *psoriasis vulgaris*. A fully developed clinical lesion of psoriasis vulgaris is a well-demarcated, red, round to oval plaque, 1 cm or longer across, surmounted by white silvery scales and overlying bony prominences. Psoriasis vulgaris assumes different appearances depending on the anatomic site involved, the activity of disease (i.e. stable, progressive, or resolving), and whether any treatment is being used. In darkly pigmented patients, the red to violet distinction is lost and lesions

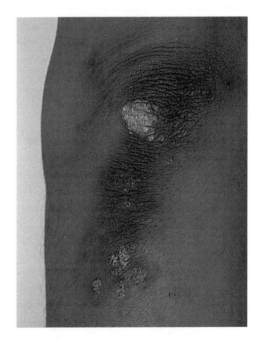

Figure 2.2 Psoriasis on the arm of a black woman.

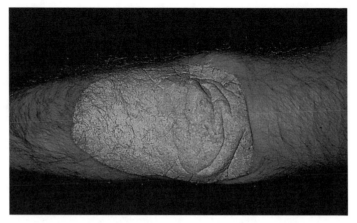

Figure 2.3 Neglected "inveterate" or "elephantine" plaque of psoriasis on an elbow.

appear hyperpigmented with various shades of brown to black, especially if they are chronically scratched or rubbed (Fig. 2.2). The scales may appear: (1) white and powdery; (2) micaceous and peeling off in thin transparent sheets; (3) "dirty" or rupioid; or, (4) ostraceous, that is, resembling an oyster shell. Thick, inveterate ("elephantine") plaques may develop gradually on the sacrum and extremities (Fig. 2.3) in some patients who neglect the care of their skin.

The primary lesion of all variants is probably a pinpoint erythematous macule, otherwise clinically nondiagnostic, that expands circumferentially, develops induration, and exfoliates. Some of the scales are adherent and may become heaped up over time if not physically or chemically dislodged. Such lesions may coalesce with each other to form large plaques with irregular (geographic) outlines. *The distinction between involved and uninvolved skin is usually sharp.* The edge of the untreated lesion is discernibly raised by palpation unless it is very early or resolving. A ring of vasoconstriction surrounding the plaque may be observed (Woronoff ring), especially during ultraviolet light and anthralin therapy. When the psoriatic plaque attains a sufficient amount of scale, the Auspitz sign may be elicited. When the adherent scale is scraped off, pinpoint bleeding becomes evident as dilated capillaries, traumatized near the skin surface, discharge their contents. Although the Auspitz sign is the clinical correlate to the histopathologic finding of a

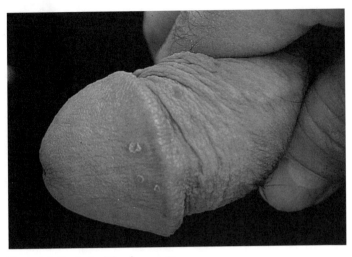

Figure 2.4 Psoriasis of the glans penis.

thinned epidermis overlying the dermal papillae between elongated tube-like rete pegs ("thin suprapapillary plate"), it lacks sensitivity and specificity.

The most common areas of involvement are the elbows, knees, scalp, sacrum, umbilicus, intergluteal cleft, and genitalia (Fig. 2.4). The latter three areas are often overlooked in a cursory examination of the skin but can be very helpful for diagnosis. The involvement is more or less symmetrical; for example, lesions may be present on both knees although they may not be exactly of the same size, configuration, or location. Of course, only one knee, one elbow, or one side of the scalp may have psoriasis.

Any one of the most common sites of predilection may also be the solitary site of psoriasis. While this is well recognized for the scalp, it also typically occurs on the male genitalia, usually the glans penis.

Differential diagnosis

Limited psoriasis on the extremities or the nape of the neck may be difficult to distinguish from subacute and chronic nummular eczema or lichen simplex chronicus. In the former, the lesions are usually not so well defined from normal skin and the scale has a yellowish to crusted appearance. In the latter, lichenification, the accentuation of the normal skin markings, is present, but is rarely seen in psoriasis. However, pruritus may occur in eczema, lichen simplex chronicus, and psoriasis. Excoriations with fissuring can be seen in psoriasis of the scalp and nape of the neck.

As plaques of psoriasis expand, they may clear centrally, spontaneously, or with treatment, especially with the systemic retinoids. This results in annular, arciform, or other bizarre patterns of psoriasis on the skin, raising a differential diagnosis that includes tinea corporis, erythema annulare centrifugum, erythema gyratum repens, and mycosis fungoides.

Genital psoriasis

Patients with genital psoriasis may fear the worst and delay presentation to their physician. Unfortunately, some general practitioners, venereologists, gynecologists and urologists are not familiar with the clinical manifestations of vulvar or penile psoriasis and may heighten concerns of sexually transmitted disease or cancer. It is not uncommon for the physician to prescribe a mild corticosteroid or antifungal cream. While neither of these medicaments or their combination will harm the psoriasis and may in fact provide some temporary relief, the patient still remains without a diagnosis, possibly without a complete skin examination or any further education about psoriasis.

The clinical history of external genital psoriasis is usually one of a mild, chronic dry scaling process that becomes redder and more apparent after sexual intercourse. It does not itch. The folds between the labia and groin may show a red raw surface with exudation or fissure. The *differential diagnosis* includes the papulosquamous disorders: lichen planus, seborrheic dermatitis, chronic eczema (irritant or contact allergic), secondary syphilis, and candidiasis. Lichen sclerosus is less likely to present in this manner. Syphilis and candidiasis can be eliminated easily with serologic testing and KOH examination of skin scrapings or fungal culture. Seborrheic dermatitis typically involves the hairy areas of the face, nasolabial folds, scalp (dandruff), the midportion of the chest, the axillae, and groin but still may be difficult to differentiate from psoriasis clinically (and histologically). The eczematous dermatoses usually itch and may be temporally related to the use of lubricants, spermicides, and latex in condoms or diaphragms. Lichen planus of the glans penis tends to be more violaceous and less scaly than psoriasis; it may be annular or have the distinctive morphology of Wickham's striae. Lichen planus (LP) of the vulva is more likely to involve the mucous membranes and may demonstrate striae or simply erythema with erosions of the introitus. The typical distribution of LP on the skin, nails, and oral mucous membranes helps to clinch the diagnosis. When there are no other signs to help clarify the diagnosis, and serology and cultures are negative, biopsy and/or allergy patch testing may be the next logical step.

Treatment

Penile psoriasis responds very well to twice daily applications of a medium potency corticosteroid ointment such as triamcinolone acetonide 0.1%, fluocinolone acetonide 0.025%, or hydrocortisone valerate 0.2% for 1–2 weeks. Thereafter, a single application following intercourse, after the penis is washed with mild soap and water, usually prevents aggravation of the condition by the isomorphic response. Employing this treatment, I have not encountered problems such as atrophy, striae, or sexual dysfunction. For intertriginous psoriasis of the vulva, the nonfluorinated topical corticosteroid creams plus a broad-spectrum antifungal imidazole cream (e.g. ketoconazole, miconazole, clotrimazole, econazole) applied once daily are usually helpful. Anthralin or coal tar products are irritants and should not be applied to the genitalia, which should also be shielded during exposure to UVB or PUVA.

Psoriasis of the palms and soles

Psoriasis of the palms and soles usually begins on the pressure-bearing areas and may not be as well demarcated as plaques on the rest of the body. Lesions are reddish brown and may not be symmetric owing to differences in use of the dominant hand or foot (see Plate 2, facing p. 34). In a survey of a large psoriasis clinic in India, all patients with unilateral palmar psoriasis had involvement of the dominant hand. Involvement may extend to the entire volar surface with paronychial and nail disease. Fissures may occur on fingertips and skin folds. Confusion of hand dermatitis with other causes is likely unless there are some typical psoriasis lesions elsewhere on the body. Tinea manum or pedis and crusted scabies are easily ruled out by KOH examinations of scales for fungal hyphae and mites.

Facial psoriasis

Facial lesions usually represent the extension of psoriasis from the scalp onto the forehead, sideburn area, ears, and postauricular area where fissuring may occur. The external auditory canal may also be affected by psoriasis, especially in erythrodermic states, and sufficient scale accumulates in this tight space to significantly reduce air conduction of sound. The desquamated skin must be irrigated and debrided as often as once per month when the disease is active, especially to maintain normal hearing in elderly patients with a preexisting deficit. Facial psoriasis has been considered to be a sign of severe or extensive disease (see Plate 3, facing p. 34). In erythrodermic psoriasis, the face may be completely covered. A few small guttate lesions may occur on the face during an acute guttate flare. Small patches of psoriasis, with more white scales than erythema, may be seen on the eyelids of patients with mild to moderate cases of psoriasis vulgaris, or may be the presenting sign. The differential diagnosis of eyelid psoriasis includes atopic dermatitis, allergic contact dermatitis (to nail polish, cosmetics, wetting solutions, etc.), and seborrheic blepharitis. If only the head is affected, the presentation may be very similar to seborrheic dermatitis. In the latter, the lesions are less discrete and the scale is yellowish and greasy rather than silvery and dry. Involvement of the nasolabial fold is typical for seborrheic dermatitis. In some patients, it is impossible to distinguish between the two, and use of the contracted terms *sebopsoriasis* or *seborrhiasis* is appropriate.

Follicular psoriasis

Psoriasis of the hair follicles is probably underreported. Erythematous scaly follicular papules on the trunk and extremities may coalesce into plaques or be associated with plaque-type psoriasis elsewhere.

Flexural or inverse psoriasis

Flexural or inverse psoriasis may also mimic seborrheic dermatitis. By definition, it occurs in the intertriginous areas: axillae, inframammary areas, groins, intergluteal cleft, and antecubital and popliteal fossae. The relative contributions of friction and resident microbiologic flora are unknown, but obese persons are particularly prone to flexural psoriasis. The appearance is that of a smooth, well-demarcated, salmon-colored macular patch. It is usually devoid of scale, moist, and superficially eroded with fissuring right at the "hinge" of the body fold. Dry areas have a "glazed-over" appearance and are frequently colonized with *Candida albicans*, staphylococci, and streptococci. Inverse psoriasis may occur alone but is more frequently accompanied by plaque psoriasis elsewhere.

Treatment

Scraping for KOH and culture for fungus and bacteria is recommended followed by the appropriate oral antibiotic coverage. Astringent (Burow's) compresses, allowing the skin to dry by air or blow-drying at a cool setting, topical antifungal creams, and non-fluorinated corticosteroids, such as hydrocortisone with iodoquinol or iodochlorhydroxyquin, are palliatives. Castellani's paint and gentian violet are still excellent traditional treatments for drying fissures and erosions in intertriginous areas. The lesions may not clear without significant weight reduction and systemic anti-psoriatic therapy.

Lines of treatment for psoriasis vulgaris

The treatments for ordinary plaque-type psoriasis are selected from the "lines" shown on Table 2.1 based on criteria covered in their respective chapters. The lines of therapy are arranged in the most likely order of adoption for psoriasis of moderate severity. Topical therapies are less toxic than light therapy, which is less toxic than systemic therapies. Line III comprises the most efficacious treatments having the greatest potential toxicity (and often the most expensive). Line IV drugs are weakly to moderately effective but have low toxic potential. It is usually safe and acceptable to combine treatments from different lines. Patients with the most severe and complicated cases of psoriasis involving arthropathy tend to accumulate in dermatology or rheumatology practices by way of consultations, self-referrals, and occasionally in-patient hospitalization. For these specialists, Line V "Innovative Systemic Therapy" and Line VI "Investigative Systemic Therapy" will be covered in Chapters 19 and 20.

Table 2.1 Lines of therapy for psoriasis.

I. *Topical therapy*
    Emollients
    Keratolytics
        Salicylic acid
        Lactic acid
        Urea
    Calcipotriene, Tacalcitol†, Calcitriol† (Ch. 18)
    Anthralin (usually short contact) (Ch. 12)
    Corticosteroids (Ch. 11)
        Topical
        Hydrocolloid occlusive dressing
        Intralesional injections
    Coal tar (Ch. 13)
    Tazarotene (Ch. 15)

II. *Light therapy* (Ch. 13)
    Natural sunlight
    Ultraviolet B (broad-band)
    Ultraviolet B + coal tar (Goeckerman regimen)
    Ultraviolet B + anthralin (Ingram regimen)
    Ultraviolet B narrow-band (311–313 nm)
    Eximer 308 nm laser

III. *Systemic therapy (high efficacy, high toxicity)*
    Photochemotherapy (PUVA) (Ch. 14)
    PUVA may be combined with UVB
    Retinoids (may be combined with UVB or PUVA) (Ch. 15)
        Etretinate†
        Acitretin
        Isotretinoin*
    Methotrexate (Ch. 16)
    Cyclosporine (Ch. 17)

IV. *Systemic therapy* * (moderate efficacy, low toxicity)
    Sulfasalazine (Ch. 19)
    Hydroxyurea (Ch. 19)
    Calcitriol (Ch. 18)
    Antibiotics

V. *Innovative systemic therapy* * (moderate efficacy, high toxicity) (Ch. 19)
    Azathioprine
    6-Thioguanine
    Mycophenolate mofetil
    Tacrolimus
    DAB(389)IL-2 fusion protein
    Alefacept (human LFA-3/IgG1 fusion protein) (FDA-approved January 2003)

Table 2.1 (*cont'd*)

VI. *Investigative systemic therapy** (Ch. 20)
Propyl thiouracil
Fumaric acid esters
Pimecrolimus
Efalizamab (anti-CD11a monoclonal antibody)++
Etanercept (anti-TNF receptor fusion protein)
Infliximab (anti-TNF monoclonal antibody)

---

*Not approved for psoriasis by the U.S. FDA.
†Not available in U.S.
++Dermatologic and Ophthalmic Drugs Advisory Committee recommended approval by FDA September 2003.

Guttate psoriasis

The clinical appearance of guttate psoriasis may be likened to splashing a pail of water on a naked body from a distance, with every drop of water that alights on the skin becoming a lesion (Fig. 2.5). This form of psoriasis most often affects children and young

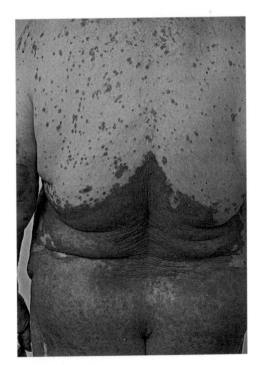

Figure 2.5 Eruptive guttate lesions of psoriasis superior to the chronic plaques.

adults. The prevalence of guttate psoriasis in the psoriatic population in general is about 18%. There is frequently a prior history of upper respiratory infection, pharyngitis, or tonsillitis. Cases of acute guttate flares of psoriasis that were believed to be precipitated by infections with Groups A, C and G streptococci have been reported.

The clinical lesions range in diameter from 0.1 to 1.0 cm and are not as indurated or scaly as the lesions of plaque-type psoriasis. They predominate on the trunk and proximal areas of the extremities and are likely to involve the face. The eruption becomes more symmetric with time. Guttate psoriasis may be the initial manifestation of psoriasis or it may represent an acute flare of preexisting chronic plaque-type psoriasis. In the latter instance, the diagnosis is secure, and a prior streptococcal infection may be suspected. When it is an initial manifestation, however, differential points must be raised. In the young child, confirmation of a streptococcal infection by culture or serology may be most helpful. A history of psoriasis in one or both parents increases the likelihood of early-onset psoriasis, especially in females. In the older child or young adult, the differential diagnosis includes pityriasis rosea, secondary syphilis, drug eruption, and guttate parapsoriasis.

Leung *et al.* found that acute guttate psoriasis following streptococcal throat infection in 10 patients was the result of streptococcal pyrogenic exotoxin C, which acts as a superantigen and stimulates VB2+ expansion of both CD4+ and CD8+ T-cells in lesional and perilesional skin. The streptococci isolated did not express any consistent M-protein type. There was no evidence for VB expansion of circulating T-cells; that is, no toxic shock-like syndrome. In the patients who then develop chronic plaque psoriasis, the activated skin-infiltrating autoreactive T-cells persist due to the abnormal recognition of specific skin antigens. Candidates for autoantigens include keratins or carbohydrates, which have cross-reactive determinants with bacterial antigens.

Treatment

In general, new-onset guttate psoriasis related to streptococcal infection involutes rapidly within a 4-week period with antibiotic treatment. In patients in whom there is familial aggregation of the disease, guttate psoriasis may evolve into localized or extensive chronic plaque-type psoriasis. In patients with chronic psoriasis who develop a guttate exacerbation, empiric treatment with antibiotics such as penicillin or erythromycin, 250 mg q.i.d. for 10–14 days, is indicated.

If guttate psoriasis does not improve within a 4-week period, if it progresses, or if it is associated with preexisting moderately severe psoriasis, outpatient UVB or natural sunlight, if available, is almost always indicated. It is difficult to justify a full Goeckerman regimen for new guttate psoriasis; however, this may be appropriate for persistent disseminated guttate lesions associated with some plaques or with flaring of stable psoriasis. The prognosis is good with outpatient therapy consisting of white petrolatum or coal tar gels applied prior to suberythmogenic UVB administered 3–5 times a week.

Pustular psoriasis

History

The pustular variants of psoriasis embody the most confusing nosology, colorful eponyms, and difficult treatment problems for the clinician. The patients with generalized disease are often among the most seriously ill, requiring hospitalization. The pustuloses can be separated into localized and generalized forms (Table 2.2). Palmoplantar pustulosis (PPP) is by far the most common pustular variant. It accounted for 1.7% of cases of psoriasis in a survey of 401 Irish patients, only one of whom had generalized pustular psoriasis (GPP).

The various forms have been recognized, reported, and embellished in the dermatologic literature spanning more than a century.

Table 2.2 Pustular psoriasis variants.

I. *Localized*
   One or more plaques with pustules
   Palmoplantar pustulosis (pustulosis palmaris et plantaris)
   Annular (? Subcorneal pustular dermatosis of Sneddon and Wilkinson)
   Acropustulosis (Acrodermatitis continua of Hallopeau)
   Keratoderma blennorhagicum (Reiter's syndrome)
   SAPHO syndrome (synovitis, acne, pustulosis, hyperostosis, osteitis)
II. *Generalized*
   von Zumbusch-type
   Impetigo herpetiformis
   Acute generalized exanthematous pustulosis

Hebra (1872) described impetigo herpetiformis as a fatal generalized pustular eruption in pregnant women. Hallopeau (1898) reported an inflammatory pustular condition of the fingers and hands related to trauma and a tendency for local destruction and generalization called acrodermatitis continua. GPP of von Zumbusch was first reported in 1910 in a patient with preexisting psoriasis vulgaris. In 1956, Sneddon and Wilkinson described a chronic benign sterile pustular disease called *subcorneal pustular dermatosis*, based on the typical histology lacking spongiosis, acantholysis, bacteria, and a deeper epidermal pustule. This condition is now considered a variant of subacute annular psoriasis by some, but enough clinical differences exist to consider subcorneal pustular dermatosis as a separate entity. In a series of publications between 1968 and 1971, Ryan and Baker reported the characteristics of 155 patients with GPP. They showed conclusively that GPP of von Zumbusch could be the final common denominator of all pustular variants, especially if the patients received systemic corticosteroids for preexisting psoriasis.

Pathomechanisms

Aberrations in the function of various leukocyte types have been found in many patients with pustular psoriasis. Patients with pustular psoriasis (including GPP, PPP, and acrodermatitis continua) had significantly higher polymorphonuclear leukocyte (PML) chemotaxis than did patients with psoriasis vulgaris. By contrast, monocyte chemotaxis is lower in pustular psoriasis than psoriasis vulgaris and not different from that in normal control subjects. The phagocytosis of IgG-coated latex particles by PMLs is significantly enhanced in patients with either psoriasis vulgaris or PPP.

In one study, natural killer cell cytotoxicity of mononuclear cells isolated from the peripheral blood of four patients with GPP was significantly reduced compared to psoriasis vulgaris and healthy control subjects. A rapid decline in the absolute number of lymphocytes was observed in 10 patients one day prior to a generalized pustular flare of psoriasis in the face of fever and leukocytosis. Nine of the patients had received systemic steroids within one month of the flare, confirming the precipitating role of these drugs. The authors (Sauder *et al.*) posited that steroid-induced stability of lysosomal membranes may have led to reactive lability when the steroids were withdrawn.

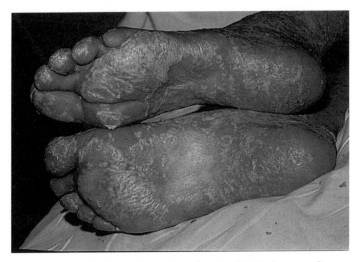

Figure 2.6 Generalized pustular psoriasis showing "lakes" of pus on soles.

A 12,000-molecular-weight PML chemotactic factor was identified and thought to be a C5-cleavage product in the stratum corneum of psoriasis vulgaris, pustular psoriasis, PPP, and subcorneal pustular dermatosis. A few cases of GPP complicated by pulmonary capillary leak syndrome have been reported, suggesting the involvement of cytokines (i.e. interleukin-1 and tumor necrosis factor).

Palmoplantar pustulosis

PPP is a chronic recurring eruption consisting of yellowish pustules on a background of redness and scaling on the thenar and hypothenar eminences or the instep of the sole and sides of the heel. Lesions are typically observed in all stages of development from vesicles to vesicopustules to frank pustules to dried brown maculopapules (Plate 4, facing p. 34). Lakes of pus are usually not seen unless the condition generalizes (Fig. 2.6). In large series of GPP, 7.9–13.5% of patients had preexisting PPP. As many as 20–30% of patients with PPP have ordinary psoriasis plaques elsewhere on the body.

Despite the reported associations with psoriasis vulgaris and GPP, some authors still consider PPP to be a separate dermatologic disorder. Szanto and Linse found evidence to support both points of view in a survey of 170 patients with PPP. The authors identified 25 patients (15%) with seronegative spondyloarthropathies similar to psoriatic arthritis. Eight of the patients were positive for HLA-B27, associated with sacroiliitis and ankylosing spondylitis, but none of the patients was positive for HLA-B13, -B17, -B37, and -Cw6 which are more closely associated with psoriasis vulgaris.

The other striking differences between PPP and psoriasis vulgaris that support separate entities are: (1) female predominance; (2) higher mean age of onset; (3) association with cigarette smoking (up to 100% of cases at onset); and, (4) consistently poor response to topical therapy. However, nail changes found in 30% of patients with PPP resemble those seen in psoriasis vulgaris and mild forms of acrodermatitis continua (vide infra). PPP often responds well to systemic lines of treatment III and IV intended for moderate to severe psoriasis.

Treatment

Recalcitrance to therapy is the rule for PPP. Topical keratolytics, corticosteroids, tars, and UVB are generally ineffective. Systemic agents, such as dapsone, sulfapyridine, colchicine, tetracyclines, trimethoprim-sulfamethoxazole, clofazimine, and methotrexate, give inconsistent results. Grenz ray treatment gives a modest temporary response.

The most effective treatments reported to date with the largest numbers of patients consist of the aromatic retinoids, etretinate or acitretin, 30–50 mg/day alone or combined with PUVA. PUVA with etretinate, 0.6 mg/kg/day, was significantly more effective than either treatment alone. Chronic maintenance therapy is required to prevent relapse. Liarozole, an imidazole-like drug, inhibits the metabolism of all-trans retinoic acid (RA), resulting in increased plasma and cutaneous levels of RA. Thus, it is retinoid-mimetic. After 12 weeks of 75 mg twice daily, liarozole was significantly more effective at reducing fresh pustule formation than placebo. Bath-water PUVA is effective and avoids the nausea and pruritus of oral 8-methoxypsoralen, systemic photosensitivity, and long-term toxicity of retinoids. Low-dose cyclosporine (1–2 mg/kg/day) is significantly more effective than placebo at suppressing the formation of new pustules.

Modifications of topical steroid therapy have been successful in remitting PPP. Goette *et al.* injected triamcinolone acetonide, 3.5–5.0 mg/ml intralesionally using a "fanning" technique. The procedure was painful but preferred by patients because clearing lasted for 3–6 months without additional treatment. Clobetasol propionate 0.05% lotion, applied under Duoderm extra-thin hydrocolloid dressings weekly, cleared the PPP lesions in 18/19 patients in 1–7 weeks. In two-thirds of patients, the PPP remained clear for 2–8 months after discontinuation of therapy. Because of the remarkable association of PPP with smoking, as shown by comparison with age- and sex-matched control subjects, some medically supervised attempt at cessation of the tobacco habit should be made.

Generalized pustular psoriasis (GPP) of von Zumbusch

The evolution of GPP, whether *de novo* or from a preexisting psoriatic state, consists of fiery red, irregular patches with round, arcuate, serpiginous borders surmounted by myriads of 1–2 mm superficial pustules. There is a predilection for flexural areas but any site may be involved. The pustules coalesce, forming lakes of pus, desquamate, and form new pustules as the border moves in waves every 24–72 hours (see Plate 5, facing p. 34). Patients are usually prostrate and febrile. Laboratory tests show leukocytosis, hypocalcemia, and hypoalbuminemia. The ionized serum calcium is usually within normal limits, but some patients with postsurgical hypoparathyroidism, hypocalcemia, and tetany have clearly responded to correction of the serum calcium level.

The average age at onset is about 50 years and the incidence by gender is approximately equal. In earlier series, the most striking finding was that one-fourth of patients had their attack of GPP within one month of first receiving or withdrawal of systemic corticosteroids. These cases were considered to be provoked by the steroid. Other precipitating factors identified included preceding infections and drugs. Some of these patients had the exanthematous type of pustular psoriasis. Among the steroid-treated patients, 67% had preexisting ordinary psoriasis compared to 56% of the entire group of 155 patients. Thirty-four of 106 patients followed up died, eight from uncontrollable GPP and nine as a complication of therapy (seven treated with steroids, two with MTX). GPP developing from acrodermatitis continua had the worst prognosis in this series. GPP evolving from PPP or atypical flexural forms of psoriasis was likely to spontaneously remit, with continuation of the original problem. GPP in 73/104 patients was treated with systemic steroids, but these patients tended to have increasingly severe GPP relapses upon withdrawal of steroids. Moreover, MTX was less efficacious in patients previously treated with steroids, and the rebound relapse after steroid withdrawal was not always controllable with methotrexate. Because spontaneous remission was common in untreated patients and the morbidity and mortality associated with steroid or MTX treatment were high (daily MTX was used at the time), Ryan and Baker advocated a conservative approach to therapy.

Zelickson and Muller generally found success with treatment with tap water or mild antiseptic wet dressings with topical steroids in a hospital setting. A variety of systemic agents (steroids, MTX, dapsone, sulfapyridine, and etretinate) or 2% crude coal tar with and without ultraviolet were needed as adjunctive therapy for the patients with the more severe relapsing recalcitrant GPP. In the seven patients who had GPP after acrodermatitis continua, the lesions resolved with few complications although more aggressive systemic therapy was needed, including cyclosporine in one patient. The most common complication of GPP was secondary infection, including septicemia which resulted in one death. Another patient died of Guillain–Barré syndrome. One patient developed a bleeding duodenal ulcer secondary to systemic steroid treatment. Hypocalcemia was found in 17 (27%) of 63 patients but, in 10 patients, this finding could be explained by hypoalbuminemia. The most common precipitating factors were believed to be upper respiratory infections (16%) and reductions in the doses of corticosteroids previously administered.

The prevalence of GPP in Japan is estimated to be 7.5 cases per million population. Two hundred and eight patients with recurrent GPP of von Zumbusch were subdivided into those with preceding ordinary psoriasis (65) and those without a history of psoriasis (43). The former group had more frequently preceding corticosteroid therapy and the latter group preceding infections. Ohkawara *et al.* concluded that there is heterogeneity of von Zumbusch type of GPP.

Treatment

Systemic retinoids can rapidly halt pustulation and decrease systemic symptoms; therefore, etretinate for men and postmenopausal women and isotretinoin or acitretin for women of childbearing potential are the treatments of choice. If conversion to MTX or PUVA for long-term maintenance is desired, the retinoid can be gradually tapered to prevent a relapse of GPP. Cyclosporine should be reserved for those patients unresponsive to or intolerant of retinoids. Low ionized calcium can be corrected rapidly by calcium infusion. Tonsillectomy was employed in 16.7% of 385 cases of GPP in Japanese hospitals. Antibiotics are usually not effective for GPP *per se*, but septicemia can occur as a complication or may have precipitated the eruption; appropriate antibiotics might be life-saving in such a situation. McFadyen and Lyell treated seven consecutive patients with GPP and coagulase positive staphylococcal septicemia with a 6-week course of antibiotics, which terminated the pustular phase in all but one patient. One patient died from antibiotic-resistant bacteria. Corticosteroids and MTX were not used. The recommendation is to perform surveillance blood cultures and cultures of pus upon admission to the hospital and treat the patients empirically if infection is suspected.

Impetigo herpetiformis

As originally described, impetigo herpetiformis refers to GPP in a pregnant woman without a prior history of psoriasis. The clinical morphology is similar to that of GPP; there are round, arcuate, polycyclic patches covered with tiny pustules in a concentric array. Lesions expand by peripheral extension. The old pustules break down, crust over, and may become vegetative in flexural areas. Lesions typically heal with hyperpigmentation. Constitutional signs and symptoms are common as are leukocytosis, hypocalcemia, and hypoalbuminemia. Most cases occur during the third trimester, but it can occur earlier. Impetigo herpetiformis recurs with increasing morbidity, with successive pregnancies, and promptly remits postpartum.

The disease has been reported in men and elderly women with hypocalcemia, but to call it "impetigo herpetiformis" obviates the need for the term. These patients have GPP. Pregnancy is a precipitating factor for generalized pustular psoriasis, therefore, patients with a prior history of psoriasis vulgaris or pustular psoriasis in whom there are flares during pregnancy should not be considered to have impetigo herpetiformis.

Treatment considerations

Prednisone, 20–60 mg daily, has been used to decrease pustulation and improve constitutional symptoms related to intense inflammation, but this treatment contradicts the negative experience with steroids in GPP. Serum calcium levels must be restored with calcium and vitamin D, and any superinfection must be treated with antibiotics. Fetal morbidity and mortality are increased. MTX, sulfones, and retinoids would, ordinarily, not be given to pregnant women. Cyclosporine may be relatively safe and effective in the third trimester, but there is a risk of fetal growth retardation and prematurity. Termination of pregnancy is the definitive treatment of impetigo herpetiformis. Depending on gestation dates, vaginal delivery by induced labor, cesarean section, or therapeutic abortion should be considered.

Exanthematous psoriasis

Ryan and Baker recognized an eruptive variant of GPP that they called *exanthematic pustular psoriasis* because it arose rapidly in the absence of preexisting psoriasis, was usually precipitated by infection or drugs, and tended to resolve spontaneously. Similar cases have probably been reported in the literature as GPP precipitated by drugs, generalized pustular dermatosis, or toxic pustuloderma. A consortium of French investigators analyzed 63 patients with so-called acute generalized exanthematous pustulosis (AGEP). They found that, in 55 patients (80%), the pustulosis could be attributed to drugs, particularly antibiotics of the penicillin and macrolide families.

The clinical appearance of AGEP is very similar to GPP with the abrupt onset of fever, pustulation, leukocytosis, and hypocalcemia within 14 days of taking the drug (less than 5 days in most patients). Polymorphous skin lesions (facial edema, purpura, vesicles, target-oid lesions) and erosions of the oral mucous membranes were recorded in about half the cases. The histology of lesions shows sub-corneal, intraepidermal or spongiform pustules. Subtle pathologic differences lead away from the diagnosis of GPP:

1 Marked papillary dermal edema.
2 Perivascular eosinophils.
3 Occasionally leukocytoclastic vasculitis.
4 Focal necrosis of keratinocytes.
5 Extravasated red blood cells.
6 Lack of psoriasiform epidermal hyperplasia.

Clinical differences that help to distinguish AGEP from GPP, even in patients with preexisting psoriasis, include:

1 Recent drug intake.
2 Higher fever.

3 Greater leukocytosis and eosinophilia.

4 Lack of arthritis.

Pustulation and fever cease within days of discontinuation of the offending drug, and erythema and desquamation resolve spontaneously within weeks. Supportive and local care is usually needed. The use of systemic corticosteroids may exacerbate or slow the resolution of AGEP and should probably be avoided or tapered rapidly if already started.

Many new cases of AGEP have been reported to be associated with commonly prescribed agents such as a cough suppressant, itraconazole, terbinafine, and calcium channel blocking agents, particularly diltiazem. For confirmation of the cause, patch testing with the suspected drugs may reproduce the clinical and histologic lesions locally in some patients. In summary, AGEP is a drug-induced reaction pattern that is more likely to occur in persons who are predisposed to psoriasis.

Erythrodermic psoriasis

The least common form of psoriasis is exfoliative dermatitis or psoriatic erythroderma, representing 1–2% of all forms. Erythroderma in general is a scaling pruritic, inflammatory process of the skin that involves all or almost all of the body surface area (see Plate 6, facing p. 34). Preexisting dermatoses are the most common cause of erythroderma, and psoriasis accounts for an average of 24% of cases in large series of erythroderma. The remaining cases are due to a variety of causes: eczematous dermatitis, seborrheic dermatitis, pityriasis rubra pilaris, drugs, lymphoma, and leukemia. Erythrodermic psoriasis usually develops gradually or acutely during the course of chronic psoriasis, but it may be the initial manifestation of psoriasis, even in children. The mean age of patients at the onset of erythroderma is about 50 years, and males outnumber females by about 2–3 : 1.

As the psoriatic erythroderma evolves, the original psoriasis plaques gradually lose their distinct outlines and surface characteristics, blending into a background of bright erythema with generalized exfoliation. The typical manifestations of psoriasis vulgaris become subtle, and without the preceding history, the diagnosis may be difficult. Sterile pustules may develop in some areas; in the most unstable cases, generalized pustular psoriasis may develop. Concomitant psoriatic arthropathy is common.

Table 2.3 Treatment-related precipitating factors for erythrodermic psoriasis.

Treatments for psoriasis	Allergic reaction to medications for other ailments
Systemic steroids	Penicillin
Topical steroid excess	Gold injection
Tar sensitivity	Chloroquine
Methotrexate withdrawal	Hydroxychloroquine
Etretinate	
PUVA burn	
PUVA + phototoxic drug	
UVB burn	

Precipitating factors for erythroderma include systemic illnesses, emotional stress, and alcoholism, but the most important ones seem to be related to treatment, especially the inappropriate use of potent topical, oral, and intramuscular corticosteroids (Table 2.3).

Complications of psoriatic erythroderma

Patients with acute erythroderma are uncomfortable, complain of feeling chilled, and may have low-grade fever. Thermoregulation is compromised because the erythrodermic skin loses more radiant and convective heat from the surface and sweats less than normal. There is increased water loss by diffusion. Protein (keratin), iron, and folic acid are lost during the profuse scaling. Resulting laboratory abnormalities may include hypovolemia, hypoalbuminemia, anemia, folic acid deficiency, and leukocytosis. In patients with a compromised cardiovascular system (the typical patient is an older male), high output cardiac failure is a risk and may be fatal during an erythrodermic flare. Lower extremity edema is common resulting from a combination of dependence, local inflammatory mediators, hypoalbuminemia, and cardiac failure. Hyperuricemia was reported in 25% of patients with psoriatic erythroderma, causing some patients with psoriatic arthritis to be misdiagnosed with gout. Boyd and Menter found that 13 (62%) of 21 patients with psoriatic erythroderma had elevated serum lactic dehydrogenase (LDH), probably a nonspecific measure of epidermal injury because isozyme LDH5 predominates in muscle and epidermis. Many seborrheic keratoses or wart-like papillomas may develop, particularly on the neck and trunk, during the course of erythroderma. Because of the compromised skin barrier and the patient's weakened state, possibly complicated by concomitant immunosuppressive drugs, septicemia, especially by *Staphylococcus aureus*, is a risk. Fatal cases of pulmonary capillary leak syndrome have occurred in this setting.

Management of erythroderma

Patients who withdraw abruptly from systemic steroids, excessive potent topical steroids, or methotrexate have the most unstable psoriasis and may develop erythroderma or pustular psoriasis. I admit such patients to the hospital for evaluation (Table 2.4) and conservative treatment (Table 2.5) until the patient is stable enough to receive more aggressive antipsoriatic therapy.

Psoriatic erythroderma can be controlled in most patients with the standard Goeckerman regimen, PUVA, etretinate, acitretin, methotrexate, or cyclosporine. The following combinations have been *successful* in small numbers of cases: acitretin plus bath PUVA;

Table 2.4 Laboratory evaluation of erythroderma.

1 Routine complete blood count, urinalysis, and chemistry profile
2 Buffy coat smear for Sézary cells
3 Chest x-ray
4 Surveillance blood and urine culture
5 Culture of pus, if any pustules are present
6 Skin biopsies from several representative sites if patient does not have firm diagnosis of preexisting psoriasis

Table 2.5 Conservative care of erythroderma.

Hospitalization
Bedrest with leg elevation
Warming blankets initially to prevent chilling
Oilated colloidal oatmeal in whirlpool bath once or twice daily
Rehydration, intravenous usually necessary upon admission followed by oral fluids
Antibiotics if necessary based on clinical impression then culture results
Multi-vitamin, folic acid, and iron supplementation
Compresses to face and flexural areas if there are fissures or exudation (saline or aluminum subsulfate)
Liberal emolliation with Aquaphor, petrolatum or Eucerin
1 or 2 1/2% hydrocortisone ointment 2 times daily
Hydroxyzine or diphenhydramine 25 mg prn itch

cyclosporine plus calcipotriene; cyclosporine plus etretinate. The disease reverts back to its pre-erythrodermic status. Kuijpers *et al.* reported the combination of cyclosporine and acitretin to be *ineffective* in three cases of psoriatic erythroderma. Systemic and potent topical steroids should be avoided. A minority of patients remain unstable and have repeated episodes of erythroderma during their lifetime.

Oral lesions

Oral lesions of psoriasis are very uncommon. There are four types of psoriatic oral lesions:
1 Minute round or oval whitish lesions that can be scraped off, leaving a bleeding surface.
2 Whitish plaques with red areas that parallel activity of skin lesions.
3 Bright red areas in pustular and erythrodermic psoriasis and Reiter's syndrome.
4 Benign migratory glossitis (BMG).

BMG, also known as *geographic tongue*, is a common inflammatory disorder of unknown etiology that affects about 2% of normal persons in the U.S. The clinical lesions are distinctive, showing well-demarcated red depapillated areas of the dorsal surface of the tongue delineated along its periphery by a slightly elevated whitish-yellow arc or annulus (see Plate 7, facing p. 34). Similar lesions also affect the lateral and ventral surfaces of the tongue. When they extend onto the labial, buccal, and soft palatal mucosa, the lesions are called *stomatitis areata migrans* (SAM). Synonyms include "ectopic geographic tongue," geographic mucositis, and erythema migrans. There is a high association of fissured tongue also called *lingua plicata* and *scrotal tongue*, with BMG (up to 20%). Geographic tongue and mucositis are usually asymptomatic and do not require any treatment. Oral candidiasis must be ruled out.

In general, the point prevalence of BMG in psoriatics is greater than that found or expected in control subjects, but the prevalence of fissured tongue (FT) is about the same as that of the general population. Further evidence of a pathogenetic relationship between psoriasis and BMG is revealed by a highly significant association of HLA-Cw6 with either condition when compared to control subjects. Zelickson and Muller noted a high prevalence of BMG (17.5%) in their patients with generalized pustular psoriasis. Pogrel and Cram observed SAM in 19 (15 on the hard palate and four on the buccal mucosa) of 100 patients admitted to a psoriasis day-care center for an acute exacerbation of psoriasis. In general, the course of SAM followed that of psoriasis. It resolved in eight patients after 3 weeks of intensive psoriasis treatment.

Morris *et al.* compared a group of 200 patients with psoriasis vulgaris to age- and sex-matched controls attending a dental clinic. The incidences of BMG and SAM was 10.3% and 5.4%, respectively, compared to 2.5% and 1.0% for the control subjects. The differences were statistically significant by chi-square analysis. There was no difference in the incidence of FT (16.7% vs. 20.3%). There was no particular association of BMG or SAM with either stable or progressive disease or correlation with the extent of body surface area involved.

Conclusions

The prevalence of BMG seems to be higher in psoriatics than the general population, and SAM is more likely to occur in patients with severe acute psoriasis. Intraoral psoriasis has a greater tendency to involve the bound keratinized tissues of the gingiva and hard palate than does SAM in nonpsoriatics. When the clinical course of the oral lesions and psoriasis parallel each other, the diagnosis of oral psoriasis is more likely.

Selected references

Arroyo M. P., Heller P., Pomeranz M. K. (2002) Generalized pustules in a healthy woman. *J Drugs Dermatol* **1**, 63–65.

Asumalahtik K., Ameen M., Suomela S. *et al.* (2003) Genetic analysis of PSORI distinguishes guttate psoriasis and palmoplantar pustulosis. *J Invest Dermatol* **120**, 627–632.

Beylot C., Doutre M. S., Beylot-Barry M. (1996) Acute generalized exanthematous pustulosis. *Sem Cut Med Surg* **15**, 244–249.

Bhalerao J., Bowcock A. M. (1998) The genetics of psoriasis: a complex skin disorder of the skin and immune system. *Hum Mol Genet* **7**, 1537–1545.

Bhushan M., Burden A. D., McElhone K. *et al.* (2001) Oral liarozole in the treatment of palmoplantar pustular psoriasis: a randomized, double-blind, placebo-controlled study. *Br J Dermatol* **145**, 546–553.

Boyd A. S., Menter A. (1989) Erythrodermic psoriasis. Precipitating factors, course, and prognosis in 50 patients. *J Am Acad Dermatol* **21**, 985–991.

Burden A. D., Kemmett D. (1996) The spectrum of nail involvement in palmoplantar pustulosis. *Br J Dermatol* **134**, 1079–1082.

Capon F., Munro M., Barker J., Trembath R. (2002) Searching for the major histocompatibility complex susceptibility gene. *J Invest Dermatol* **118**, 745–751.

Christophers E., Henseler T. (1991) Psoriasis type 1 and type 2 as subtypes of nonpustular psoriasis. In: Roenigk H. H. Jr, and Mailbach H. I. (eds) *Psoriasis*, 2nd edn. Marcel Dekker, New York, 15–21.

Cupuano M., Lesnon la Parola I., Masini C. *et al.* (1999) Immunohistochemical study of the early histopathologic changes occurring in trauma-injured skin of psoriatic patients. *Eur J Dermatol* **9**, 102–106.

Elder J. T., Nair R. P., Henseler T. *et al.* (2001) The genetics of psoriasis 2001: The odyssey continues. *Arch Dermatol* **137**, 1447–1454.

Errko P., Granlund H., Remitz A. *et al.* (1998) Double-blind placebo-controlled study of long-term low-dose cyclosporine in the treatment of palmoplantar pustulosis. *Br J Dermatol* **139**, 997–1004.

Farber E. M., Nall L. (1991) Epidemiology: natural history and genetics. In: Roenigk H. H. Jr, and Mailbach H. I. (eds) *Psoriasis*, 2nd edn. Marcel Dekker, New York, 209–258.

Finch T. M., Tan C. Y. (2000) Pusutlar psoriasis exacerbated by pregnancy and controlled by cyclosporin A (Letter to editor). *Br J Dermatol* **142**, 582–584.

Flugman S. L., McClain S. A., Clark R. A. (2001) Transient eruptive seborrheic keratoses associated with erythrodermic psoriasis and erythrodermic drug eruption: report of two cases. *J Am Acad Dermatol* **45**(Suppl 6), S:212–214.

Goette D. K., Morgan A. M., Fox B. J., Horn R. T. (1984) Treatment of palmoplantar pustulosis with intralesional triamcinolone injections. *Arch Dermatol* **120**, 319–323.

Gonzaga H. F. S., Torres E. A., Alchorne M. M. A., Gerbase-Delima M. (1996) Both psoriasis and benign migratory glossitis are associated with HLA-Cw6. *Br J Dermatol* **135**, 368–370.

Gudjonsson J. E., Karason A., Antonsdottir A. A. *et al.* (2002) HLA-Cw6-positive and HLA-Cw6-negative patients with psoriasis vulgaris have distinct clinical features. *J Invest Dermatol* **118**, 362–365.

Henseler T. (1998) Genetics of psoriasis. *Arch Dermatol Res* **290**, 463–476.

Kastelan M., Gruber F., Cecuk-Jelicic E. *et al.* (2003) A new extended haplotype CW*0602-B57-DRB1*0701-DQB1*0201 associated with psoriasis in the Croatian population. *Clin Exp Dermatol* **28**, 200–202.

Kokelj F., Plozzer C., Torsello P., Trevisan G. (1998) Efficacy of cyclosporine plus etretinate in the treatment of erythrodermic psoriasis (three case reports). *J Eur Acad Dermatol Venereol* **11**, 177–179.

Kuijpers A. L., van Dooren-Greebe J. V., van de Kerkhof P. C. (1997) Failure of combination therapy with acitretin and cyclosporin A in 3 patients with erythrodermic psoriasis. *Dermatol* **194**, 88–90.

Kumar B., Saraswat A., Kaur I. (2002) Palmoplantar lesions in psoriasis: a study of 3065 patients. *Acta Dermato-Venereol* **82**, 192–195.

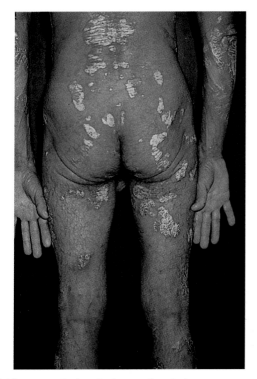

Plate 1 Fairly symmetric chronic plaques of psoriasis.

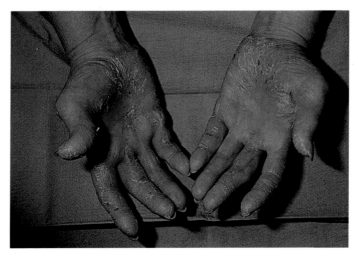

Plate 2 Psoriasis of the palms.

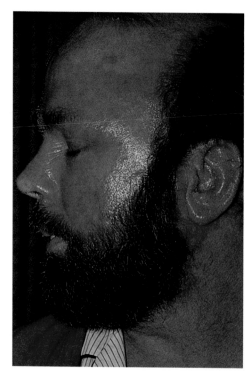

Plate 3 Psoriasis of the face indicates severe psoriasis elsewhere on the body.

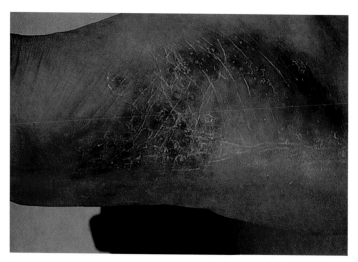

Plate 4 Palmoplantar pustulosis demonstrates lesions in all stages of development: vesicles, pustules, and dried brown scaly macules and papules.

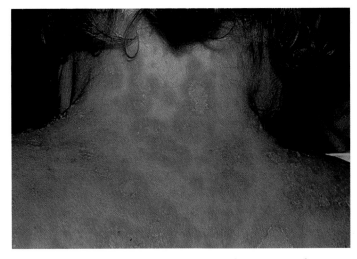

Plate 5 Generalized pustular psoriasis showing coalescence, central desquamation, and centrifugal spread of tiny pustules.

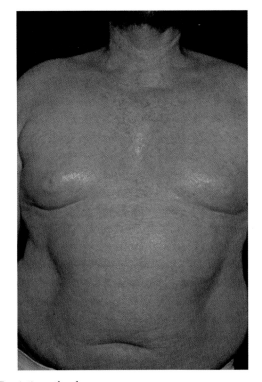

Plate 6 Psoriatic erythroderma.

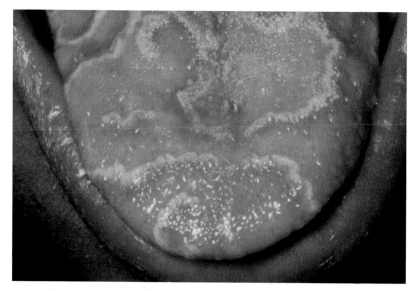

Plate 7 Benign migratory glossitis (geographic tongue).

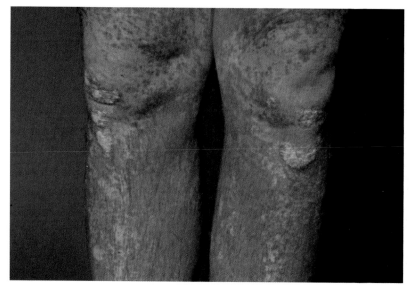

Plate 8 Coexistence of vitiligo and psoriasis. Note that psoriasis occurs within vitiliginous skin.

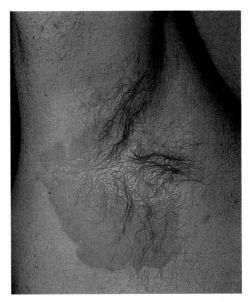

Plate 9 Inverse psoriasis of the axilla in an HIV-positive patient.

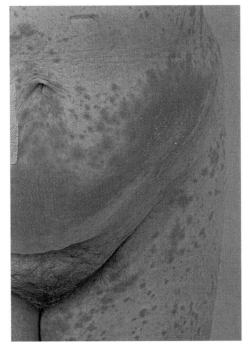

Plate 10 Acute generalized exanthematous pustulosis induced by diltiazem.

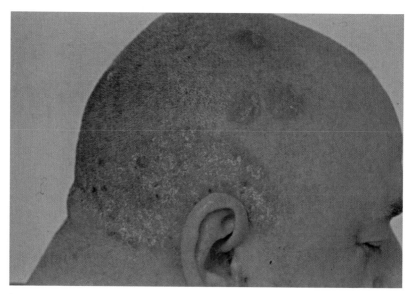

Plate 11 Psoriasis of the scalp involves ear and posterior auricular area. The patient shaved his head in order that natural sunlight could improve his skin.

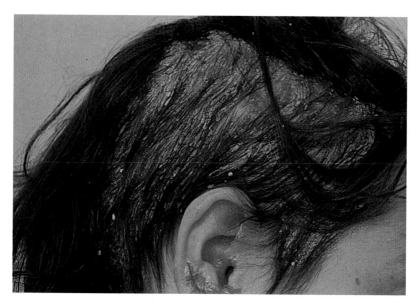

Plate 12 Adherent, thick scales suggest pityriasis amiantacea, but the patient has typical psoriasis elsewhere. Note the hair loss and ear involvement.

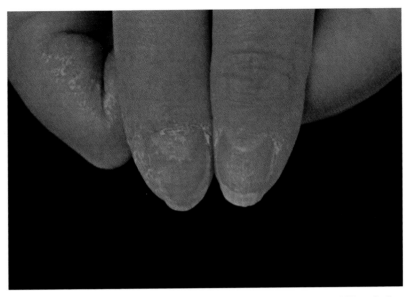

Plate 13 Pitting of the nail plate and psoriasis of the lateral nailfolds and side of the finger.

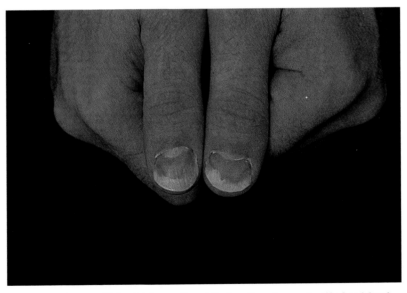

Plate 14 Yellowish-brown line at the junction of normal nail bed and distal onycholysis is very suggestive of psoriasis.

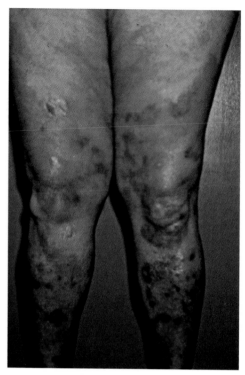

Plate 15 Anthralin-induced inflammation and staining of uninvolved skin surrounding psoriatic plaques.

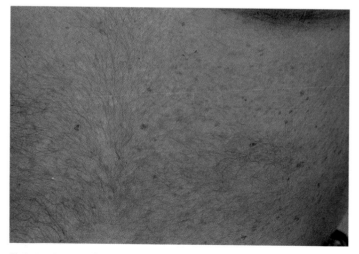

Plate 16 PUVA-induced pigmented macules (lentigines).

Leung D. Y., Travers J. B., Giorno R. *et al.* (1995) Evidence for a streptococcal superantigen-driven process in acute guttate psoriasis. *J Clin Invest* **96**, 2106–2112.

Mallon E., Bunce M., Savoie H. *et al.* (2000) HLA-C and guttate psoriasis. *Br J Dermatol* **143**, 1177–1182.

Morris L. F., Phillips C. M., Binnie W. H. *et al.* (1992) Oral lesions in patients with psoriasis: a controlled study. *Cutis* **49**, 339–344.

Ohkawara A., Yasuda H., Kobayashi H. *et al.* (1996) Generalized pustular psoriasis in Japan: two distinct groups formed by differences in symptoms and genetic background. *Acta Derm Venereol* **76**, 68–71.

Ozawa A., Ohkido M., Haruki Y. *et al.* (1999) Treatment of generalized pustular psoriasis: a multicenter study in Japan. *J Dermatol* **26**, 141–149.

Ploysangam T., Mutasim D. F. (1997) Follicular psoriasis: an under-reported entity. A report of five cases. *Br J Dermatol* **137**, 988–991.

Pogrel M. A., Cram D. (1988) Intraoral findings in patients with psoriasis with a special reference to ectopic geographic tongue (erythema circinata). *Oral Surg Oral Med Oral Pathol* **66**, 184–189.

Robinson C. M., DiBiase A. T., Leigh I. M. *et al.* (1996) Oral psoriasis. *Br J Dermatol* **134**, 347–349.

Ryan T. J., Baker H. (1971) The prognosis of generalized pustular psoriasis. *Br J Dermatol* **85**, 407–411.

Sauder D. N., Steck W. D., Bailin P. L., Krakauer R. S. (1981) Lymphocyte kinetics in pustular psoriasis. *J Am Acad Dermatol* **4**, 458–460.

Schmitt-Egenolf M., Eiermann T. H., Boehncke W.-H. *et al.* (1996) Familial juvenile onset psoriasis is associated with the human leukocyte antigen (HLA) Class I side of the extended haplotype Cw6-B57-DRB1*0701-DQA1*0201-DQB1*0303: A population- and family-based study. *J Invest Dermatol* **106**, 711–714.

Sneddon I. B., Wilkinson D. S. (1956) Subcorneal pustular dermatosis. *Br J Dermatol* **68**, 385–394.

Swanbeck G., Inerot A., Martinsson T. *et al.* (1995) Age at onset and different types of psoriasis. *Br J Dermatol* **133**, 768–773.

Szanto E., Linse U. (1991) Arthropathy associated with palmoplanter pustulosis. *Clin Rheumatol* **10**, 130–135.

Whittam L. R., Wakelin S. H., Barker J. N. W. N. (2000) Generalized pustular psoriasis or drug-induced toxic pustuloderma? The use of patch testing. *Clin Exp Dermatol* **25**, 122–124.

Wohl Y., Bergman R., Sprecher E., Brenner S. (2003) Stress in a case of SAPHO syndrome. *Cutis* **71**, 63–67.

Wong S. S., Tan K. C., Goh, C. L. (2001) Long-term colchicine for recalcitrant palmoplantar pustulosis: treatment outcome in 3 patients. *Cutis* **68**, 216–218.

Zelickson B. D., Muller S. A. (1991) Generalized pustular psoriasis. A review of 63 cases. *Arch Dermatol* **127**, 1339–1345.

3   Histopathology of psoriasis

Charles Camisa

Introduction

A skin biopsy is not always helpful in the diagnosis of psoriasis because many of its histopathologic features are shared with other skin diseases. In the overwhelming majority of cases, it is preferable to make a clinical diagnosis unless a pharmacologic study is being conducted. The clinician has the luxury of knowing the family and personal history, the anatomic distribution of lesions, and the varying morphology of lesions of different ages and whether nail changes are present. The pathologist is at a disadvantage because he or she receives only a minuscule sample of a dynamic process frozen at a random time point. The classic histopathology of psoriasis may only be seen in a lesion that is one week to one month old. Unfortunately, it may not be possible to histologically distinguish with confidence a clinically typical lesion of psoriasis from "chronic dermatitis" or "psoriasiform dermatitis."

Psoriasis vulgaris

Glabrous skin

Dermatopathology textbooks emphasize the rapidly evolving nature of the psoriatic lesion and the changing histologic picture. For example, the earliest pinhead-sized macule shows nonspecific findings: slight epidermal hyperplasia, erythrocytes packed in dilated capillaries and extravasated in dermal papillae, and a sparse perivascular lymphocytic infiltrate.

When neutrophils enter the picture, a more definitive diagnosis can be made. The neutrophils move rapidly because the earliest diagnostic lesion, a small smooth-surfaced papule, shows mounds

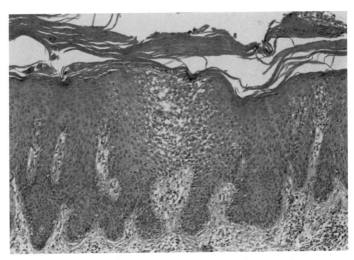

Figure 3.1 Biopsy specimen from a developed lesion of psoriasis shows epidermal hyperplasia, mounds of parakeratosis containing neutrophils, and early spongiform pustules.

of parakeratosis containing neutrophils, the earliest manifestation of Munro microabscesses. The older scaly lesions show aggregations of neutrophils in the upper stratum spinosum, which form small spongiform pustules of Kogoj while mononuclear cells remain confined to the lower epidermis (Fig. 3.1). Meanwhile, the epithelium becomes increasingly hyperplastic, more mitotic figures are seen above the basal cell layer, and the epidermis develops the characteristic "psoriasiform" appearance.

The term "psoriasiform" refers to regular elongation of rete ridges that are thick with bulbous tips and a tendency to coalesce (Fig. 3.2). The dermal papillae are correspondingly widened at their summits, appear edematous, and contain dilated tortuous capillaries with extravasated erythrocytes. The suprapapillary epidermis is thinned. A fully developed lesion may show confluent parakeratosis, but many biopsies show orthokeratosis admixed with parakeratosis, either in a focal vertical column or in alternating layers attesting to the episodic nature of the psoriatic process. Where there is parakeratosis there is usually a reduction of keratohyaline granules and a diminished or absent stratum granulosum underlying it. A resolving plaque of psoriasis shows compact orthokeratosis and return of the granular layer. For studies of therapeutic agents, a simple, mathematically-weighted system of grading the spectrum of

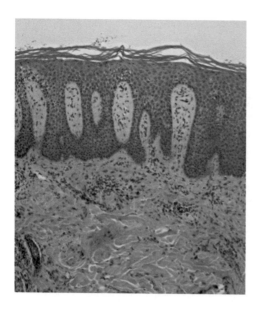

Figure 3.2 Psoriasiform hyperplasia demonstrates tendency of bulbous rete ridges to coalesce.

Table 3.1 Histopathologic features of a fully-developed lesion of psoriasis.

1 Psoriasiform epithelial hyperplasia
2 Elongation and edema of dermal papillae
3 Thinned suprapapillary plates with occasional spongiform pustule (Kogoj)
4 Diminution or absence of the granular layer
5 Continuous or alternating parakeratosis
6 Neutrophils in the stratum corneum (Munro microabscesses)

microscopic features in biopsy specimens has been developed, including thickness of the stratum malpighii.

In summary, a fully developed lesion of psoriasis, when sampled at the active margin of an enlarging plaque or from a more raised erythematous area with yellowish scale (a "hot spot") within a stable plaque, shows characteristic features (Table 3.1).

Scalp skin

The histopathologic description of scalp psoriasis is the same as glabrous skin except that mounds of parakeratosis may flank the follicular openings (Fig. 3.3). This change is also suggestive of seborrheic dermatitis, especially when there is associated spongiosis

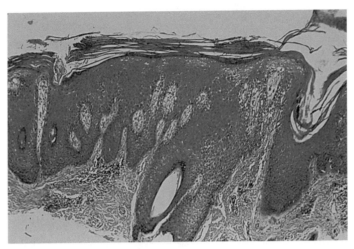

Figure 3.3 Biopsy specimen of scalp psoriasis shows mounds of parakeratosis around the follicular openings.

of the infundibulum, the chief differential diagnosis for psoriasis. Other less common scaling conditions of the scalp are easier to distinguish histologically from psoriasis: dermatomyositis, mycosis fungoides, and histocytosis-X.

A new approach to scalp biopsy involves processing of tissue by horizontal sections (as opposed to the standard vertical), thereby increasing the number of hair follicles evaluated. A study of involved and uninvolved scalp in 28 psoriatic patients was performed by this method, and revealed no evidence of alopecia in involved scalp. Hair follicles may have been smaller with a decreased hair shaft size, however. Sebaceous glands were also decreased in size.

Light microscopy of hair bulbs reveals increased percentages of telogen and catagen hairs in psoriatic plaques compared to uninvolved areas and normal controls. A localized telogen effluvium may occur in some patients with scalp psoriasis. Scarring alopecia may rarely be associated with scalp psoriasis when other causes have been excluded.

Nail unit

Psoriasis of the proximal nail fold shows essentially the same microscopic features of the disease as elsewhere on the skin, but psoriasis of the matrix and nailbed is somewhat different. Elongation of the

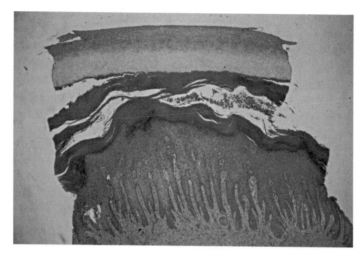

Figure 3.4 Biopsy specimen of nail unit psoriasis shows epidermal hyperplasia, focal hypergranulosis, and parakeratosis in the horny layer of the nail bed below the nail plate.

rete ridges is seen along with mounds of parakeratosis in the nail plate and small Munro's abscesses (Fig. 3.4). Because the changes of psoriasis may be indistinguishable from those of onychomycosis unless fungal elements are found, the tissue must be stained with periodic acid–Schiff (PAS) or silver methenamine in addition to hematoxylin–eosin.

PAS-positive diastase resistant globules may be seen between cells of the horny layer in biopsy samples taken from the yellowish greasy-appearing lesions with subungual hyperkeratosis. The matrix and nail bed normally lack a granular layer, but in psoriasis and acrodermatitis continua of Hallopeau they paradoxically develop one. The finding of a focal granular layer and keratohyaline granules aids in the diagnosis of psoriasis, but it is considered a nonspecific reaction to different inflammatory insults because it is also present in lichen planus and spongiotic trachyonychia. Nailbed biopsies of long-standing or traumatized psoriatic nails show changes more in keeping with lichen simplex chronicus: thin elongated rete ridges, compact orthokeratosis, and hypergranulosis with vertical streaks of fibrosis in the papillary dermis.

A simpler and more practical diagnostic method is to submit atraumatically avulsed or debrided onycholytic nail plate for hematoxylin–eosin and fungal stains. The nail plate may demonstrate mounds of parakeratosis and neutrophilic microabscesses. If nail bed epithelium is attached, diagnostic spongiform pustules of Kogoj may be present. Immersing the nail plate in cedar oil for 3 days softens it and produces superior sections compared to routine processing.

In acropustulosis, neutrophils accumulate in the superficial epithelium followed by spongiosis and necrosis of keratinocytes. As the process extends into the parakeratotic horny layer, Munro abscesses form, and the nail plate separates. Biopsy specimens of acropustulosis and Reiter's syndrome are similar to samples of skin lesions of pustular psoriasis. In Reiter's syndrome, extravasation of red blood cells is more prominent.

Pustular psoriasis

In the pustular variants of psoriasis, generalized pustular psoriasis of von Zumbusch, acrodermatitis continua of Hallopeau, impetigo herpetiformis, and possibly even Reiter's disease, the microscopic spongiform pustule of Kogoj enlarges to form a macropustule. The neutrophils aggregate within the interstices of a sponge-like network formed by degenerated and thinned epidermal cells. As the neutrophils move up in the horny layer, they become pyknotic and assume the appearance of large Munro abscesses (Fig. 3.5). The epidermal changes are similar to those seen in psoriasis vulgaris. In some patients with generalized or annular pustular psoriasis and acute generalized exanthematous pustulosis, the macropustules may assume a subcorneal position, causing some investigators to consider subcorneal pustular dermatosis of Sneddon and Wilkinson to be a variant of pustular psoriasis (Fig. 3.6).

Palmoplantar pustulosis

In patients with localized palmoplantar pustulosis, some of whom have ordinary psoriasis elsewhere, the fully developed lesion is a large intraepidermal unilocular pustule that is rounded on both sides. Spongiform pustules may be seen in the epidermal walls of the macropustule. The earliest lesion shows spongiosis with mononuclear cells in the lower epidermis and tips of the dermal papillae, followed by an intraepidermal vesicle containing primarily

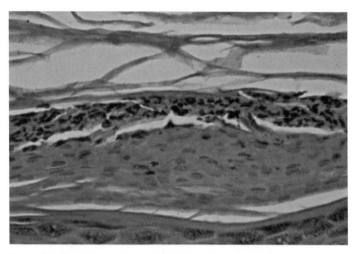

Figure 3.5 Aggregation of neutrophils in the stratum corneum (Munro microabscess).

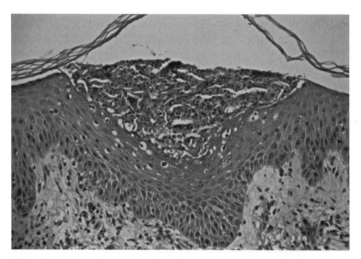

Figure 3.6 Biopsy of acute generalized exanthematous pustulosis shows pustule formation in a subcorneal location.

mononuclear cells. As the cavity expands, the stratum corneum becomes the roof, and neutrophils invade and transform the vesico-pustule into a pustule. Older lesions of keratoderma blennorrhag-icum may be differentiated from pustular psoriasis by the presence of a greatly thickened horny layer.

Erythrodermic psoriasis

When erythrodermic psoriasis is acute, it usually shows enough of the characteristics in Table 3.1 to allow the diagnosis to be established. In a study of 56 cases of erythroderma of all causes, the highest correlation rate between a blinded pathological diagnosis and the final discharge diagnosis was observed for psoriasis (80%). Tomasini *et al.* determined that, in 45 cases of psoriatic erythroderma, the histopathologic features were specific for psoriasis in 88%, but these were most often the features of early eruptive guttate lesions rather than fully developed plaques. The most consistent finding was the dilated tortuous capillaries in the papillary dermis. Notwithstanding, exfoliative dermatitis due to any cause including drug eruptions, eczema, pityriasis rubra pilaris, cutaneous T-cell lymphoma, and psoriasis, may sometimes be interpreted as "chronic nonspecific dermatitis" or "psoriasiform dermatitis." Biopsy samples may have to be taken from several locations at different times during the course of erythroderma in order to establish the correct diagnosis.

Oral psoriasis

The histopathology of benign migratory glossitis and erythema migrans is identical to that of psoriasis: epithelial hyperplasia, spongiosis, and exocytosis of neutrophils and lymphocytes (Fig. 3.7).

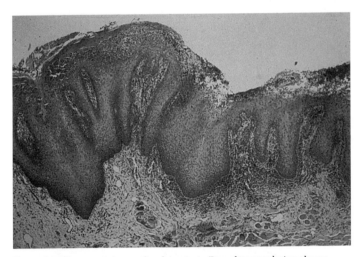

Figure 3.7 Biopsy specimen of oral psoriasis. Dorsal tongue lesion shows psoriasiform epithelial hyperplasia and spongiform pustules.

However, fungal stains must rule out candidiasis. It is important to remember that parakeratosis and psoriasiform hyperplasia are normal findings for the dorsal surface of the tongue.

Selected references

Altman E. M., Kamino H. (1999) Diagnosis: psoriasis or not? What are the clues? *Sem Cutan Med Surg* **18**, 25–35.

Bardazzi F., Fanti P. A., Orlandi C. *et al.* (1999) Psoriatic scarring alopecia: Observations in four patients. *Int J Dermatol* **38**, 765–768.

Botella-Estrada R., Sanmartin O., Oliver V. *et al.* (1994) Erythroderma. A clinicopathological study of 56 cases. *Arch Dermatol*, **130**, 1503–1507.

Elder D., Elenitsas R., Jaworsky C., Johnson B. (eds) (1997) *Lever's Histopathology of the Skin*, 8th edn. Lippincott-Raven, Philadelphia, 424.

Grammer-West N. Y., Corvette D. M., Giandoni M. B., Fitzpatrick J. E. (1998) Clinical pearl: Nail plate biopsy for the diagnosis of psoriatic nails. *J Am Acad Dermatol* **38**, 260–262.

Headington J. T., Gupta A. K., Goldfarb M. *et al.* (1998) A morphometric and histologic study of the scalp in psoriasis. *Arch Dermatol* **125**, 639–642.

Scher R. K., Daniels R. C. (1990) *Nails: Diagnosis, Therapy, Surgery*, WB Saunders, Philadelphia.

Schoorl W. J., van Baar H. J., van de Kerkhof P. C. (1992) The hair root pattern in psoriasis of the scalp. *Acta Derm Venereol* **72**, 141–142.

Tomasini C., Aloi F., Solaroli C., Pippione M. (1997) Psoriatic erythroderma: a histopathologic study of forty-five patients. *Dermatol* **194**, 102–106.

Trozak D. J. (1994) Histologic grading system for psoriasis vulgaris. *Int J Dermatol* **33**, 380–381.

van de Kerkhof P., Chang A. (1992) Scarring alopecia and psoriasis. *Br J Dermatol* **126**, 524–525.

Zip C., Murray S., Walsh N. M. G. (1993) The specificity of histopathology in erythroderma. *J Cutan Pathol* **20**, 393–398.

4 Pathogenesis of psoriasis

Charles Camisa

The *pathogenesis* of psoriasis is unknown, but more is known about the *pathophysiology* of psoriasis than any other skin disease.

Psoriasis is the result of hyperproliferation of the epidermis, concomitant inflammation and vascular changes, which occur in response to the proper combination of genetic and environmental pressures.

Psoriatic epidermis has 26.6% of the proliferative cells in the DNA synthesis (S) phase compared to 7.8% of normal skin. The growth fraction increases from 60 to 100% and the size of the population of proliferative cells is doubled, but the main defect in epidermal kinetics is the overall eight-fold increase in the germinative cell cycle compared to that occurring in normal skin.

The result is a cell cycle shortened from 311 to 36 hours and an epidermal turnover time, that is, the time it takes a basal cell to reach the stratum corneum, accelerated from 27 to 4 days. These experimentally derived time periods help to explain how scales can redevelop within 24 hours of removal. Interestingly, hyperproliferation of psoriatic keratinocytes cannot be duplicated under the conditions of cell culture techniques. In xenografts of psoriasis lesions to genetically immunodeficient mice, the psoriasiform epidermal hyperplasia persists in the absence of leukocytic infiltration, suggesting that the pathogenic elements for psoriasis reside in the dermis or the circulation or both.

The identification of aberrant cell kinetics in psoriasis has been exploited in the development of therapy. Treatments in this category include the antimetabolites methotrexate, hydroxyurea, azathioprine, 6-thioguanine, 5-fluorouracil, and mycophenolate mofetil, as well as photochemotherapy with 8-methoxypsoralen plus ultraviolet A (PUVA).

Another pathomechanism involved in psoriasis is abnormal keratinocyte *differentiation*, in contrast to *proliferation*. Histopathologically, the granular cell layer is reduced or absent, and hyperkeratosis and parakeratosis develop. Cytokeratin expression is altered compared to normal skin. Involucrin and membrane-bound transglutaminase appear prematurely in psoriatic epidermis. Involved psoriatic skin reveals little or no reaction of anti-filaggrin antibody in the stratum corneum or granular layer. Involucrin staining appears paradoxically in the lower cell layer. The uninvolved epidermis of psoriatic patients shows the same staining pattern as normal skin. In psoriatic epidermis, there is apparently a downregulation of cytokeratins K1 and K10 and an upregulation of K6 and K16. These quantitative differences in cytokeratins result from a delay in the differentiation of the basal cell layer in psoriatic epidermis. Thus, the earliest sign of epidermal differentiation that has been detected to date, the appearance of K1 and K10 in the suprabasal cell compartment, is delayed in psoriasis.

These findings have prompted interest in vitamin D_3 and analogues in the therapy of psoriasis because they promote the terminal differentiation of cultured murine epidermal cells. Moreover, 1,25-dihydroxyvitamin D_3 inhibits growth and DNA synthesis in a dose-dependent fashion in cell cultures of normal, psoriatic involved and uninvolved keratinocytes.

Cyclic adenosine monophosphate (cAMP) has been implicated as a modulator of cellular growth and differentiation in many cell systems and was thought to be involved in the pathogenesis of psoriasis because of the reduced levels measured in involved skin. Later, epidermal levels were shown to be normal or higher overall, with a relative reduction in the basal proliferative compartment. Basal cAMP levels were significantly lower in cultured psoriatic compared to control fibroblasts. Stimulation by beta-adrenergic agonists had a much less stimulatory effect and addition of phosphodiesterase inhibitor had no effect.

The cAMP-dependent protein kinases are deficient in cultured fibroblasts and uncultured red blood cells (RBCs), and the binding of cAMP to the regulatory subunits of protein kinase A in fibroblasts and erythrocytes is abnormal. Mitogen-activated protein kinase activity is significantly higher in psoriatic fibroblasts than normal fibroblasts.

Polymorphonuclear leukocytes

Because of the identification of polymorphonuclear leukocytes (PMLs) in histologic sections of psoriasis and the development of pustular variants, the role of circulating PMLs in the pathogenesis of psoriasis has been studied intensively. The PML and monocyte functions evaluated by numerous investigators included chemokinesis (random migration); chemotaxis (directed migration); lysosomal enzyme release; morphology; adherence; generation of oxidation intermediates such as superoxide anion, hydroxyl radical, and hydrogen peroxide; phagocytosis; chemiluminescence; and antibody-dependent cytotoxicity. Various stimuli were used, and cells were incubated with buffer or serum from psoriatics or normal controls. Unfortunately, the results were inconsistent and of little practical value to the clinician. When PML functions are evaluated before and after clearing of psoriasis in response to therapy, such experiments may help to answer whether the abnormalities identified are intrinsic to the disease process. There appears to be normalization of increased chemotaxis for PMLs and monocytes and the enhancing effect of psoriatic plasma after PUVA treatment.

Long-term methotrexate treatment normalizes enhanced PML and mononuclear cell (MNC) chemotaxis before clinical resolution of psoriasis is noted. Conversely, lithium increases migrational activity of PMLs, possibly by lowering cAMP levels, and can induce psoriasis or exacerbate preexisting disease. Basal cyclic AMP and guanosine monophosphate (GMP) levels are normal in psoriatic PMLs and MNCs.

Some reasonable conclusions that can be drawn from experimental evidence found in this large body of work are:

1 PMLs from psoriatics may be more sensitive to the usual chemoattractants employed in experimental assays.

2 Potent chemoattractants are passively trapped or produced de novo in the psoriatic epidermis. Candidates include immune complexes detected in the stratum corneum by direct immunofluorescence; serine proteinases; cytokines produced by MNC such as tumor necrosis factor; granulocyte-macrophage colony-stimulating factor; a 12-kDa chemotactic factor found in psoriatic scales; C5-cleavage products; leukotriene B4, and interleukin (IL)-8.

3 Psoriatic serum may contain high levels of chemoattractants, the result of diffusion from the skin or generated in the circulation by activated PMLs and MNCs.

4 Treatment of psoriasis may be successful in part by reducing the epidermal synthesis of chemoattractants and proinflammatory mediators, or by inactivating them, thereby preventing the accumulation of stimulated PMLs in the skin.

5 Pustular psoriasis, a model of exaggerated PML accumulation in skin, is appropriate for closer scrutiny because more homogeneous groups of patients in terms of activity (severe) and extent (generalized, localized, or palmoplantar) can be stratified and compared.

Neuropeptides

The effect of stress or worry may be considered an "endogenous Koebner phenomenon" if inflammation and proliferation is evoked by the release of peptides from cutaneous nerve fibers. While it has been proposed that extirpation of abnormal microvasculature or dermal growth factors are the mechanisms by which CO_2 laser vaporization or keratome excisions "cured" psoriasis, it is also plausible that severing nerve endings contributed to the result.

Biochemical and histochemical data have been sought. Vasoactive intestinal peptide (VIP) and substance P (SP) were detected in suction blisters induced over psoriatic plaques. Two studies demonstrated that the immunocytochemical localization of neuropeptides were similar for lesional, nonlesional, and control skin. There was a low but similar frequency of nerve fibers: SP was found in dermal papillae parallel to the dermoepidermal junction and VIP was found in the deeper dermis around eccrine glands and parallel to the skin surface. Nerve growth factor, which promotes growth of nerves and upregulation of SP, was detected in greater numbers of keratinocytes (KC) from biopsies of psoriasis compared to uninvolved psoriatic skin, normal skin, and lichen planus.

Plasma levels of these neurotransmitters measured by RIA in active and stable psoriatics and normal controls were not different. There was no correlation between the plasma level and the area of body surface involvement suggesting that, if neutrotransmitters play any role in the pathogenesis of psoriasis, it is probably at the local level.

Using double-labeling immunohistochemical stains, Naukkarinen *et al.* found that both mast cells and mast cell-nerve contacts were markedly more frequent in the basement membrane zone and papillary dermis of psoriatic lesional skin in comparison to healthy control skin. There was increased contact between mast cells and sensory nerves containing SP in lesional compared to nonlesional skin. The corresponding contact values for VIP were decreased. Neurogenic stimuli mediated by SP can degranulate mast cells that release proinflammatory substances.

The levels of SP and VIP measured in skin biopsies of psoriasis (picomoles per gram weight tissue) have been inconsistent. Rabier *et al.* showed that VIP stimulated KC proliferation in culture in a dose-dependent fashion; SP did not stimulate growth and blocked VIP-induced proliferation. An imbalance in the quantity of VIP and SP in vivo, taken together with disparate effects on KC proliferation in vitro, suggests that neurotransmitters are probably involved in the pathogenesis of psoriasis by exerting modulatory influences on growth and inflammatory mediators.

Capsaicin depletes nerve endings of SP and other peptides and prevents their reuptake. Topical capsaicin cream 0.25% produced modest overall clinical improvement compared to the vehicle cream. Scaling and erythema were diminished. Burning, stinging, itching, and redness were experienced by nearly half the subjects upon initial application of the capsaicin cream.

Various hypotheses have been advanced suggesting that psoriasis is under the neuroendocrine control of human growth hormone (HGH), prolactin, epidermal growth factor (EGF), insulin-like growth factor 1 (IGF-1, somatomedin-C), and insulin. Serum growth hormone levels are not elevated in psoriasis, nor are those of IGF-1 through which HGH effects are mediated. Any association between psoriasis and acromegaly or pituitary hyperplasia is coincidental. Somatostatin (SOM) and its analogue octreotide have improved psoriasis and psoriatic arthritis but not via HGH or IGF-1. In lesional skin, SOM-positive dendritic cells are found mainly in the dermis, and some cells extend dendritic processes into the epidermis. The number of SOM-positive cells was significantly reduced after healing of psoriasis by conventional topical therapies. Plasma EGF levels were reduced by SOM treatment in one series. SOM inhibits the release of many pituitary and gastrointestinal hormones, including insulin, producing mild carbohydrate intolerance. Carbohydrate metabolism is otherwise normal in psoriatics, but serum insulin levels were significantly higher than controls during the oral glucose tolerance test in one study. The development of a prolactinoma in three women correlated with a flare of plaque-type psoriasis. Bromocriptine, a dopamine agonist that suppresses the secretion of prolactin, improved psoriasis in all three patients.

IGF-1 receptors are confined to the basal cell layer where proliferative cells normally reside. IGF-1 or high dose insulin transmodulates the expression of EGF receptors by cultured KC via the IGF-1 receptor, increasing EGF binding 1.8 times. There are qualitative differences between the EGF/EGF receptor regulatory system of KC derived from normal skin and lesional skin. Interleukin-6 enhanced EGF-dependent growth of normal KC but had no effect on psoriatic KC. EGF receptor is markedly expressed in normal-appearing skin at the margin of relapsing psoriasis. Inhibition of IGF-1 receptor expression in lesional skin may reverse hyperproliferation of psoriatic epithelium. Inhibitory antisense oligonucleotides, which target messenger RNA, injected into psoriasis lesions grafted onto nude mice, caused normalization of the hyperplastic epidermis.

In summary, no effective treatment for psoriasis has yet emerged from the neurotransmitter hypothesis. Topical capsaicin produces intolerable local reactions and seems to be only weakly active against psoriasis. Native somatostatin, octreotide, and bromocriptine have unacceptable side-effect profiles and probably should not be used outside of carefully controlled trials. Future directions might include the development of VIP antagonists and antisense oligonucleotides for topical use.

Arachidonic acid metabolites

Arachidonic acid (AA) is found esterified to certain phospholipids that constitute the lipid bilayer of the cell membrane. The membrane-bound enzyme phospholipase A2 (PLA2) cleaves the esterified AA from the phospholipids, and now free AA can be metabolized to either the prostaglandins and thromboxanes or the leukotrienes and eicosanoids via the cyclooxygenase pathway or via a series of lipoxygenase enzymes, respectively. Several lines of evidence have suggested that these enzymes and their resulting inflammatory mediator products may cause development of the psoriatic lesion.

First, PLA2 activity in keratome slices is significantly elevated in both involved and uninvolved psoriatic specimens compared to normal controls. Involved and uninvolved psoriatic specimens also show increased transformation of AA via 5-lipoxygenase and 12-lipoxygenase. Leukotriene B4 (LTB4), a 5-lipoxygenase product, increases both random and directed migration of human neutrophils in vitro at physiologic concentrations (10^{-9} to 10^{-7} M), and is as potent as C5a. Neutrophils have specific receptors for LTB4. Application of LTB4 to normal or uninvolved psoriatic skin produced heavy collections of neutrophils in the epidermis (Munro microabscesses) within 24 hours. A proliferative response of keratinocytes was also observed 72–96 hours after LTB4 application. No difference, however, was observed in the effects between psoriatics and healthy controls. The dramatic appearance of numerous microabscesses compared to their relative paucity in chronic plaques of psoriasis suggests that the former is an interesting experimental artifact. That PLA2 is elevated in both uninvolved and involved skin implies that an important piece of the puzzle is missing or that inhibitors of the enzyme are active in vivo.

Meclofenamate and indomethacin are nonsteroidal anti-inflammatory drugs (NSAIDs) that are potent inhibitors of cyclooxygenase and modest inhibitors of 5-lipoxygenase activity. After an initial anecdotal report that meclofenamate cleared psoriasis, a 4-week double-blind placebo-controlled trial was performed and showed that there was no difference in the response of psoriasis between the group taking meclofenamate and the group taking the placebo. The authors (Ellis *et al.*) concluded that it is therefore an appropriate choice for psoriatic arthritis. Based on the combined experience of the Cleveland Clinic rheumatology and dermatology services, I do not hesitate to recommend the use of any NSAID for psoriatic arthropathy or other concomitant disease if it is indicated.

Benoxaprofen, a potent inhibitor of 5-lipoxygenase, was very effective in about 75% of patients with severe psoriasis, but is no longer available. Two topical 5-lipoxygenase inhibitors have been tested in treating psoriasis. Both lonapalene and R68151 2% ointments were statistically superior to their respective vehicles after 4 weeks. In fluid samples taken from skin chambers from lonapalene-treated sites, leukotriene B4 levels were significantly reduced compared to vehicle-treated and untreated sites at 4 days prior to the attainment of a clinically therapeutic effect.

MK-886 inhibits leukotriene biosynthesis by preventing the translocation and activation of 5-lipoxygenase. MK-886 potently inhibited the activity of calmodulin-dependent phosphodiesterase in vitro. Calmodulin is a calcium binding protein that is elevated in involved psoriatic epidermis and falls to normal levels after various palliative treatments. At nontoxic concentrations, MK886 had no effect on keratinocyte proliferation in culture. The oral administration of MK886 for 10 days had no clinical effect on psoriasis and did not change lesional LTB4 levels, but there was a slight reduction of PML in the epidermis. A novel oral LTB4 receptor antagonist, VML295, was ineffective in the treatment of psoriasis or in the prevention of relapse after clearing of the skin by other means. Flow cytometric markers of differentiation, inflammation, and proliferation were unchanged.

Based on the finding of increased levels of free AA, 12-HETE, PGE_2, PGF_2 alpha, and LTB4, LTC4, LTD4, an attempt was made to modify the metabolism of AA by supplementing the diet of psoriatic patients with fish oil containing large amounts of eicosapentaenoic acid (EPA), an omega-3 fatty acid relative of AA. It was hoped that free EPA might compete with AA as substrate and lead to the formation of less "psoriagenic" metabolites. Unfortunately, two double-blind placebo-controlled trials of fish oil and evening primrose oil as dietary supplements demonstrated no clinical effects on chronic stable plaque psoriasis or activity of psoriatic arthritis. However, the concept was proved by the intravenous infusion of an omega-3 fatty acid-based lipid emulsion containing EPA and docosahexaenoic acid. It resulted in a rapid rise in the plasma-free concentration of EPA, EPA derived 5-lipoxygenase products, and overall improvement in the severity of psoriasis.

Immunology/cytokine network

The development of cyclosporin A as an effective immunosuppressive agent (that is neither cytotoxic nor myelosuppressive) and its efficacy in treating the most recalcitrant cases of psoriasis has placed T-cell activation center-stage and focused attention on psoriasis as a putative autoimmune disease. Routine histopathology of psoriasis does not resemble a cell-mediated immune reaction and cannot distinguish specific immunoreactive cell-types nor identify their products. The obstacles inherent with proving that psoriasis is caused by chronic T-cell activation were overcome by technologic advances, such as immunohistochemistry and flow cytometry employing monoclonal antibodies, sensitive immunoassays of secreted products, messenger RNA transcripts coding for cytokines by Northern analysis, reverse transcriptase-polymerase chain reaction, and in situ hybridization.

Animal models of psoriasis potentially aid in the understanding of the pathogenesis of psoriasis. They can be divided into four broad categories:

1 Mice with spontaneous mutations, e.g. asebia (ab) and flaky-skin (fsn), which result in psoriasiform phenotypes of unclear pathogenesis.

2 Transgenic mice with cutaneous over-expression of cytokines such as IFN-gamma, IL-1-alpha, TGF-alpha, and vascular endothelial growth factor for studying the effects of isolated cytokines on the pathogenesis of the psoriatic phenotype.

3 Severe combined immunodeficiency (scid) mice reconstituted with dysregulated T-cells that induce psoriasiform abnormalities.

4 Xenotransplantation of human skin onto immunodeficient mice which allows the effects of individual cell types, cytokines, and therapeutic agents to be studied.

Topical clobetasol, and anti-CD11a monoclonal antibody and cyclosporine, both administered by intraperitoneal injection, reduced the epidermal thickness of psoriatic skin xenografts. Autologous immunocytes may be injected into transplanted uninvolved psoriatic skin. CD4+ but not CD8+ T-cells produced psoriatic lesions and the appearance of CD4+ and CD8+ T-cells that express natural killer (NK) cell receptors. The injection of autologous *natural killer cells* into uninvolved psoriatic xenografts induced classic psoriasis histology with epidermal expression of HLA-DR, ICAM-1, and K-16. These experiments suggest that the psoriasis phenotype is the result of a cutaneous defect that is triggered by autoreactive immunocytes.

Cyclosporine and tacrolimus target calcineurin and suppress inflammation and immune-based reactions in a generic fashion by diminishing the activation of genes encoding for proinflammatory cytokines such as IL-2, IL-4, and interferon gamma. IL receptor messenger RNA transcription is not directly affected by cyclosporine, nor does it specifically target any unique autoreactive T-cell clones. Cyclosporine is thus clinically useful in many inflammatory skin diseases, e.g. psoriasis, chronic graft vs. host reaction, lichen planus, atopic dermatitis, and pyoderma gangrenosum.

Cytokines are potent multifunctional glycoproteins, capable of influencing their target cell by binding to specific cell surface receptors at picomolar concentrations. The term *cytokines* encompasses lymphokines, monokines, interleukins, interferons, and growth factors. Keratinocytes, T-lymphocytes, and macrophages (antigen-presenting cells) communicate by a complex, bidirectional, functional cascade that is distinct for psoriasis. Some investigators believe that psoriasis is an autoimmune disease caused by a genetic defect in one or more of these three cell types. The isolation of the gene defect and the antigen-specific T-cells (with the exception of Vβ2+ T-cells in acute guttate psoriasis mediated by the streptococcal superantigen exotoxin C) have remained elusive. However, independent laboratories confirmed that certain T-cell receptor rearrangements are preferentially expanded and associated with lesional epidermis. It can be inferred that T-cell clones are specifically recruited and activated in psoriasis skin due to the recognition of psoriatic antigens. Analysis of the T-cell receptor in skin and synovial lesions of three patients demonstrated the same Vbeta CDR3 sequences, indicating that T-cells with identical T-cell receptors are present at two sites of chronic inflammation. The recombinant fusion protein, alefacept, targets memory-effector T-lymphocytes. The leukocyte-function-associated antigen type 3 (LFA-3) portion of the molecule binds to CD2 on the surface of the activated T-cell and the IgG1 portion binds with a receptor on the natural killer cell leading to T-cell apoptosis. That the defect lies with the immunocyte is supported by the numerous reports of patients with severe psoriasis and arthritis and leukemia or lymphoma who achieved and maintained complete remissions after allogeneic bone marrow transplantation. The role of mixed chimerism is uncertain but, to some degree, graft-vs.-host disease seems necessary in order to achieve graft-vs.-autoimmunity effects.

In the early phase of developing psoriasis lesions, macrophages appear first within the epidermis followed by lymphocytes, predominantly CD8+ T-cells. The macrophages are bone-marrow derived, HLA-DR+, non-Langerhans' cell CD1a⁻, antigen-presenting cells (APCs). Cells expressing natural killer markers were most commonly found in the papillary dermis just below the dermoepidermal junction. Nickoloff posited that the APC is the pivotal cell involved because of its strategic anatomic location between epidermal KC and dermal microvascular endothelial cells (EC) and their intercommunication (Table 4.1). The genesis of an immune reaction such as psoriasis may be initiated by nonspecific proinflammatory stimuli but the specific immune-mediated reaction includes activation of T-cells subsets with unique expression of cutaneous lymphocyte antigen which contact adhesion molecules (ICAM-1 and E-selectin) on endothelial cells. Efalizumab, a humanized anti-CD11a monoclonal antibody, binds to the alpha subunit of LFA-1 and blocks the activation of memory T-cells, binding of T-cells to endothelial cells, and T-cell trafficking into the skin. Efalizumab is effective in the treatment of plaque-type psoriasis and will be covered in detail in

Table 4.1 Model for the immunopathogenesis of psoriasis. (Adapted from Nickoloff BJ. (1991) The cytokine network in psoriasis. *Arch Dermatol* 127, 871–874.)

I. Response to nonspecific injury: induction of acute-phase inflammatory reactants
II. Recruitment of leukocytes: cytokine induction of adhesion molecules, chemotaxins
III. Regenerative wound-healing response: induction of growth factors
IV. Revelation of psoriasis mutation: interaction between cytokine-activated quiescent basal stem cells in the proliferative compartment of epithelium and T-cells with return to the circulation of autoreactive memory T-cells
V. Repetition of II–IV with propagation of lesions both locally and at remote sites via skin-seeking (epidermotropic) autoreactive memory–T-cells

Chapter 22. E-selectin is involved in adhesion of PML, monocytes and T-cell subsets; it is upregulated by IL-1 and TNF-alpha. Humanized monoclonal antibody to E-selectin was *not* effective in the treatment of moderate to severe psoriasis. However, the human TNF-receptor fusion protein, etanercept, and the chimeric monoclonal antibody that binds to TNF-alpha, infliximab, are very effective therapeutic agents for psoriasis (see Chapter 22). The T-cell can bind to the macrophage via the CD3 molecular complex and to cytokine-activated KC by the accessory surface molecules CD2 and CD18. Transforming growth factor (TGF) alpha, which acts via EGF receptors and has effects on angiogenesis, is elevated in psoriatic epidermis compared to nonlesional skin. Elevated IL-6 is expressed in psoriatic but not normal epidermis. IL-6 receptor has been demonstrated only in the transitional zone. Interleukin-8 is increased 50 times in psoriatic scales compared to normal callus. It has potent chemotactic activity for PML and T-cells and promotes epidermal cell proliferation. There was, however, no correlation between serum IL-8 levels and disease severity.

The activated T-cell inflammatory response in psoriasis is dominated by type 1 cytokines: IL-2, interferon-gamma, IL-8, TNF-alpha. The shift toward type 1 differentiation bias is found in both lesional skin and peripheral blood T-cells. Both CD8+ and C4+ T-cells, Tc1 and Th1, respectively, are affected. Few cells express the type 2 cytokines, IL-4 or IL-10. This imbalance most likely contributes to the sustained immune-activation of T-cells in patients with psoriasis.

IFN-gamma is present in high levels in psoriatic lesions and stimulates KC to express ICAM-1 and HLA-DR. Psoriatic KC are not as inhibited by IFN gamma as normal KC. CD4+ and C8+IFN-gamma+ T-cells were both significantly elevated in psoriatic epidermis compared to normal skin. Serum IFN-gamma levels were elevated and rapidly returned to normal with etretinate or cyclosporine treatment before any clinical improvement was documented. Psoriatic lesions developed at the site of intradermal IFN gamma and IFN alpha injections. Systemic administration of interferons may improve or aggravate psoriasis. Psoriasis and psoriatic arthritis have been exacerbated or induced by systemic IFN alpha, beta, or gamma therapy.

In an attempt to skew the autoreactive IFN-gamma and TNF-alpha-producing T-helper cells (Th1) toward a Th2 phenotype, psoriasis patients have been treated with immunosuppressive and anti-inflammatory type 2 cytokines. Treatment of psoriasis with recombinant human IL-10 was initially successful in short-term studies, but a randomized 12-week, double-blind, placebo-controlled trial showed no improvement in spite of a reduction in the ratio of type 1 to type 2 cytokine production. Interleukin-4 treatment also showed promise in open-label pilot studies for 6 weeks. IL-4 treatment reduced the concentration of IL-8 and the IFN-gamma: IL-4 ratio in psoriatic lesions. IL-4 treatment must be put to the same test as IL-10. The mechanism of action of narrow-band UVB was recently elucidated: IFN-gamma messenger RNA production decreased by 60% and IL-4 mRNA increased by 82% in irradiated psoriatic lesions.

Gottlieb *et al.* studied the relative contributions of epidermal proliferation and immunologic activation to the maintenance of active psoriatic lesions by examining the specific effects of cyclosporine treatment on these cells in vivo. Cyclosporine treatment reduced the number of 1L-2R positive T-cells in plaques, decreased HLA-DR expression in KC, and decreased interferon-gamma-induced protein-10 (chemoattractant and mitogenic cytokine). On the other hand, markers of KC growth activation, TGF-alpha and IL-6, did not change after 1–3 months of cyclosporine treatment. Five of eight patients continued to express the keratin marker of hyperproliferation, K16, after cyclosporine treatment. Petzelbauer *et al.* reported slightly different results after 2 weeks of cyclosporine treatment. HLA-DR expression by KC was not altered, but ICAM-1 expression by endothelial cells lining the blood vessels within the tips of dermal papillae was markedly reduced in most patients who improved clinically but persisted in those who failed to respond.

In four patients who had transient improvement of severe psoriasis after two weeks of treatment by murine CD4 monoclonal antibody infusion, there was a decrease in the keratinocytes expressing ICAM-1 and HLA-DR and a decrease in intraepidermal CD4+ and CD8+ T-cells. Epidermal Langerhans' cells were restored to normal numbers. The density of CD3, CD4, and CD8 cells did not change. In patients responding to PUVA, mRNA expression of IL-2, 6, 8, 10, TNF-α and IFN-γ declined compared to baseline levels. In a non-responder, IFN-γ increased above pretreatment levels.

The predominant in vivo effect of cyclosporine is to decrease immune activation; KC growth activation is less sensitive. The inability of cyclosporine treatment to decrease TGF-alpha and IL-6 levels in plaques, as well as the persistence of K16, help to explain the recurrence of disease to pretreatment activity after cessation of cyclosporine. Moreover, cyclosporine does not inhibit IL-8 synthesis or secretion by monocytes. The structurally unrelated macrolide immunosuppressant, tacrolimus, reduced IL-1β, IL-6, and IFN-γ transcripts in lesional biopsies and made IL-8 undetectable. The foregoing studies indicate that immune activation is important in the pathogenesis of psoriasis and that agents which interfere with T-cell activation and inhibit the secretion of key proinflammatory cytokines will continue to play a major role in the future therapy of psoriasis. In subsequent chapters, the details of clinical experience and current recommendations for the use of systemic cyclosporine and tacrolimus and biologic agents for the treatment of moderate to severe psoriasis will be covered.

Selected references

Adkins D. R., Abidi M. H., Brown R. A. *et al.* (2000) Resolution of psoriasis after allogenic bone marrow transplantation for chronic myelogenous leukemia: late complications of therapy. *Bone Marrow Transplantation* **26**, 1239–1241.

Austin L. M., Ozawa M., Kikuchi T. *et al.* (1999) The majority of epidermal T cells in Psoriasis vulgaris lesions can produce type 1 cytokines interferon-gamma, IL-2, and tumor necrosis factor-alpha, defining TCI (cytotoxic T lymphocyte) and THI effector populations: a type 1 differentiation bias is also measured in circulating blood T cells in psoriatic patients. *J Invest Dermatol* **113**, 752–759.

Bata-Csorgo Z., Hammerberg C., Voorhees J. J., Cooper K. D. (1995) Intralesional T-lymphocyte activation as a mediator of psoriatic epidermal hyperplasia. *J Invest Dermatol* **105** (Suppl), 89S–94S.

Bhushan M., Bleiker T. O., Ballsdon A. E. *et al.* (2002) Anti-E-selectin is ineffective in the treatment of psoriasis: a randomized trial. *Br J Dermatol* **146**, 824–831.

Bjorntorp E., Wickelgren R., Bjarnason R. *et al.* (1997) No evidence for involvement of the growth hormone/insulin-like growth factor-1 axis in psoriasis. *J Invest Dermatol* **109**, 661–665.

Borgato L., Puccetti A., Beri R. *et al.* (2002) The T cell receptor repertoire in psoriatic synovitis is restricted and T lymphocytes expressing the same TCR are present in joint and skin lesions. *J Rheumatol* **29**, 1914–1919.

Cameron A. L., Kirby B., Fei W., Griffiths C. E. (2002) Natural killer and natural killer-T cells in psoriasis. *Arch Dermatol Res* **294**, 363–369.

Castelijns F. A., Gerritsen M. J., Van Vlijmen-Willems I. M. *et al.* (1999) The epidermal phenotype during initiation of the psoriatic lesion in the symptomless margin of relapsing psoriasis. *J Am Acad Dermatol* **40**, 901–909.

Chakrabarti S., Handa S. K., Bryon R. J. *et al.* (2001) Will mixed chimerism cure autoimmune diseases after a nonmyeloablative stem cell transplant? *Transplantation* **72**, 340–342.

Christophers E. (1996) The immunopathology of psoriasis. *Int Arch Allergy Immunol* **110**, 199–206.

Ellis C. N., Goldfarb M. T., Roenigk H. H. Jr *et al.* (1986) Effects of oral meclofenamate therapy in psoriasis. *J Am Acad Dermatol* **14**, 49–52.

Ghoreschi K., Thomas P., Breit S. *et al.* (2003) Interleukin-4 therapy of psoriasis induces Th2 responses and improves human autoimmune diseases. *Nature Med* **9**, 40–46.

Gilhar A., Ullmann Y., Kerner H. *et al.* (2002) Psoriasis is mediated by a cutaneous defect triggered by activated immunocytes: induction of psoriasis by cells with natural killer receptors. *J Invest Dermatol* **119**, 384–391.

Gottlieb A. B., Grossman R. M., Khandke L. *et al.* (1992) Studies of the effect of cyclosporine in psoriasis in vivo: combined effects of activated T lymphocytes and epidermal regenerative maturation. *J Invest Dermatol* **98**, 302–309.

Hegemann L., Hatzelmann A., Grewig S., Schmidt B. H. (1995) Potent antagonism of calmodulin activity *in vitro*, but lack of antiproliferative effects on keratinocytes by the novel leukotriene biosynthesis inhibitor MK-886. *Br J Dermatol* **133**, 41–47.

Henderson W. R. (1994) The role of leukotrienes in inflammation. *Ann Intern Med* **121**, 684–697.

Kimball A. B., Kawamura T., Tejura K. *et al.* (2002) Clinical and immunologic assessment if patients with psoriasis in a randomized double-blind, placebo-controlled trial using recombinant human interleukin 10. *Arch Dermatol* **138**, 1341–1346.

Lemster B. H., Carroll P. B., Rilott R. *et al.* (1995) 1L-8/1L-8 receptor expression in psoriasis and the response to systemic tacrolimus (FK506) therapy. *Clin Exp Immunol* **99**, 148–154.

Lin W. J., Norris D. A., Achziger M. *et al.* (2001) Oligoclonal expansion of intraepidermal T cells in psoriasis skin lesions. *J Invest Dermatol* **117**, 1546–1553.

Mayser P., Grimm H., Grimminger F. (2002) N-3 fatty acids in psoriasis. *Br J Nutrition* **87** (Suppl), 577–582.

Mommers J. M., Van Rossum M. M., Kooijmans-Otero M. E. *et al.* (2000) VML 295 (LY-293111), a novel LTB4 antagonist, is not effective in the prevention of relapse in psoriasis. *Br J Dermatol* **142**, 259–266.

Mozzanica N., Cattaneo A., Vignati G., Finzi A. (1994) Plasma neuropeptide levels in psoriasis. *Acta Dermatovenereol* **186**, 67–68.

Naukkarinen A., Jarvikallio A., Lakkakorpi J. *et al.* (1996) Quantitative histochemical analysis of masT cells and sensory nerves in psoriatic skin. *J Pathol* **180**, 200–205.

Nickoloff B. J., Wrone-Smith T. (1999) Injection of pre-psoriatic skin with CD4+ T cells induces psoriasis. *Am J Pathol* **155**, 145–158.

Olaniran A. K., Baker B. S., Paige D. G. *et al.* (1996) Cytokine expression in psoriatic skin lesions during PUVA therapy. *Arch Dermatol Res* **288**, 421–425.

Oyama N., Sekimata M., Nihei Y. *et al.* (1998) Different growth properties in response to epidermal growth factor and interleukin-6 of primary keratinocytes derived from normal and psoriatic lesional skin. *J Dermatol Sci* **16**, 120–128.

Petzelbauer P., Stingl G., Wolff K., Volc-Platzer B. (1991) Cyclosporin A suppresses ICAM-1 expression by papillary endothelium in healing psoriatic plaques. *J Invest Dermatol* **96**, 362–369.

Prens E. P., van Joost T., Hegmans J. P. *et al.* (1995) Effects of cyclosporine on cytokines and cytokine receptors in psoriasis. *J Am Acad Dermatol* **33**, 947–953.

Rabier M. J., Farber E. M., Wilkinson D. I. (1993) Neuropeptides modulate leukotriene B4 mitogenicity toward cultured human keratinocytes. *J Invest Dermatol* **100**, 132–136.

Raychaudari S. P., Jiang W. Y., Farber E. M. (1998) Psoriatic keratinocytes express high levels of nerve growth factor. *Acta Derm Venereol* **78**, 84–86.

Raychaudhuri S. P., Dutt S., Raychaudari S. K. *et al.* (2001) Severe combined immunodeficiency mouse-human skin chimeras: a unique animal model for the study of psoriasis and cutaneous inflammation. *Br J Dermatol* **144**, 931–939.

Rizova H., Nicolas J.-F., Morel P. *et al.* (1994) The effect of anti-CD4 monoclonal antibody treatment on immunopathological changes in psoriatic skin. *J Dermatol Sci* **7**, 1–13.

Sanchez Regana M., Umbert Millet P. (2000) Psoriasis in association with prolactinoma: Three cases. *Br J Dermatol* **143**, 864–867.

Schon M. P. (1999) Animal models of psoriasis—what we can learn from them? *J Invest Dermatol* **112**, 405–410.

Slavin S., Nagler A., Varadi G., Or R. (2000) Graft vs autoimmunity following allogenic non-myeloablative blood stem cell transplantation in a patient with chronic myelogenous leukemia and severe systemic psoriasis and psoriatic polyarthritis. *Exp Hematol* **28**, 853–857.

Sticherling M., Sautier W., Schroder J. M., Christophers E. (1999) Interleukin-8 plays its role at 10 cal level in psoriasis vulgaris. *Acta Derm Venereol* **79**, 4–8.

Szabo S. K., Hammerberg C., Yoshida Y. *et al.* (1998) Identification and quantification of interferon-gamma producing T cells in psoriatic lesions: localization to both CD4+ and CD8+ subsets. *J Invest Dermatol*, **111**, 1072–1078.

Talme T., Schultzberg M., Sundquist K.-G., Marcusson J. A. (1999) Somatostatin- and factor XIIIa- immunoreactive cells in psoriasis during clobetasol propionate and calcipotriol treatment. *Acta Derm Venereol* **79**, 44–48.

Veale D. J., Torley H. I., Richards I. M. *et al.* (1994) A double-blind placebo controlled trial of Efamol Marine on skin and joint symptoms of psoriatic arthritis. *Br J Rheumatol* **33**, 954–958.

Vollmer S., Menssen A., Prinz J. C. (2001) Dominant lesional T cell receptor rearrangements persist in relapsing psoriasis but are absent from nonlesional skin: evidence for a stable antigen-specific pathogenic T cell response in psoriasis vulgaris. *J Invest Dermatol* **117**, 1296–1301.

Walters I. B., Ozawa M., Cardinale I. *et al.* (2003) Narrowband (312-nm) UVB suppresses interferon gamma and interleukin (IL) 12 and increases IL-4 transcripts differential regulation of cytokines at the single-cell level. *Arch Dermatol* **139**, 155–161.

Wraight C. J., White P. J., Mckean S. C. *et al.* (2000) Reversal of epidermal hyperproliferation in psoriasis by insulin-like growth factor I receptor antisense olignucleotides. *Nature Biotechnol* **18**, 521–526.

Xia Y. P., Li B., Hylton D. *et al.* (2003) Transgenic delivery of VEGF to mouse skin leads to an inflammatory condition resembling human psoriasis. *Blood* **102**, 161–168.

Zeigler M., Chi Y., Tumas D. B. *et al.* (2001) Anti CD-11a ameliorates disease in the human psoriatic skin—SCID mouse transplant model: comparison of antibody to CD11a with cyclosporine A and clobetasol propionate. *Lab Invest* **81**, 1253–1261.

5   Conditions associated with psoriasis

Charles Camisa

Almost any other disease or condition can coexist with psoriasis. Common pathogenetic factors help to explain the relationships among psoriasis, peripheral arthropathy, Reiter's syndrome, sacroileitis, ankylosing spondylitis, uveitis, and inflammatory bowel diseases (Table 5.1). In a case-control study, the prevalence of psoriasis was significantly higher in patients with ulcerative colitis (5.7%) and Crohn's disease (11.2%) compared to the control group (1.5%). Diseases like palmoplantar pustulosis (PPP) and subcorneal pustular dermatosis are highly associated with ordinary psoriasis and may alternate between the original state and generalized pustular psoriasis.

The "autoimmune" diseases, such as systemic lupus erythematosus and the bullous diseases, occur infrequently in association with psoriasis.

Because of the past and present treatment of patients with potential and known carcinogens [arsenic, ionizing radiation, sunlight, artificial ultraviolet B (UVB) light, coal tar, and psoralen with ultraviolet A (PUVA)], the relative risks of all types of cancers have been sought in patients with psoriasis. Smoking and ethanol drinking patterns may be influenced by the disease or be causally related to the activity of psoriasis and increase the risk of serious comorbidity from respiratory cancers and liver cirrhosis, respectively.

As most patients with severe or complicated psoriasis are cared for by dermatologists, concurrent cutaneous conditions are more likely to be noted after long-term observation of the entire body skin. Patients who present unusual diagnostic or treatment dilemmas are more likely to be reported. On the other hand, common skin diseases that occur in association with psoriasis are probably underreported. For example, almost every case of psoriasis coexisting with pemphigus vulgaris is described in the literature, while it is doubtful

Table 5.1 Diseases coexisting with psoriasis.

Probable pathogenetic relationship
Psoriatic arthritis
Reiter's syndrome
Sternoclavicular arthro-osteitis (SAPHO* syndrome)
Palmoplantar pustulosis
Subcorneal pustular dermatosis
Geographic tongue
Inflammatory bowel diseases
   Crohn's disease
   Ulcerative colitis

Possible pathogenetic relationship
Bullous diseases
   Bullous pemphigoid
   Novel autoimmune 200-kDa subepidermal blistering disease ("psoriasis bullosa
     acquisita")
   Pemphigus vulgaris
   Pemphigus foliaceus
   Benign familial chronic pemphigus
Systemic amyloidosis, secondary
HIV infection

Remote pathogenetic relationship
Atopic dermatitis
Vitiligo
Lichen planus
Lichen striatus
Reticular erythematous mucinosis
Erythema annulare centrifugum
Chronic actinic dermatitis
Other autoimmune diseases
   Alopecia areata
   Systemic and discoid lupus erythematosus
   Hashimoto's thyroiditis
   Myasthenia gravis
   Systemic sclerosis and morphea
   Sjögren's syndrome

---

*Synovitis, acne, pustulosis, hyperostosis, and osteitis.

that any cases of concomitant acne or atopic eczema would be published as such.

Bullous diseases

Most patients with psoriasis reported in association with autoimmune bullous diseases have bullous pemphigoid (BP) with circulating antibodies directed against 230-kDa or 180-kDa basement membrane zone (BMZ) antigens (Fig. 5.1). In all cases, psoriasis preceded BP. Therefore, anti-psoriatic treatment that is proinflammatory including radiation therapy, PUVA, UVB, sun exposure, tar, anthralin, and salicylic acid has been implicated as the cause. The order of occurrence, based on the mean age of onset of psoriasis (28 years) and BP (60 years), is to be expected. An almost equal number of cases of coexisting psoriasis and BP have been reported without a suspected cause. Blisters may occur on psoriatic and uninvolved skin. Psoriasis can arise as a Koebner response to a pemphigoid lesion, or blisters may be confined to psoriatic plaques. The treatment of BP in these circumstances is problematic because an effort has to be made to avoid systemic steroids in psoriasis. In one patient with long-standing psoriatic arthritis without skin

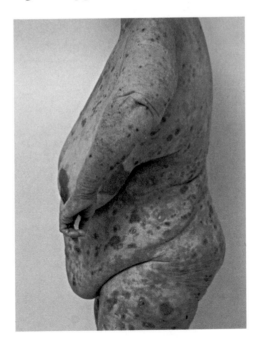

Figure 5.1 Coexistence of bullous pemphigoid and psoriasis.

lesions who developed BP, psoriatic plaques appeared for the first time after oral steroid therapy was withdrawn. If topical steroids and erythromycin or tetracycline plus niacinamide are unsuccessful at preventing blisters, dapsone 100 mg daily may be effective. Methotrexate, azathioprine, cyclosporine, mycophenolate mofetil, and acitretin may all be effective at controlling both diseases without oral steroids. BP has a tendency to remit spontaneously before psoriasis. Further associations with arthritis and auto-immune thyroid disease should be sought in these patients.

A new bullous disease, reported in six patients with psoriasis, consists of a subepidermal blister containing neutrophils, circulating antibodies directed against a 200-kDa antigen located in the lower lamina lucida. The disease is immunologically distinct from epidermolysis bullosa acquisita and bullous pemphigoid. Indirect immunofluorescence testing of salt-split skin demonstrates IgG on the *floor* of the induced blister. It was recently proposed to name this disease "psoriasis bullosa acquista."

Individual cases of classic epidermolysis bullosa acquisita (290-kDa antigen) and linear IgA bullous dermatosis (97-kDa antigen) were reported to coexist with psoriasis vulgaris. Aside from the prior treatments of psoriasis, another plausible explanation for the pathogenesis of autoimmune subepidermal blistering diseases in patients with psoriasis is that the large numbers of mast cells found along the BMZ may degranulate in response to neurogenic stimuli via substance P. Tryptase can degrade basement membrane components, perhaps making them more immunogenic in the process.

The blisters of the superficial forms of pemphigus, foliaceus and erythematosus, occur in a subcorneal location and may clinically resemble subcorneal pustular dermatosis, pustular psoriasis, or psoriasis vulgaris when the lesions appear dry, red and scaly. These diseases have been reported in association with psoriasis. Scalp involvement is very common in both conditions; however, biopsy and immunofluorescence studies can usually differentiate all forms of autoimmune pemphigus and psoriasis. If systemic steroids are used to treat pemphigus, and they are often indicated, a steroid-sparing agent may be required to prevent a rebound flare of psoriasis. A suppressor T-cell deficit or dysfunction in psoriasis has been proposed as the mechanism that allows the production of autoantibodies in coexisting bullous diseases. Plasminogen activator, which is believed to be crucial in the development of acantholysis, is found to be markedly increased in the involved epidermis of psoriasis, BP, and benign familial chronic pemphigus (Hailey–Hailey disease). Plasminogen activator activity is normal or modestly elevated in pemphigus vulgaris or foliaceus.

In Hailey–Hailey disease, the intertriginous exudative lesions may be confused with atypical inverse psoriasis. Phototherapy may aggravate it. A positive family history or histopathology showing acantholysis is necessary for the diagnosis. Immunofluorescence studies are negative. The course of benign familial chronic pemphigus may be altered by topical steroids and antimicrobials, broad spectrum systemic antibiotics, or dapsone. In a recent case report, both diseases responded well to suberythemogenic UVB phototherapy.

Common skin diseases

Among common skin diseases, urticaria and candidiasis showed an excess rate in psoriasis patients, but in the past, psoriasis was believed to be mutually exclusive of atopic dermatitis, vitiligo, and lichen planus. In a large prospective study, systematic examinations in a dermatology clinic revealed that 16.7% of atopic dermatitis patients had psoriasis and 9.5% of psoriatic patients had atopic dermatitis. A survey of over 9000 children born in 1958 revealed that of 354 with visible eczema, 1.4% had visible psoriasis, and 1.0% of patients without visible eczema had psoriasis. Clearly, the two diseases frequently coexist or occur consecutively in the same individual. Chronologically, the atopic dermatitis generally precedes the onset of psoriasis, and both diseases respond well to similar treatments.

Vitiligo was also thought to be rarely associated with psoriasis until reports in 1982 and 1983 showed it to be as prevalent in psoriasis patients as in the general population (0.55%). The converse was also true. Vitiligo usually appeared first. Psoriasis lesions were randomly distributed with respect to the depigmented skin. Occasionally, psoriasis lesions are limited to areas of preexisting vitiligo (see Plate 8, facing p. 34), suggesting the effect of the Koebner phenomenon. The coexistence of vitiligo with psoriasis apparently increases the incidence of additional putative autoimmune diseases: arthritis, thyroid disease, diabetes, ulcerative colitis, pernicious anemia, lupus, and alopecia areata. Occasionally, both vitiligo and psoriasis will respond to potent topical steroids, but PUVA is an ideal treatment for both diseases if one of the conditions is extensive enough to warrant the time, expense, and risks involved. Vitiligo developed in the sites of resolving psoriasis plaques in two patients during treatment with topical PUVA with trimethoxalen cream and with narrow band UVB phototherapy. A patient with coexisting scalp lesions of psoriasis and alopecia areata can be treated with intralesional injections of triamcinolone acetonide, 5 mg/ml.

Considering the high prevalence of psoriasis and lichen planus (LP) in dermatology practices, their coexistence does seem under-represented in the literature. A case was reported in which long-standing psoriasis improved during the development of LP, and exacerbation of psoriasis was associated with resolution of LP. The authors suggested that the two diseases might be mutually exclus-ive because of immunologic and pathogenetic interrelationships. For example, local production of interferon-gamma by lymphocytes in the inflammatory infiltrate is believed to play a role in the expres-sion of HLA-DR on keratinocytes, which is more marked in LP than in psoriasis. The epidermal kinetics are vastly different with hyper-proliferation in psoriasis and markedly reduced proliferation in LP, resulting in the characteristic histologic picture of hypergranulosis and orthokeratosis. One similarity, however, is that both diseases demonstrate the classic Koebner phenomenon. One patient with psoriasis developed bullous LP localized to an old skin donor graft site. Naldi *et al.* demonstrated in a case-control study that psoriasis and LP coexist at the expected frequency. Of 711 patients with LP, 12 (1.7%) reported a diagnosis of psoriasis. Among the control subjects with skin disease other than LP, 2.7% reported a diagnosis of psoriasis. The difference between the two groups was not statistic-ally significant. Among 19 reported cases of lichen striatus in chil-dren, three patients had psoriasis, including one with an unusual eruptive variant on the contralateral side. Erythema annulare cen-trifugum may also coexist with psoriasis vulgaris.

Secondary systemic amyloidosis

A rare but serious complication of long-standing severe inflam-matory plaque or pustular psoriasis, almost always associated with deforming arthritis, is secondary systemic amyloidosis. About 40 cases have been reported. Deposition of fibrillar amyloid protein is seen in the kidneys, heart, and gastrointestinal tract. In the skin, the deposits are found in the reticular dermis around appendages and in blood vessel walls, and in subcutaneous fat. Nephrotic syndrome, chronic renal failure, and cardiac dysfunction may supervene and culminate in death. Colchicine treatment for 57 months successfully reversed nephrotic syndrome in a patient affected by psoriatic erythroderma and arthropathy. A similar result was reported with oral chlorambucil in a patient with severe psoriatic arthritis. There is a trend toward a decreasing incidence of secondary amyloidosis associated with inflammatory joint diseases in Finland. This may be the result of the earlier and more frequent therapeutic use of cytotoxic drugs.

Lupus erythematosus

Based on their prevalence in the population, the coexistence of all forms of lupus with psoriasis seems to be less than expected. Dubois reported that 0.6% of 520 patients with systemic lupus erythematosus (SLE) had concurrent psoriasis. The coexistence of psoriasis and lupus raises issues of diagnosis and treatment. Forty-three percent of patients with SLE are photosensitive, and 80% of patients with psoriasis show improvements with sunlight. However, a subset of "photosensitive psoriasis" accounts for about 5.5% of all cases. These patients have a significantly higher frequency of skin type I, and 30–50% have preceding polymorphous light eruption developing into psoriasis. Subacute cutaneous lupus erythematosus (SCLE) lesions may be either annular or psoriasiform. Biopsy, immunofluorescence, and serologic testing are necessary to distinguish SCLE from psoriasis. Some of these patients, especially those with circulating Ro (SS-A) antibodies, are exquisitely photosensitive. The action spectrum for lupus is generally considered to be UVB, but in some patients the disease may flare after UVA exposures received in tanning salons or from sunlight filtered through window glass.

The control of systemic lupus erythematosus often requires systemic steroids, especially for renal and central nervous system involvement. A rebound flare of psoriasis is possible upon withdrawal of steroids. Antimetabolites used as steroid-sparing agents may prevent this as well as improve psoriasis. Phototherapy is contraindicated in patients with lupus, but PUVA is indicated for "photosensitive psoriasis" if it is severe. Screening for anti-nuclear antibodies including SS-A, SS-B, and double-stranded DNA is necessary prior to treating any photosensitive patient with light. Antimalarials are now the drugs of choice in the treatment of the cutaneous and joint manifestations of lupus, but chloroquine and hydroxychloroquine may precipitate drug reactions or flares of psoriasis. The retinoids, isotretinoin, etretinate, and acitretin, have been used successfully to treat cutaneous lupus erythematosus in open trials. Double-blind trials confirmed the efficacy of acitretin (50 mg/day) or hydroxychloroquine (400 mg/day) in 50% of cases of cutaneous LE. Therefore, retinoids may help both diseases in patients who are so affected. Alternative drugs that may amelior-ate one disease without aggravating the other are dapsone, thalido-mide, mycophenolate mofetil, and azathioprine.

Alcohol consumption

In a Swedish population study including 372 psoriatics, liver cir-rhosis and alcoholism showed excess rates in both genders. After 10 years of prospective study of a cohort of 1380 American patients treated with PUVA, there were more deaths caused by cirrhosis than expected in the general population (11% vs. 2.9%). The invest-igators found that having two alcoholic drinks per day increased the risk of death threefold whereas prior MTX treatment was not a risk factor.

Alcohol consumption has been investigated in recall question-naire-type surveys using patients with other skin diseases as con-trols. A study of Finnish men found a striking increase during the last year in the daily consumption of alcohol by 129 psoriatics (55 g vs. 20 g) and the annual frequency of intoxication (58 vs. 37) compared to 238 control subjects. In a similar but larger ($n = 215$) Italian study, there was a trend for increased relative risk of psoriasis: 1.3 for 1–2 drinks daily and 1.6 for three or more drinks daily compared to nondrinkers. A survey of 789 Chinese psoriatics and 789 control subjects revealed that there was a significant asso-ciation of smoking and alcohol use in men, but not women, with psoriasis. In Finnish women, although the relative risk of develop-ing psoriasis was 3.3 for those smoking 20 cigarettes/day compared to nonsmokers, the extent of body surface involvement was signi-ficantly associated with alcohol consumption and not smoking or negative life events. I suggest that smoking is a risk factor for the development of psoriasis and alcohol worsens it.

Smoking cigarettes

In a study of 216 patients with palmoplantar pustulosis (PPP), 80% were smokers at the onset of disease compared to 36% of control subjects, an odds ratio of 7.2. Of 50 patients with PPP, 96% were smokers at the time of the survey. Mills *et al.* studied 108 psoriatics including 16 with PPP. There were 46.2% current smokers compared to 23.6% among matched control subjects. The relative risk of psoriasis was greatest (5.3) for those currently smoking more than 20 cigarettes/day. This was confirmed by Naldi *et al.* who reported that current smokers were at higher risk of psoriasis than "never-smokers" and that the relative risk became significant (2.1) for people smoking 15 or more cigarettes per day. The risk of pustular lesions was 10.5 in patients currently smoking more than 15 cigarettes per day. Smoking more than 10 cigarettes per day was associated with greater severity of psoriasis involving the forearms, hands, and feet; that is, the distal portions of extremities.

The dose–response relationship between the number of cigarettes smoked daily and the development of psoriasis have suggested a "cause and effect" relationship. The relationship between the smoking and the drinking habit is difficult to unravel. For example, in a case-control study of 404 patients, there was no *overall* association with alcohol consumption, but a moderate association was found in men. The higher prevalence of current smoking among psoriatics is probably an indicator of a stressful life-style. Whatever the rationale, it is clear that these patients take on the additional risks of cardiovascular diseases, respiratory ailments, and certain cancers.

Internal cancers

Stern *et al.* found no increase in cardiovascular disease in their PUVA-treated cohort. A study of 372 psoriatics from a defined population of 159,200 Swedes showed a significant association with lung cancer in women. In another Swedish population of 20,328 living persons with psoriasis, there was no increase in the overall number of internal cancers or lung cancers. In a more selective series of 4799 PUVA-treated patients in Sweden (which probably includes some of the same patients from the two previously cited studies), respiratory cancer in both genders, kidney and colonic cancer in women, and pancreatic cancer in men were significantly increased. Stern's group found increased colonic cancer in their PUVA cohort during the first decade but not in the second decade. They also noted a significantly increased incidence of female breast, thyroid, and central nervous system cancers in 20 years. The overall incidence of noncutaneous cancer and death was not increased in this study, suggesting that PUVA is not a risk factor and that the three internal cancers that were increased represent a statistical artifact or a selection bias in the study population. A Danish study of patients with psoriasis followed for 9.3 years after discharge from the hospital revealed excesses of lung cancer in both genders, and cancer of the larynx and pharynx in men. A Scottish study reported the same incidence of lung cancer and bladder cancer (another neoplasm linked to smoking) among 8400 psoriatics diagnosed between 1968 and 1979 as expected in the general population. The PUVA cohort did not show an increased risk of lymphoma or leukemia, but a study of conditions associated with adult acute leukemias revealed that patients with lymphoblastic leukemia were three times more likely to have psoriasis than healthy controls. Follow-up of 5687 Finnish psoriatic patients discharged from the hospital between 1973 and 1984 revealed a higher than expected incidence of laryngeal cancer, Hodgkin's disease, and non-Hodgkin's lymphoma.

The concordance of the findings of excess numbers of respiratory cancers in both genders and possibly lymphoproliferative cancers, especially in the nonoverlapping national studies, is worrisome. It is possible that the genetic makeup of individuals with psoriasis, related behavioral patterns including diet, smoking, and alcohol consumption, and the various treatments used contributed to these risks. More prospective case-control studies are needed to resolve these questions.

Skin cancer

Long-term studies of patients with severe psoriasis in diverse population groups consistently show that the overall risk of developing malignancy is between one and two times that of the general population, owing predominantly to an excess risk of squamous cell carcinoma (SCC). When the PUVA cohort is selected out of the Swedish series, the relative risk of cutaneous SCC increases from 1.48 to six-fold. Men who received >1200 J/cm^2 cumulative dose or >200 PUVA treatments had 27–30 times the incidence of SCC in the general population. In the American PUVA cohort of 1380 patients first treated in 1975–6, the relative risk for developing SCC or basal cell carcinoma (BCC) after >200 PUVA treatments was 37–62 and 5–7, respectively. The overall risk of developing malignant melanoma was 2.3, but the risk increased significantly in patients who received ≥250 PUVA treatments (3.1) or if more than 15 years passed since their first treatment (3.8). In the Danish cohort of 795 psoriatics discharged from the hospital, the standardized incidence risk (SIR) of nonmelanoma skin cancer was 2.5. There was a tendency for BCCs to occur in multiple sites in young women. SCCs occur frequently on the lower extremities. In a similar Finnish cohort of 5687 patients, the SIR of SCC was 3.2. A U.S. study of patients in three states determined the relative risk of developing malignancy in several diseases, assuming the risk in hypertensive patients as unity. The risk ratio was 1.78 for severe psoriasis and 2.12 for patients with a "history of organ transplantation," accounted for mostly by nonmelanoma skin cancers and lymphoproliferative cancers.

Diet and obesity

Diet and obesity may contribute to the development and severity of psoriasis (Fig. 5.2). On average, patients with psoriasis are about 15% heavier than their ideal body weight. In a survey of patients diagnosed during the last 2 years, the risk of psoriasis increased with increasing body mass index (BMI) and was inversely related to consumption of carrots, tomatoes, and fresh fruit when compared to control subjects with other skin diseases. After controlling for

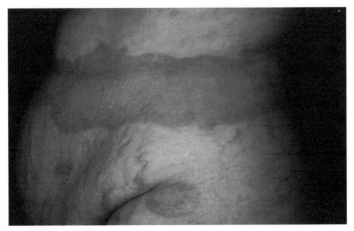

Figure 5.2 Severe inflammatory plaque-type psoriasis in an obese female patient.

socioeconomic status, alcohol consumption, and cigarette smoking, the association of psoriasis with increased BMI remained significant. In the Swedish population study, there was an excess of obesity in women with psoriasis. Restricted calorie (weight reduction) or vegetarian diets are likely to contribute to the improvement of psoriasis in over-weight individuals.

The serologic markers of celiac disease, IgA antigliadin antibodies (AGA), have been variably positive in psoriatics (0–16%), but anti-endomysium antibodies (EMA) have been consistently absent. In some patients with AGA, the psoriasis improved after 3 months of a gluten-free diet (GFD). A survey of 114 patients with psoriasis and arthropathy revealed that five (4.4%) patients had coexisting celiac disease. After excluding these patients, the serum level of IgA AGA was significantly higher than that of a reference group. The IgA AGA concentration was correlated with significantly higher erythrocyte sedimentation rate and duration of morning joint stiffness. Further studies of GFD would be worthwhile to determine whether the diet influences the inflammatory activity of psoriasis.

Human immunodeficiency virus infection

The incidence of psoriasis in persons infected with human immuno-deficiency virus (HIV) is about the same as the general population, 1–3%. The sudden onset of a psoriasiform dermatitis or exacerbation of preexisting psoriasis may suggest screening for HIV infection in patients with appropriate risk factors. If it occurs in patients with known HIV infection, then it is recommended to check CD4 counts and viral load and to consider initiating highly active antiretroviral therapy. Psoriasis in HIV-positive patients may be mild or severe, localized or generalized, but there is a distinct tendency for the disease to resist all of the usual topical remedies. There is also a tendency for inverse psoriasis of the axillae (see Plate 9, facing p. 34) and groins resembling seborrheic dermatitis and acral involvement of the palms and soles with hyperkeratotic plaques or pustules (Fig. 5.3). In the latter case, when there is concomitant asymmetric polyarthritis, the patients are diagnosed with either psoriatic arthritis or Reiter's syndrome. The incidence of Reiter's syndrome in HIV infection is 0.5–10%, and 75% of these patients are HLA-B27-positive.

The pathogenesis of psoriasis in HIV infection is unknown but it may be related to predominant suppressor/cytotoxic effects of

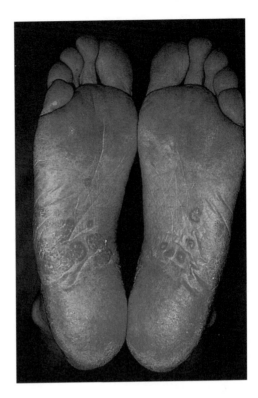

Figure 5.3 Psoriasis of the soles
in an HIV-positive patient
resembling keratoderma
blennorrhagicum.

T-cells due to the reduction of functional T-helper cells or to the reduced number of epidermal Langerhans' cells in lesions, which results in clinical deterioration.

Treatment of HIV-associated psoriasis is difficult because topical therapy is mostly ineffective and some of the more effective systemic therapies which are putatively immunosuppressive (i.e. methotrexate, PUVA, cyclosporine) may not be used. Treatments that have been tested for HIV-associated psoriasis and are shown to be safe and effective at temporarily improving more than half the patients are zidovudine (AZT, Retrovir), 1200 mg/day (see reference by Duvic *et al.*) UVB phototherapy (see Chapter 13); etretinate, and acitretin (see Chapter 15).

Other organ systems

A striking overlap exists within psoriasis patients and family members of rheumatological, gastroenterological, and ocular diseases.

The high prevalence of psoriasis in association with inflammatory bowel diseases (IBD) and possibly celiac disease was mentioned earlier in this chapter. For example, patients with ankylosing spondylitis and IBD have a higher prevalence of psoriasis or iritis than control subjects. Ankylosing spondylitis precedes the secondary disorders.

Gastrointestinal tract

Subtle inflammatory abnormalities of the gut that were asymptomatic have been detected by biopsy in patients with psoriasis. Some patients have circulating IgG and IgA antigliadin antibodies without celiac disease. Recurrent cholestatic jaundice, due to neutrophilic cholangitis, was reported in two cases of generalized pustular psoriasis. In a registry of patients with nonalcoholic steatohepatitis, three patients had psoriasis. The association may be fortuitous, but the risk of hepatotoxicity in such patients from methotrexate treatment is self-evident.

Kidney

A variety of renal abnormalities have been infrequently reported in association with psoriasis, including IgA nephropathy (the most common glomerular disease in the world), membranous nephropathy, and glomerulonephritis. In a study of 73 patients with psoriatic arthritis, 17 (23.3%) had subclinical abnormalities of creatinine clearance or urinary albumin excretion unassociated with treatment of their underlying disease.

Eye

Approximately 10% of patients with psoriasis have some form of ocular involvement: lids, conjunctiva, cornea, and anterior uveal tract. Subtle abnormalities of conjunctival cytology and tear film function were detected in 50% of psoriatics compared to 5% of age and sex-matched control subjects. Seronegative spondyloarthritis is frequently complicated by episcleritis or uveitis. Three patients with palmoplantar pustulosis and arthro-osteitis (SAPHO syndrome) were reported with associated episcleritis. A retrospective cohort study of 71 patients with psoriatic arthritis identified 13 (18%) with uveitis. The best predictors of the development of uveitis were extensive axial involvement (bilateral sacroileitis and syndesmophytes) and HLA-DR13-positivity. There was a less significant association with HLA-B27. The uveitis is more likely to be of insidious onset, with posterior pole involvement.

A rare but serious ocular complication of connective tissue disorders and other autoimmune diseases, called the *peripheral corneal melting syndrome*, has also been reported in association with a small number of cases of psoriasis. The prognosis of corneal melting is grave because it can lead to destruction of one or both corneas. An ophthalmology consultation is recommended for psoriasis patients who complain of a painful red eye in addition to aggressive therapy of the skin disease.

Selected references

Secondary amyloidosis

Kagan A., Husza'r M., Frumkin A., Rapoport J. (1999) Reversal of nephrotic syndrome due to AA amyloidosis in psoriatic patients on long-term colchicine treatment. Case report and review of the literature. *Nephron* **82**, 348–353.

Laiho K., Tiitinen S., Kaarela K. *et al.* (1999) Secondary amyloidosis has decreased with inflammatory joint disease in Finland. *Clin Rheumatol* **18**, 122–123.

Mpofu S., Teh L. S., Smith P. J. *et al.* (2003) Cytostatic therapy for AA amyloidosis complicating psoriatic spondyloarthropathy. *Rheumatol* **42**, 362–366.

Wittenberg G. P., Oursler J. R., Peters M. S. (1995) Secondary amyloidosis complicating psoriasis. *J Am Acad Dermatol* **32**, 465–468.

Bullous diseases

Chen K. -R., Shimizio S., Miyakawa S. *et al.* (1996) Coexistence of psoriasis and an unusual IgG-mediated subepidermal bullous dermatitis: identification of a novel 200-kDa lower lamina lucida target antigen. *Br J Dermatol* **134**, 340–346.

Hayakawa K., Shiohara T. (1999) Coexistence of psoriasis and familial benign chronic pemphigus. *Br J Dermatol* **140**, 374–375 (Letter to Editor).

Kirtschig G., Chow E. T. Y., Venning V. A., Wojnarowska F. T. (1996) Acquired subepidermal bullous diseases associated with psoriasis: a clinical immunopathological and immunogenetic study. *Br J Dermatol* **135**, 738–745.

Kobayashi T. T., Elston D. M., Libow L. F., David-Bajar K. (2002) A case of bullous pemphigoid limited to psoriatic plaques. *Cutis* **70**, 283–286.

Morita E., Amagai M., Tanaka T. *et al.* (1999) A case of herpetiform pemphigus coexisting with psoriasis vulgaris. *Br J Dermatol* **141**, 754–755.

Morris S. D., Mallipeddi R., Oyama N. *et al.* (2002) Psoriasis bullosa acquisita. *Clin Exp Dermatol* **27**, 665–669.

Panzarella K., Camisa C. (1996) Coexistence of superficial pemphigus and psoriasis. *Cutis* **57**, 414–418.

Tomasini D., Cerri A., Cozzani E., Berti E. (1998) Development of pemphigus foliaceus in a patient with psoriasis: a simple coincidence? *Eur J Dermatol* **8**, 56–59.

Skin cancer

Stern R. S., Vakeva L. H. (1997) Noncutaneous malignant tumors in the PUVA follow-up study: 1975–1996. *J Invest Dermatol* **108**, 897–900.

Stern R. S., Nichols K. T., Vakeva L. H. (1997) Malignant melanoma in patients treated for psoriasis with methoxsalen (psoralen) and ultraviolet A radiation (PUVA). *N Engl J Med* **336**, 1041–1045.

Diet and obesity

Krueger G. G., Duvic M. (1994) Epidemiology of psoriasis: clinical issues. *J Invest Dermatol* **102**, 145–185.

Naldi L., Parazzini F., Peli L. *et al.* (1996) Dietary factors and the risk of psoriasis. Results of an Italian case-control-study. *Br J Dermatol* **134**, 101–106.

HIV infection

Buccheri L., Katchen B. R., Karter A. J., Cohen S. R. (1997) Acitretin therapy is effective for psoriasis associated with HIV infection. *Arch Dermatol* **133**, 711–715.

Duvic M., Crane M. M., Conant M. *et al.* (1994) Zidovudine improves psoriasis in HIV-positive males. *Arch Dermatol* **130**, 447–451.

Fotiades J., Lim H. W., Jiang S. B. *et al.* (1995) Efficacy of UVB phototherapy for psoriasis in patients infected with human immunodeficiency virus. *Photodermatol Photoimmunol Photomed* **11**, 107–111.

Maurer T. A., Zackheim H. S., Tuffanelli L., Berger T. G. (1994) The use of methotrexate for treatment of psoriasis in patients with HIV infection. *J Am Acad Dermatol* **31**, 372–375.

McAleer P., Chu P., White S. M. *et al.* (2001) Psoriasis associated with human immuno-deficiency virus in an infant. *Pediatr Dermatol* **18**, 87–89.

Romani J., Puig L., Baselga E., de Moragas J. M. (1996) Reiter's syndrome-like pattern in AIDS-associated psoriasiform dermatitis. *Int J Dermatol* **35**, 484–488.

Zemelman V., VanNeer F., Roberts N. *et al.* (1994) Epidermal Langerhans cells, HIV-1 infection and psoriasis. *Br J Dermatol* **130**, 307–311.

Internal cancer

Frentz G., Olsen J. H. (1999) Malignant tumours and psoriasis: a follow-up study. *Br J Dermatol* **140**, 237–242.

Hunnuksela-Svahn A., Pukkala E., Laara E. *et al.* (2000) Psoriasis, its treatment, and cancer in a cohort of Finnish patients. *J Invest Dermatol* **114**, 597–590.

Margolis D., Bilker W., Hennessy S. *et al.* (2001) The risk of malignancy associated with psoriasis. *Arch Dermatol* **137**, 778–783.

Autoimmune diseases

Bilen N., Apaydin R., Ercin C. *et al.* (1999) Coexistence of morphea and psoriasis responding to acitretin treatment. *J Eur Acad Dermatol Venereol* **13**, 113–117.

Dubois E. L. (1974) *Lupus Erythematosus*, 2nd edn. University of Southern California, Los Angeles.

Sahoo B., Kamar B. (2002) The coexistence of photosensitive psoriasis and chronic actinic dermatitis. *Dermatol* **204**, 77–79.

Watanabe M., Shinohara M., Katayama I. (1998) Association of psoriasis vulgaris with Sjogren's syndrome. *J Dermatol* **25**, 349–350.

Yamamoto T., Katayama I., Nishioka K. (2002) A rare association of systemic sclerosis with psoriasis vulgaris. *J Dermatol* **27**, 346–349.

Braphy S., Pavy S., Lewis P. *et al.* (2001) Inflammatory eye, skin, and bowel disease in spondyloarthritis: genetic, phenotypic, and environmental factors. *J Rheumatol* **28**, 2667–2673.

Ikegawa S., Urano F., Suzuki S. *et al.* (1999) Three cases of pustulotic arthro-osteitis associated with episcleritis. *J Am Acad Dermatol* **41**, 845–846.

Eye

Karabulut A. A., Yalvac I. S., Vahaboglu H. *et al.* (1999) Conjunctival impression cytology and tear-film changes in patients with psoriasis. *Cornea* **18**, 544–548.

Queiro R., Torre J. C., Blezunegui J. *et al.* (2002) Clinical features and predictive factors in psoriatic arthritis-related uveitis. *Semin Arthritis Rheum* **31**, 264–270.

Varma S., Woboso A. F., Lane C., Holt P. J. A. (1999) The peripheral corneal melting syndrome and psoriasis: coincidence or association? *Br J Dermatol* **141**, 344–346.

Gastrointestinal

Allez M., Roux M. E., Bertheau P., Erlinger S. *et al.* (2000) Recurrent cholestatic jaundice associated with generalized pustular psoriasis: evidence for a neutrophilic cholangitis. *J Hepatol* **33**, 160–162.

Cardinali C., Degl'innocenti D., Caproni M., Fabbri P. (2002) Is the search for serum antibodies to gliadin, endomysium and tissue transglutaminase meaningful in psoriatic patients? Relationship between the pathogenesis of psoriasis and celiac disease. *Br J Dermatol* **147**, 187–188. (Letter to editor).

Li S. P., Tang W. Y., Lam W. Y., Wong S. N. (2000) Renal failure and cholestatic jaundice as unusual complications of childhood pustular psoriasis. *Br J Dermatol* **143**, 1292–1296.

Lindquidt U., Rusander A., Bostrom A. *et al.* (2002) IgA antibodies to gliadin and celiac disease in psoriatic arthritis. *Rheumatol* **41**, 31–37.

Lonardo A., Loria P., Carulli N. (2001) Concurrent non-alcoholic steato hepatitis and psoriasis. Report of three cases from the POLISTENA study. *Digest Liver Dis* **33**, 86–87.

Scarpa R., Manguso F., D'Arienzo A. *et al.* (2000) Microscopic inflammatory changes in colon of patients with both active psoriasis and psoriatic arthritis without bowel symptoms. *J Rheumatol* **27**, 1241–1246.

Kidney

Ahuja T. S., Funtanilla M., de Groot J. J. *et al.* (1998) IgA nephropathy in psoriasis. *Am J Nephrol* **18**, 425–429.

Alenius G. M., Stegmayr B. G., Dahlquist S. R. (2001) Renal abnormalities in a population of patients with psoriatic arthritis. *Scand J Rheumatol* **30**, 271–274.

Sirolli V., Bonomini M. (2000) Glomerulopathies associated with psoriasis: a report of three cases. *Nephron* **86**, 89–90.

Smoking and alcohol

Mills C. M., Srivastava E. D., Harvey I. M. *et al.* (1992) Smoking habits in psoriasis: a case control study. *Br J Dermatol* **127**, 18–21.

Naldi L., Peli L., Parazzini F. (1999) Association of early-stage psoriasis with smoking and male alcohol consumption: evidence from an Italian case-control study. *Arch Dermatol* **135**, 1479–1484.

Poikolainen K., Reunala T., Karvonen J. (1994) Smoking, alcohol, and life events related to psoriasis among women. *Br J Dermatol* **130**, 473–477.

Zhang X., Wang H., Te-Shao H. *et al.* (2002) Frequent use of tobacco and alcohol in Chinese psoriasis patients. *Int J Dermatol* **41**, 659–662.

Common skin diseases

Goodwin R. G., Finlay A. Y., Anstey A. V. (2001) Vitiligo following narrow-band TL-01 phototherapy for psoriasis. *Br J Dermatol* **144**, 1264–1265 (Letter to Editor).

Hakin C., Hann S.-K., Kauh Y. C. (1997) Vitiligo following the resolution of psoriatic plaques during PUVA therapy. *Int J Dermatol* **36**, 534–536.

Papadavid E., Yu R. C., Munn S., Chu A. C. (1996) Strict anatomical coexistence of vitiligo and psoriasis vulgaris—a Koebner phenomenon? *Clin Exp Dermatol* **21**, 138–140.

Serhat Inaloz H., Patel G., Holt P. J. A. (2001) Bullous lichen planus arising in the skin graft donor site of a psoriatic patient. *J Dermatol* **28**, 43–46.

6 Drugs that induce or exacerbate psoriasis

Charles Camisa

Some anti-psoriatic treatments have the potential to exacerbate psoriasis by irritating uninvolved skin (coal tar, anthralin), with ultraviolet-induced burns (sunlight, ultraviolet B (UVB), psoralen with ultraviolet A (PUVA)), or by causing flares upon their reduction or withdrawal (superpotent topical and systemic corticosteroids).

When psoriasis flares upon the withdrawal of potent systemic agents like methotrexate, etretinate and cyclosporine, it usually represents a return to the natural course of a severe skin disease. Therefore, if it is necessary to stop such potent treatment, it is advisable to taper the dose and convert to another treatment simultaneously. Whenever possible, systemic corticosteroids should be avoided in psoriatic patients. Their use accounts for most cases of extremely unstable psoriasis and the conversion of ordinary psoriasis into generalized pustular and erythrodermic variants. Moreover, systemic corticosteroids are not particularly effective in treating the most severe forms of psoriasis.

The nonsteroidal anti-inflammatory drugs (NSAIDs), cyclooxygenase inhibitors, are widely used for fever, pain, and inflammation. Specifically, they are effective in stabilizing or diminishing the activity of peripheral psoriatic arthropathy. The implication that NSAIDs exacerbate psoriasis is anecdotal and not substantiated by literature or by experience. In fact, the only double-blind studies of these drugs in psoriasis showed no effect (meclofenamate) or significant improvement (benoxaprofen).

Based on reviews and cumulative case reports to the present, four classes of drugs have been implicated in the induction or aggravation of preexisting psoriasis. These are beta-adrenergic blockers, lithium carbonate, antimalarials, and interferons. The fifth category is "miscellaneous drugs." No prospective controlled studies of the effects of any of these drugs on psoriasis have ever been published, so the information is necessarily anecdotal and contro-versial. There are, however, hypothetical reasons to explain the putative associations as well as some supporting but inconclusive biochemical and immunological data.

Beta-blocking drugs

Both the cardioselective (beta-1-adrenergic receptor) and the non-selective (beta-1- and beta-2-adrenergic receptor) blocking agents can cause various cutaneous eruptions, described as maculopapu-lar, lichenoid, eczematous, and psoriasiform, in patients without psoriasis after an average 10–12 months of therapy. The appear-ance of a psoriasiform rash or aggravation of psoriasis occurs within several weeks to months in patients with established psoriasis. Many of the earlier cases occurred with treatment with practolol, a beta-2 blocker that has been withdrawn from the market. When oral rechallenge tests were done, the cutaneous eruption recurred within 5 days. A generalized pustular flare of chronic plaque-type psoriasis occurred 3 days after propranolol (prototype of nonselect-ive blockade of beta-1- and beta-2-receptors) was taken, and on the occasion of two oral provocation tests.

When propranolol, 0.1 mg/day, was fed to guinea pigs and injected intradermally along with Freund's complete adjuvant, the animals developed a psoriasiform dermatitis that resembled psori-asis but lacked many of the characteristic histopathologic features. This model has potential for studying other drugs that cause psoriasiform reaction patterns.

In a retrospective study of 26 selected patients receiving UVB or PUVA in 1986–7, there was a total of 29 exposures to beta-blocking drugs and 21 (72%) self-reported exacerbations of psoriasis.

The beta-blockers have many uses in medicine today: angina, arrhythmias, hypertension, postmyocardial infarction, migraine headache prophylaxis, open-angle glaucoma, essential tremor, and thyrotoxicosis. Therefore, they are not contraindicated in patients with concomitant psoriasis. When consulting on a patient with a new psoriasiform eruption or flaring of stable psoriasis who is also taking a beta-blocker, one should ask if it is feasible to switch from a nonselective beta-adrenergic blocker to a cardioselective (beta-1) blocking agent. If the patient is already taking a beta-1 blocker, he or she can be switched to another drug in that class as they may not cross-react.

Lithium

Lithium carbonate is used in the treatment of manic disorders and for the prophylaxis and treatment of psychotic depression. Lithium is a cation that substitutes incompletely for other extracellular and intracellular cations, notably sodium, in metabolic reactions. It also interferes with cyclic adenosine monophosphate (cAMP)-mediated processes. Cutaneous reactions, particularly folliculitis and acneiform eruptions, are common with lithium. The first cases of preexisting psoriasis exacerbated by lithium were reported in 1972. This finding was confirmed in 1976 with the report of three patients showing flares after a few weeks and a new case of psoriasis appearing a few months after the patient started taking lithium. The largest single series reported from Denmark included 12 patients who developed psoriasis de novo during lithium therapy. The mean latency period was 10 months (range, 1–24 months). Oral provocation with lithium induced the reappearance of psoriasis in two patients after 5 and 21 days when the original latency was 7 and 15 months, respectively. In three patients, preexisting mild to moderate psoriasis was aggravated and became treatment resistant after 1 week, 1 month, and 6 months, respectively. Thus, it would seem that the latency period is shorter for aggravating preexisting psoriasis or provoking a recurrence of psoriasis upon oral rechallenge than for inducing psoriasis for the first time. Because psoriasis has been associated with psychic factors, it should be emphasized that the new onset and exacerbation of psoriasis in patients taking lithium generally occurred without relation to changes in mood or after the mental illness had actually improved. Notwithstanding, lithium carbonate is not contraindicated in patients with psoriasis. It does not aggravate all cases of preexisting psoriasis, but if it does, an attempt should be made to lower the dose before discontinuing lithium and substituting another drug. The antidepressant fluoxetine, which selectively inhibits serotonin reuptake, reportedly induced psoriasis in two patients. The latency period was 6 months and 1 year; one patient improved after the dose of fluoxetine was reduced.

Mechanisms of beta-blockers and lithium carbonate

These chemically diverse compounds may induce or aggravate psoriasis by different mechanisms through a final common pathway.

Human keratinocytes have beta-2-adrenergic receptors. Pharmacologic blockade of the beta-adrenergic pathway may lead to a decrease in the adenylate cyclase-cAMP cascade and decreased intracellular cAMP and free calcium, which is associated with increased rates of proliferation and insufficient epidermal differentiation, both features of psoriasis. The adenyl cyclase system of psoriatic involved skin has a markedly decreased response to epinephrine and prostaglandin E_2 in vitro. Lithium carbonate inhibited adenyl cyclase stimulation by epinephrine in pig epidermis. Basal levels of cAMP were not altered after 24 hour incubation with lithium. The authors (DiGiovanna *et al.*) also showed that the involved and uninvolved epidermis from a psoriatic patient taking lithium carbonate generated less cAMP compared to the mean values of patients not on lithium therapy. The ability of lithium to inhibit the same adenyl cyclase receptors that are defective in lesional epidermis may amplify the defect and produce flares of psoriasis. Lithium carbonate also increases the total mass of polymorphonuclear leukocytes (PMLs) in the circulation. Decreases in intracellular cAMP can enhance mobility and phagocytosis of PMLs. The increased migration of activated PMLs into the skin and their products may attract more PMLs and stimulate epidermal hyperproliferation.

Lithium probably also affects the cytokine network in psoriasis. When lithium was added to psoriatic keratinocytes in coculture with HUT 78 lymphocytes, the secretion of transforming growth factor and interleukin-2 was increased 150% and that of interferon was decreased 180%. It may be that endogenous interferon mediates the psoriagenic effects of lithium (vide infra).

Antimalarials

All of the antimalarial drugs currently used to treat dermatologic and rheumatologic diseases, quinacrine, chloroquine, and hydroxychloroquine, have been associated with drug eruptions and aggravation of preexisting psoriasis. The structurally related antiarrhythmic agent quinidine may also exacerbate psoriasis, although this occurs rarely. The antimalarials are indicated for lupus erythematosus and rheumatoid arthritis, but are used for many other purposes, including psoriatic arthritis.

In the 1950s and 60s, there was an accumulation of evidence that the antimalarials caused acute flares of psoriasis, sometimes exfoliative dermatitis, and were to be avoided in the treatment of psoriatic arthritis. There was a resurgence in the use of hydroxy-chloroquine for psoriatic arthritis after a report treating 50 patients showed no exacerbation of psoriasis, but four patients (8%) experienced generalized maculopapular eruptions. In this study, 34 (68%) patients achieved remission, improvement, or stabilization of psoriatic arthritis after therapy for 3–4 months.

Isolated cases of exacerbation of psoriasis, exfoliative erythroderma, and a new case of pustular psoriasis associated with hydroxychloroquine continue to be reported, however. Slagel and James critically reviewed the literature on the subject and found that 18% of patients had "worsening of psoriasis" within one month of taking the antimalarial drug, which was most commonly chloroquine. Quinacrine was responsible for the greatest frequency of acute generalized eruptions. A new case of psoriasis with pustules developed three weeks after treating a man with quinacrine for chronic actinic dermatitis. A markedly lower incidence of worsening psoriasis and drug eruptions was found with hydroxychloroquine. Malarial prophylaxis is not contraindicated for psoriatics traveling to endemic areas. Hydroxychloroquine may be used with caution in the treatment of psoriatic arthritis because the risk of flare-ups of skin disease recalcitrant to conventional therapy is low.

The mechanism of action of antimalarials in all diseases, with the possible exception of porphyria cutanea tarda, is unknown. Anti-inflammatory (stabilization of lysosomal membranes and inhibition of PML chemotaxis) and immunosuppressive (inhibition of lymphocyte response to mitogens) effects have been observed in vitro with chloroquine. Recently, investigators showed that chloroquine impaired the allostimulatory properties of fresh normal epidermal antigen-presenting cells (EAPCs) to activate T-cells, but had no such effect on these cells from psoriatic skin. In fact, the investigators noted that, in some experiments, the chloroquine-treated psoriatic EAPCs displayed significantly enhanced abilities to activate allogeneic T-cells. This constitutive difference between normal and psoriatic EAPCs may be relevant to the exacerbation of psoriasis experienced by some patients while receiving chloroquine. It has also been hypothesized that the mechanism of action of triggering of psoriasis by hydroxychloroquine is by modulation of epidermal transglutaminase activity. It caused concentration-dependent inhibition of enzyme activity in skin explant cultures.

Interferons

All forms of interferon can induce or aggravate psoriasis and psoriatic arthritis. Psoriatic lesions developed at the site of intradermal IFN-alpha and IFN-gamma injections. Interferon-alpha, now more commonly prescribed for hepatitis C virus infection, can aggravate preexisting and cause new onset psoriasis and psoriatic arthritis. The new disease may not improve after interferon is stopped; it may recur following rechallenge. Recombinant serine-substituted interferon-beta used to treat multiple sclerosis caused a pustular flare of usually mild psoriasis.

The new development of psoriasis in patients receiving interferon-alpha-2a for erythrodermic cutaneous T-cell lymphoma provides further support for the concept that psoriasis is a disease predominated by Th1 cells which secrete interleukin-2, interferon-gamma and tumor necrosis factor-alpha. Th2 clones secrete interleukin-4, -5, and -10. Interferon-gamma apparently influences the cytokine cascade toward increased Th1 expression.

Miscellaneous drugs

Alcohol

In the previous chapter, I mentioned that alcohol consumption is associated with worsening psoriasis in women. It also produces a poorer outcome of anti-psoriatic therapy in men. One possible explanation for this is that ethanol influences cytokine expression by psoriatic keratinocytes in cocultures with HUT 78 lymphocytes. Transforming growth factor-alpha and interferon-gamma levels were increased 150% and 175%, respectively, by the addition of ethanol, but interleukin-6 levels were unaffected.

Calcium channel blockers

Acute generalized exanthematous pustulosis (AGEP) is probably a distinct drug-induced entity that may occur at higher frequency in psoriatic patients. Although antibiotics are thought to be the chief cause of AGEP, calcium channel blockers are also prominent on the expanding list of provocative agents (see Plate 10, facing p. 34). Psoriasiform eruptions and exacerbation of preexisting psoriasis have been reported which were resolved or easily controlled after discontinuation of the drugs, which included diltiazem, dihydropy-ridine, nifedipine, felodipine, amlodipine, nisoldipine, and nicardip-ine. A retrospective case-control study of 150 patients admitted to the hospital for psoriasis or psoriasiform eruptions revealed that 18 were taking calcium channel blockers. The association with new or flaring psoriasis was statistically significant ($p = 0.018$).

Other drugs that are possibly associated with development of de novo or exacerbation of psoriasis include the antihypertens-ive angiotensin converting enzyme inhibitors (e.g. captopril) or angiotensin II receptor antagonists, and the oral antifungal, ter-binafine. Bupropion, used in the management of smoking cessa-tion, was associated with severe pustular or erythrodermic flares of preexisting psoriasis in three patients.

Selected references

Cohen A. D., Kagen M., Friger M., Halevy S. (2001) Calcium channel blockers intake and psoriasis: a case-control study. *Acta Derm Venereol* **51**, 347–349.

Cox N. H., Gordon P. M., Dodd H. (2002) Generalized pustular and erythrodermic psoriasis associated with bupropion treatment. *Br J Dermatol* **146**, 1061–1063.

DiGiovanna J.J., Aoyagi T., Taylor J.R., Halprin K.M. (1981) Inhibition of epidermal adenyl-cyclase by lithium carbonate. *J Invest Dermatol* **76**, 259–263.

Downs A. M., Dunnill M. G. (2000) Exacerbation of psoriasis by inter-feron-alpha therapy for hepatitis C. *Clin Exp Dermatol* **25**, 351–352.

Gordon M. M., Sturrock R. D. (2000) Antimalarials in the management of psoriatic arthritis. *Clin Exp Rheumatol* **20**, 117.

Gupta A. K., Sibbald R. G., Knowles S. R. *et al.* (1997) Terbinafine therapy may be associated with the development of psoriasis de novo or its exacerba-tion: Four case reports and a review of drug-induced psoriasis. *J Am Acad Dermatol* **36**, 858–862.

Kitamura K., Kanasashi M., Suga C. *et al.* (1993) Cutaneous reactions induced by calcium channel blocker: high frequency of psoriasiform eruptions. *J Dermatol* **20**, 279–286.

Marquart-Elbaz C., Lipsker D. (2002) Sartans, angiotensin II receptor antagonists, can induce psoriasis. *Br J Dermatol* **147**, 617–618.

Ockenfels H. M., Wagner S. N., Keim-Maas C. *et al.* (1996) Lithium and psoriasis: cytokine modulation of cultured lymphocytes and psoriatic keratinocytes by lithium. *Arch Dermatol Res* **288**, 173–178.

Slagel G.A., James W.D. (1985) Plaquenil-induced erythroderma. *J Am Acad Dermatol* **12**, 857–862.

Taylor C., Burns D. A., Wiselka M. J. (2000) Extensive psoriasis induced by interferon alfa treatment for chronic hepatitis C. *Postgrad Med* **76**, 365–367.

Wolf R., Ruocco V. (1999) Triggered psoriasis. *Adv Exp Med Biol* **455**, 221–225.

Wolf R., Shechter H., Brenner S. (1994) Induction of psoriasiform changes in guinea pig skin by propanolol. *Int J Dermatol* **33**, 811–814.

Wolfe J. T., Singh A., Lessin S. R. *et al.* (1995) De novo development of psoriatic plaques in patients receiving interferon alfa for treatment of erythrodermic cutaneous T-cell lymphoma. *J Am Acad Dermatol* **32**, 887–893.

7   Evaluation of psoriasis symptoms and disability

Charles Camisa

The task of critically interpreting therapeutic studies is made diffi-cult by the bewildering array of evaluation scoring and assessment systems currently in use.

One of these, the psoriasis area and severity index or PASI, was introduced for studies of the synthetic retinoids in 1978 (Fig. 7.1). It has been employed in numerous clinical trials to assess differences before and after treatment in a fairly rigorous and consistent man-ner that is reproducible between investigators.

Figure 7.1 *PASI score determination*

The four main anatomic sites are assessed: the head (h), upper extremities (u), trunk (t) and lower extremities (l) roughly corresponding to 10%, 20%, 30% and 40% of body surface area, respectively. The PASI score is calculated from:

$$PASI = 0.1(E_h + I_h + D_h)A_h + 0.2(E_u + I_u + D_u)A_u$$
$$+ 0.3(E_t + I_t + D_t)A_t + 0.4(E_l + I_l + D_l)A_l$$

where E = erythema, I = induration, D = desquamation and A = area. E, I, and D are assessed according to a 4-point scale where 0 = no symptoms, 1 = slight, 2 = moderate, 3 = marked, and 4 = very marked. A is assigned a numerical value based on the extent of lesions in a given anatomical site: 1(<10%); 2(10–29%); 3(30–49%); 4(50–69%); 5(70–89%); 6(90–100%). The PASI varies in steps of 0.1 units from 0.0 to 72.0. The highest score represents complete erythroderma of the severest possible degree.

The PASI is most useful for the hospital inpatient, day treatment center, or pharmaceutical research setting. Such a complex and detailed assessment is neither practical nor necessary in an ordinary office-based practice. The PASI score is good but not infallible for the following reasons:

1 Experienced clinicians may differ in their estimates of body surface area involved which could alter the resulting PASI and render comparisons to the same study performed in other centers or in the literature invalid.

2 There is high interobserver variability in the calculation of the area involved. The same clinician must calculate the PASI score for a given patient throughout the entire study or treatment period.

3 PASI does not apply as well to the less common but more severe forms of psoriasis such as erythroderma and pustular compared to plaque-type disease. For example, erythroderma with moderate erythema, slight induration, and scaling could have the same score as chronic plaque-type psoriasis involving 10–30% of body surface area with marked erythema, induration and desquamation. (Patients with variants of psoriasis other than plaque-type are usually excluded from clinical pharmaceutical studies.)

4 The evaluation of the physical signs or parameters of psoriatic lesions is purely subjective on the part of the investigator.

5 The PASI score does not take into account the patient's subjective symptoms such as itching or pain and the level of disability. Modifications of the PASI scoring method may be used for evaluation of specific anatomic sites (scalp, palms and soles) or treatment modalities (Dead-Sea climatotherapy).

The Wake Forest University Psoriasis Study group developed and meticulously evaluated a simple PASI-like instrument for patients to complete. It consists of an anatomic diagram for patients to shade in affected areas and three questions to evaluate redness, thickness, and scaliness of an average lesion on a visual analog scale 120 mm in length with extremes and intermediate grades labeled, e.g. no thickness, feels firm, raised, thick, very thick (Fig. 7.2). The self-administered PASI (SAPASI) was demonstrated to be valid by showing a significant correlation between SAPASI and PASI scores for all four parameters measured on the same day. Retest reliability within 2 days was high; inter-rater reliability among five raters for estimating the percentage of involved body surface area from the diagram was very high. The SAPASI decreased over time as the psoriasis improved and correlated with changes in PASI scores.

How bad is your psoriasis **TODAY**?

Name:_____
Date:_____

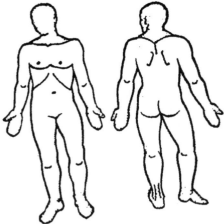

1. As best you can, please shade in on the drawing exactly where you have psoriasis.

2. Answer each question with a mark on the line to show how red, thick, and scaly an average spot of your psoriasis is (see example).

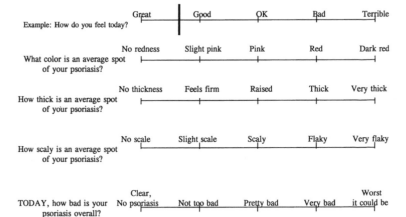

	Great	Good	OK	Bad	Terrible
Example: How do you feel today?					

	No redness	Slight pink	Pink	Red	Dark red
What color is an average spot of your psoriasis?					

	No thickness	Feels firm	Raised	Thick	Very thick
How thick is an average spot of your psoriasis?					

	No scale	Slight scale	Scaly	Flaky	Very flaky
How scaly is an average spot of your psoriasis?					

	Clear, No psoriasis	Not too bad	Pretty bad	Very bad	Worst it could be
TODAY, how bad is your psoriasis overall?					

Copyright 1993

Figure 7.2 SAPASI score determination.

Based on the patient-completed shading of anatomic diagram, an investigator assigns a numeric value of 0 to 6 where 0 indicates no involvement, 1 is <10%, 2 is 11–30%, 3 is 31–50%, 4 is 51–70%, 5 is 71–90%, and 6 is 91–100% of head (h), upper extremities (u), trunk (t) and lower extremities (l). The SAPASI score is calculated from:

$$\text{SAPASI} = \frac{[(0.1 \times A_h) + (0.2 \times A_u) + (0.3 \times A_t) + (0.4 \times A_l)] \times 4 \, (\text{VAS}_E + \text{VAS}_I + \text{VAS}_S)}{\text{VAS length (mm)}}$$

Where A corresponds to investigator numeric score 0–6 representing area, VAS = visual analog scale, E = erythema, I = induration, and S = scale. All VAS scores are in mm.

Note: The SAPASI is a copyright instrument. Permission to use this instrument may be obtained only by contacting Dr Steven R. Feldman or Dr Alan Fleischer at the Bowman Gray School of Medicine of Wake Forest University, Dept of Dermatology, Medical Center Blvd, Winston-Salem, NC 27157-1071.

The SAPASI may be utilized in multicenter studies. The SAPASI was also significantly related to measures of psoriasis comorbidity: pruritus, skin soreness, joint pain.

To highlight the wide variation in assessment methods of psoriasis, Marks *et al.* analyzed 30 articles published in 1985 and 1986:

1 Seven different formulae distinct from the PASI were used resulting in a wide range of incompatible and noncomparable totals.

2 The definition of "clearing" differed widely.

3 The percentage area of body involvement was estimated in nine of the 30 studies.

4 None of the 30 studies objectively measured the three common physical signs of psoriasis: erythema (redness), scaling (desquamation), thickness (induration).

5 The symptom of pruritus was recorded in only four of the 30 studies.

The "gold standard" for measuring involved body surface area is computerized image analysis of traced plaque outlines (planimetric method). The human eye is more likely to overestimate the area involved especially when assessing patients with small-plaque disease (overestimated 3.8 times) compared to large-plaque psoriasis (overestimated 1.7 times). The estimates of individual observers were consistent on two consecutive days, suggesting that the estimates have clinical value if recorded sequentially by the same observer. Computer image analysis (CIA) of whole body digital photographs based on color segmentation gave results similar to those achieved by the planimetric method. The human eye estimates were usually higher when the PASI was less than 15, and changes in the PASI before and after treatments differed significantly between the human eye and the CIA determinations. The CIA system offers an objective measurement of involved surface in patients with psoriasis.

There are alternative objective methods of quantifying the other parameters of psoriasis. The decrease in erythema due to the reduction of vasodilation and skin blood flow during anti-psoriatic therapy can be measured by laser Doppler velocimetry or reflectance spectrophotometry. There is significant correlation between visual scores and the instrumental evaluations. Thickness or induration of psoriatic plaques can be evaluated by high frequency 40–50 MHz ultrasound imaging systems. The width of a nonechogenic region corresponds to the elongated rete ridges and the edematous papillary dermal papillae with congested vessels. The width of this band correlates best with the clinical severity score, and the change in activity correlates best with change in the thickness of this band. The images were of high resolution and reproducible by different investigators. Recovery of barrier function properties and formation of efficient stratum corneum results in decreased transepidermal water loss as measured by an evaporimeter. Nitric oxide (NO) production (measured by a noninvasive chemiluminescence technique) is significantly greater in lesional vs. nonlesional skin and is reduced by effective anti-psoriatic treatment. More sophisticated quantification of multiple parameters can be obtained before and after treatments by flow cytometry of skin biopsies which evaluates epidermal proliferation, differentiation, and inflammation.

Pruritus is an important symptom of psoriasis. About 70–80% of patients report moderate to severe itching during flares of psoriasis. Because uninvolved skin does not itch, the sensation is probably due to the physical effects of dry scales with their rough, irritating edges. The scalp is most frequently affected by pruritus, which may be severe and paroxysmal at night. Itching leads to scratching and even this injury may provoke the isomorphic response and exacerbation of psoriasis.

Evaluation of disability

Depression

There is a strong association between subjective self-reported levels of anxiety and depression and the degree of pruritus. Patients with three different itchy disorders, psoriasis, urticaria, and atopic dermatitis, were evaluated by the Carroll Rating Scale for Depression. A direct correlation was found between pruritus severity and the depressive psychopathology score. Using the same scale, Gupta *et al.* (1998) demonstrated that patients who experienced social rejection by people avoiding touching them, had higher depression scores than the nonstigmatized psoriatic control group. There was no difference in the psoriasis severity scores between the two groups. Beck depression scores were significantly higher in subjects with psoriasis vulgaris and lichen planus compared to control subjects. The PASI scores *were* correlated with the depression scores in this study.

Instruments to evaluate quality of life

Distillation of various questionnaires administered to outpatients before and at 3 months of treatment revealed that the two most useful questions were: (1) Does the state of your psoriasis affect your life in any way? and (2) Have you had to stop your usual sports or hobbies because of your skin? The combined responses to these questions were the best predictors of overall disease severity scores in the judgment of the patient or doctor. The severity score was derived by asking the patient to grade the following six features of their psoriasis on a scale of 0–4 (none to severe): (1) amount of body with psoriasis; (2) degree of itch; (3) degree of pain or discomfort; (4) amount of scaliness; (5) level of embarrassment; and (6) how much it stops the patient from doing what he or she wants to do. The authors (McHenry and Doherty) found that about one-third of patients considered their symptoms of itch, irritation, or scaliness to be the worst aspect of their psoriasis.

The U.K. Sickness Impact Profile (SIP), a questionnaire with 136 questions that evaluates how disease affects patients' physical and emotional states, registered the same score regardless of extent or severity of psoriasis. Psychosocial activities were most severely impaired whereas physical ability was least impaired. Psoriasis had a major impact on patients' ability to sleep, work, manage their homes, and participate in recreational activities. Their overall quality of life was adversely affected to about the same degree as that for patients with cardiovascular disease. This finding was confirmed by Rapp *et al.* using the nondisease-specific health-related quality of life (HRQL) instrument known as the Short Form Health Survey Questionnaire (SF-36). Commonly employed coping strategies, i.e. covering lesions and avoiding people, are associated with reduction in HRQL. Patients with medical conditions, e.g. myocardial infarction, unrelated cancer, spinal cord injury, employ certain coping strategies with a frequency similar to that of psoriasis.

There was good correlation between SIP score and the Psoriasis Disability Index (PDI), a more compact questionnaire consisting of 15 questions answered on a linear analogue scale from 1 ("not at all") to 7 ("very much"). Overall PDI scores, but not overall SIP scores, correlated well with PASI scores. The PDI provides a practical way of monitoring the effect of treatment on functional impairment together with visual documentation of psoriasis morphology and extent. Since unemployment is an important issue among psoriatic patients, return to work may be a more critical and attainable goal than clearing of psoriasis.

A self-completed 29-item questionnaire consisting of items grouped into four psychosocial (embarrassment, despair, irritableness, distress) and four activity subscales (everyday, summer, social, sexual) is called the Dermatology Quality of Life Scales (DQOLS). It was tested on psoriasis and acne patients showing good short-term test-retest reliability. The results indicated that acne had a greater psychosocial impact but lesser impact on activities compared with psoriasis. The results also confirmed that both conditions had a greater psychosocial impact for women than for men.

The DQOLS were refined further by Finlay and Khan in the U.K. to 10 self-administered questions covering daily activities, personal relationships, leisure, work, and treatments. It is called the Dermatology Life Quality Index (DLQI). The DLQI scores are higher for patients with psoriasis and atopic dermatitis than for acne and basal cell carcinoma. The DLQI has been validated in Scandinavian and U.S. dermatology patients. In the latter group, examined in the outpatient clinic at Indiana University Medical Center, patients were able to complete the form within 3 minutes; the results could be stratified by severity of disease as evaluated by a separate instrument. A cartoon version of the DLQI for children is now available.

In an audit of consultations for psoriasis in two teaching hospitals, most of the case notes lacked an estimation of extent or distribution of lesions including routine use of an anatomic diagram (Fig. 7.3), as well as any reference to the patients' symptoms or disability. It was also unclear as to whose assessment of treatment was being recorded at follow-up visits; the patient's or the physician's. Without baseline documentation of extent of disease, symptoms, and disability, it is impossible to compare the outcome of different treatment strategies.

Many physicians and their assistants use the SOAP—subjective, objective, assessment, plan—method for documenting patient encounters, which includes the patient's symptoms, perceived disability, and reference to current and previously used medications. The objective, or O, part includes the morphologic description of rash, the distribution, and an estimation of percentage of body area involved. The use of self-sticking labels or rubber stamps of anatomic diagrams facilitates the graphic representation of this information (see Fig. 7.3). The assessment, or A, part is the

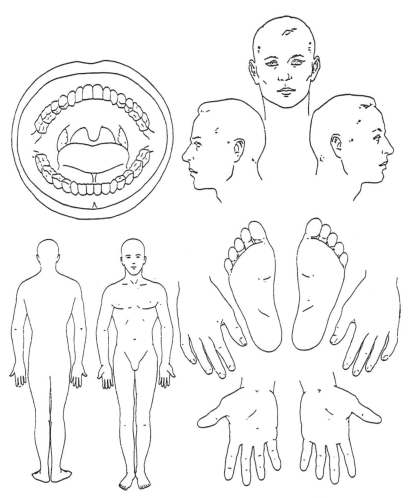

Figure 7.3 Anatomic diagram used for documenting percentage of body surface area involved with psoriasis in the Cleveland Clinic Department of Dermatology.

diagnosis, determination of psoriasis variant, and the physician's impression of whether the disease is mild, moderate, or severe.

To estimate percentage of body surface area involved, the "rule of nines" or "modified rule of nines" may be used (Table 7.1). The area of the side of a flat closed hand has been used to estimate 1% of body surface area (BSA), but the actual value calculated by the planimetric method was 0.70–0.76% of BSA.

Table 7.1 Estimation of body surface area involvement.

Rule of nines		Modified rule of nines	
Head	9%	Head	3%
Anterior trunk		Scalp	6%
Upper	9%	Anterior trunk	14%
Lower	9%	Posterior trunk	16%
Posterior trunk		Genitalia	1%
Upper	9%	Leg	16% each
Lower	9%	Dorsum foot	2% each
Legs	18% each	Sole	2% each
Arms	9% each	Arm	7% each
		Dorsum hand	1.5% each
		Palm	1.5% each
Total	99%		100%

By incorporating quality of life parameters into the assessment of psoriasis severity, the traditional definitions now call for an overlapping of estimates of involved BSA:
- Mild psoriasis; generally less than 5% BSA
- Moderate psoriasis; generally 2–20% BSA
- Severe psoriasis; generally more than 10% BSA

On follow-up visits the subjective aspect includes the *patient's* subjective assessment of progress, and the assessment is the *physician's* impression of progress based on integration of the patient's symptoms and results of the physical examination *compared to the previous one.*

The plan, or **P**, includes the choice of medical or physical therapies and documentation of any verbal or written information dispensed about the disease or its treatment [e.g. The American Academy of Dermatology pamphlet on psoriasis (*www.aad.org*), the manufacturer's brochure on acitretin (*www.soriatane.com*), or the National Psoriasis Foundation's booklet on systemic treatments (*www.psoriasis.org*)]. If a consultant is involved, a copy of a brief summary report to the referring physician or agency should be maintained in the record. Medical record keeping is held to high standards in a cost-conscious and litigious society; the case notes are important for clinical documentation, for outcome research, and also for quality assurance, legal, and economic concerns.

Stressful life events have been estimated to affect the course of psoriasis (initiate or exacerbate) in 40–80% of patients.

Patients were more likely to report that one or more stressful events predated the onset and exacerbation of their psoriasis than were patients with other skin diseases. For psoriasis, the most common types of major life events were family upsets (deaths, arguments, children leaving home) followed by personal illness or injury, work or school pressures (more responsibilities or examinations), hormonal changes (childbirth and puberty), and financial concerns. A questionnaire survey of 870 Korean psoriasis patients seen between 1982 and 1995 confirmed a statistically significant correlation between the extent of the psoriasis and the percentage of patients stating that their disease flared during the times of psychological stress.

The chronic daily low-grade stress arising from the cosmetic disfigurement and social stigma of psoriasis may adversely affect the course of the disease. The Psoriasis Life Stress Inventory (PLSI), which consists of 15 items rated from 0 to 3 (not at all, slight, moderate, a great deal), selects for more cosmetically disfiguring psoriasis, more flare-ups, and greater pruritus severity if the score is 10 or higher (Table 7.2). Thus, the recurrent stress of living with psoriasis may be a more accurate indicator of psychosocial disability associated with psoriasis. Patients who believe their psoriasis is exacerbated by stress may be more susceptible to the effect of stress. The patients' views of the severity of their disease are related to both disability and to psychological distress. Social disability is the mediator between severity and distress. Perceived severity affects a patient's willingness to engage in common social activities which in turn results in distress. Visible or "emotionally charged" areas of involvement such as face, neck, hands, and genitalia increase self-rated severity although the extent may be limited. Genital involvement is particularly relevant for the stigmatization experience. A group in Salford, U.K. (Kirby *et al.*, 2000), advocates the use of a complex 3-figure index analogous to the TNM (tumor, lymph nodes, metastases) classification of malignancies. The three figures incorporate PASI score, psychosocial disability, and interventions.

Biofeedback training, stress management, relaxation exercises, guided imagery, psychotherapy, psychopharmaceuticals, and hypnosis have all been suggested as helpful adjuncts to the traditional medical treatments of psoriasis. Psychological interventions can help patients to reinterpret major stressful life events and develop

Table 7.2 Psoriasis Life Stress Inventory.

---

1 Inconvenienced by the shedding of your skin

2 Feeling self-conscious among strangers

3 Feeling that you have to set aside a large part of your time to take care of your psoriasis

4 Not going to a public place (e.g. swimming pool, health club, restaurant) when you would have liked to

5 Wearing unattractive or uncomfortable clothes in order to cover certain regions of the body

6 Having to avoid sunbathing in the company of others

7 Fear of having serious side-effects from medical treatments

8 People treating you as if your skin condition is contagious

9 Avoiding social situations

10 Strangers (children or adults) making rude or insensitive remarks about your appearance

11 Not enough money to pay medical bills

12 Feeling like an "outcast" or "social misfit" a great deal of the time

13 People making a conscious effort not to touch you

14 Hairdresser or barber appearing reluctant to cut your hair

15 People implying that your skin condition may be due to AIDS, leprosy or a venereal disease

---

Note: Items are rated 0, not at all; 1, slight; 2, moderate; 3, a great deal. A total of 10 or more correlates with greater disfigurement, pruritus, and more flare-ups.

strategies for coping with the psychosocial disability associated with psoriasis.

Group meetings of psoriatic patients led by a dermatologic nurse or physician are fairly easy to organize in existing psoriasis treatment centers. Such groups become forums for dissemination of general information about psoriasis and its treatments and for discussion of anecdotal experience with the disease, social situations, specific treatments, and professional staff. Familiarity with the environment, clinic, staff, and other people with psoriasis presumably reduces anxiety and any sense of stigmatization. It is valuable for patients to learn what areas of their life are stressful, how to reduce stressful issues, and cope with them more effectively (i.e. develop defense mechanisms).

In one study, patients who took part in group therapy sessions were taught relaxation techniques including self-hypnosis and were encouraged to practice these at home and whenever they were under stress. Their anxiety scores decreased after the group sessions, and the decreased scores persisted at the 6-month follow-up visit. The control group showed no change. The authors noted a paradoxical significant negative correlation between anxiety and severity of disease, suggesting that a patient's anxiety may be out of proportion to the extent of disease. Group therapy sessions had no demonstrable clinical benefit on the clearing of psoriasis compared to the control group. Patients with extensive disease may become better adjusted to its chronicity than those with mild disease who may have unrealistic expectations of a cure. A questionnaire survey of 162 patients attending a tertiary referral clinic indicated that, while 82% responded that psoriasis is "likely to be permanent," 32% believed that "treatments will be effective in curing it."

In another study, improvement in the symptoms of scalp psoriasis was obtained in a few patients who were meditating, leading the authors to conclude that stress reduction techniques should be a component of the overall treatment of psoriasis. Interestingly, perceived stress increased the most in psoriatics during the stressor exposure but tended to normalize faster in psoriatics compared to control groups of atopic dermatitis patients or healthy subjects. Coping style and other cognitive factors were found to be more significant discriminators between the groups than were psychosocial stress and the specific skin disease. Stress apparently affects skin reactivity but cognitive factors modulate these effects. Subjective and objective (cutaneous blood flow) measures improved slightly but significantly in patients receiving seven individual psychotherapy sessions in 12 weeks. Routine psychological consultation is not indicated for psoriatic patients unless requested by the individual patient or if a patient demonstrates unusual aggressiveness or suicidal ideation. Completion of one or more questionnaires to evaluate baseline disability or stress is recommended, with periodic repetition as treatment progresses. Group discussions with patients and the health care professional team leader are beneficial.

A telephone survey of 500 members of the National Psoriasis Foundation revealed that psoriasis patients felt embarrassed when people viewed their psoriasis (81%), felt unattractive (75%), and felt depressed (54%). A mail-survey of the entire membership garnered 17,434 responders. Sixty-seven (0.4%) reported that psoriasis negatively affected sexual activity and 20 (0.1%) contemplated suicide.

While the disease does not overtly affect established social relationships, it can certainly interfere with the social development of children, and adults who are initiating sexual relationships. Because the genitalia are so often affected by psoriasis, an explanation that it is not a venereal disease is usually required. Children may become withdrawn, angry, and frustrated if their self-image is poor. They may not be able to benefit from exposure to natural sunlight because of avoidance of public pools and beaches for fear of stares and questions concerning contagion (stigmatization).

The sexual relations of married couples may be adversely affected during flares when ointments and other dressings must be worn to bed or when scales accumulate between the sheets and on the floors of the bedroom and bathroom. Perhaps because there is a greater emphasis on female beauty in western culture, women appear to be more emotionally disturbed by psoriasis than men. Patients might avoid sexual relations altogether until remission occurs.

If the physician is comfortable and sympathetic in discussing emotional and sexual problems, a special longer session, possibly together with the patient's partner, should be arranged for more open communication. If either the physician or patient is uncomfortable discussing these matters, then referral to a psychologist, sex therapist, or psychiatrist is indicated. Supportive group therapy would be ideal for discussing feelings of shame or guilt, isolation, and appearing sexually unattractive because these emotions are probably common to most psoriasis patients at some time during the course of their disease. In group and private sessions, advice and treatment concerning abuse of tobacco, caffeine, alcohol and other substances, and irregular eating habits which can theoretically increase stress and aggravate psoriasis should be dispensed. Aerobic exercise should be promoted to help obese patients lose weight, improve the cardiovascular system, increase high-density lipoprotein cholesterol levels, and improve their self-image.

In conclusion, calculation of the PASI score is far too cumbersome for ordinary office practice, but the SAPASI provides a more practical alternative that employs patient participation and communication. However, as a minimum, the clinician should include in the evaluation an estimate of the percentage of body surface area involved or a diagrammatic display of this (a record of symptoms such as pruritus, skin pain, joint pain, and arthritis) and a determination of the level of disability by way of directed verbal queries or administration of one or more of the self-completed questionnaires discussed in this chapter.

Selected references

Akay A., Pekcanlar A., Bozdag K. E. *et al.* (2002) Assessment of depression in subjects with psoriasis vulgaris and lichen planus. *J Eur Acad Dermatol Venereol* **16**, 347–352.

Al'Abadil M. S., Kent G. G., Gawkrodger D. J. (1994) The relationship between stress and the onset and exacerbation of psoriasis and other skin conditions. *Br J Dermatol* **130**, 199–203.

Berardesca E., Vignoli G. P., Farinelli N. *et al.* (1994) Non-invasive evaluation of topical calcipotriol versus clobetasol in the treatment of psoriasis. *Acta Derm Venereol* **74**, 302–304.

Feldman S. R., Fleischer A. B., Reboussin D. M. *et al.* (1996) The self-adminis-tered psoriasis area and severity index is valid and reliable. *J Invest Dermatol* **106**, 183–186.

Finlay A. Y., Kelly S. E. (1987) Psoriasis—an index of disability. *Clin Exp Dermatol* **12**, 8–11.

Finlay A. Y., Khan G. K., Luscombe D. K., Salek M. S. (1990) Validation of sick-ness impart profile and psoriasis disability index in psoriasis. *Br J Dermatol* **123**, 751–756.

Finlay A. Y., Khan G. K. (1994) Dermatology Life Quality Index (DLQI)—a simple practical measure for routine clinical use. *Clin Exp Dermatol* **19**, 210–216.

Fleischer A. B., Feldman S. R., Rapp S. R. *et al.* (1996) Disease severity meas-ures in a population of psoriasis patients: The symptoms of psoriasis corre-late with self-administered psoriasis area severity index scores. *J Invest Dermatol* **107**, 26–29.

Fortune D. G., Main C. J., O'Sullivan T. M., Griffiths C. E. M. (1997) Quality of life in patients with psoriasis: the contribution of clinical variables and psoriasis-specific stress. *Br J Dermatol* **137**, 755–760.

Fortune D. G., Richards H. L., Main C. J. *et al.* (1998) What patients with psori-asis believe about their condition. *J Am Acad Dermatol* **39**, 196–201.

Fortune D. G., Richards H. L., Main C. J., Griffiths C. E. (2002) Patients' strat-egies for coping with psoriasis. *Clin Exp Dermatol* **27**, 177–184.

Fried R. G., Friedman S., Paradis G. *et al.* (1995) Trivial or terrible? The psy-chosocial impact of psoriasis. *Int J Dermatol* **33**, 101–105.

Gaston L., Crombez J. C., Lassonde M. *et al.* (1991) Psychological stress and psoriasis: experimental and prospective correlational studies. *Acta Derm Venereol* **156** (Suppl.), 37–43.

Glade C. P., van Erp P. E., Werner-Schlenzka H., Van de Kerkhof P. C. (1998) A clinical and flow cytometric model to study remission and relapse in psori-asis. *Acta Derm Venereol* **78**, 180–185.

Gupta A. K., Turnbull D. H., Harasiewicz K. A. *et al.* (1996) The use of high-frequency ultrasound as a method of assessing the severity of a plaque of psoriasis. *Arch Dermatol* **132**, 656–662.

Gupta M. A., Gupta A. K., Schork N. J., Ellis C. N. (1994) Depression modulates pruritus perception: A study of pruritus in psoriasis atopic dermatitis, and chronic idiopathic urticaria. *Psychosomatic Med* **56**, 36–40.

Gupta M. A., Gupta A. K., Watteel G. N. (1998) Perceived deprivation of social touch in psoriasis is associated with a greater psychologic morbidity: an index of the stigma experience in dermatologic disorders. *Cutis* **61**, 339–342.

Gupta M. A., Gupta A. K. (1995) The psoriasis life stress inventory: a preliminary index of psoriasis-related stress. *Acta Dermatovenereol* **75**, 240–243.

Hahn H. B., Melfi C.A., Chuang T. Y. *et al.* (2001) Use of the Dermatology Life Quality Index (DLQI) in a Midwestern US urban clinic. *J Am Acad Dermatol* **45**, 44–48.

Harari M., Shani J., Hristakieva E. *et al.* (2000) Clinical evaluation of a more rapid and sensitive Psoriasis Assessment Severity Score (PASS), and its comparison with the classic method of Psoriasis Area and Severity Index (PASI), before and after climatotherapy at the Dead-Sea. *Int J Dermatol* **39**, 913–918.

Holme S. A., Man I., Sharpe J. L. *et al.* (2003) The Children's Dermatology Life Quality Index: validation of the cartoon version. *Br J Dermatol* **148**, 285–290.

Mork C., Wahl A., Moum T. (2002) The Norwegian version of the dermatology, life quality index: a study of validity and reliability in psoriatics. *Acta Derm Venereol* **82**, 347–351.

Kirby B., Fortune D. G., Bhyshan M. *et al.* (2000) The Salford psoriasis index: an holistic measure of psoriasis severity. *Br J Dermatol* **142**, 728–732.

Krueger G., Koo J., Lebwohl M. *et al.* (2001) The impact of psoriasis on quality of life: results of a 1998 National Psoriasis Foundation patient-membership survey. *Arch Dermatol* **137**, 280–284.

Krueger G. G., Feldman S. R., Camisa C. *et al.* (2000) Two considerations for patients with psoriasis and their clinicians: What defines mild, moderate, and severe psoriasis? What constitutes a clinically significant improvement when treating psoriasis? *J Am Acad Dermatol* **43**, 281–285.

Marks R., Barton S. P., Shuttleworth D., Finlay A. Y. (1989) Assessment of disease progress in psoriasis. *Arch Dermatol* **125**, 235–240.

McHenry P. M., Doherty V. R. (1992) Psoriasis: an audit of patient's views on the disease and its treatment. *Br J Dermatol* **127**, 13–17.

Modell J. G., Boyce S., Taylor E., Katholi C. (2002) Treatment of atopic dermatitis and psoriasis vulgaris with bupropion-SR: A pilot study. *Psychosom Med* **64**, 835–840.

Morgan M., McCreedy R., Simpson J., Hay R. J. (1997) Dermatology quality of life scales—a measure of the impact of skin diseases. *Br J Dermatol* **136**, 202–206.

Moum T. (2002) The Norwegian version of the dermatology life quality index: a study of validity and reliability in psoriatics. *Acta Derm Venereol* **82**, 347–351.

Ormerod A. D., Dwyer C. M., Weller R. *et al.* (1997) A comparison of subjective and objective measures of reduction of psoriasis with the use of ultrasound, reflectance colorimetry, computerized video image analysis, and nitric oxide production. *J Am Acad Dermatol* **37**, 51–57.

Park B. S., Youn J. I. (1998) Factors influencing psoriasis: an analysis based upon extent of involvement and clinical type. *J Dermatol* **25**, 97–102.

Rapp S. R., Cottrell C. A., Leary M. R. (2001) Social coping strategies associated with quality of life decrements among psoriasis patients. *Br J Dermatol* **145**, 610–616.

Rapp S. R., Feldman S. R., Exum M. L. *et al.* (1999) Psoriasis causes as much disability as other major medical diseases. *J Am Acad Dermatol* **41**, 401–407.

Savolainen L., Lontinen J., Alatalo E. *et al.* (1998) Comparison of actual psoriasis surface area and psoriasis area and severity index by the human eye and machine vision methods in following the treatment of psoriasis. *Acta Derm Venereol* **78**, 466–467.

Schmid-Ott G., Kuensebeck H. W., Jaeger B. *et al.* (1999) Validity study for the stigmatization experience in atopic dermatitis and psoriasis patients. *Acta Derm Venereol* **79**, 443–447.

Suh D. H., Kwon T. E., Kim S. D. *et al.* (2001) Changes of skin blood flow and color on lesional and control sites during PUVA therapy for psoriasis. *J Am Acad Dermatol* **44**, 987–994.

Thaci D., Daiber W., Boehncke W. H., Kaufmann R. (2001) Calcipotriol solution for the treatment of scalp psoriasis: Evaluation of efficacy, safety and acceptance in 3396 patients. *Dermatol* **203**, 153–156.

Zachariae R., Oster H., Bjerring P., Kragballe K. (1996) Effects of psychologic intervention on psoriasis: A preliminary report. *J Am Acad Dermatol* **34**, 1008–1015.

8   Scalp psoriasis

Thomas N. Helm
Charles Camisa

Introduction

Psoriasis of the scalp is common and may occur with or without cutaneous involvement elsewhere. Although scalp psoriasis may be concealed by the hair in mild cases, severe cases can cause discomfort, embarrassment and emotional distress to patients. Concomitant pruritus, hair loss or secondary infection may prompt patients to seek medical attention. This chapter will address the clinical manifestations of scalp psoriasis and its treatment.

Epidemiology

About 50% of all psoriatics have scalp involvement. Most patients with generalized plaque type psoriasis will develop scalp involvement at some time during their lives. Scalp involvement is less common in guttate psoriasis, and more common in pustular and erythrodermic forms. Scalp psoriasis in the absence of other cutaneous or nail findings is uncommon.

Clinical findings

The cutaneous changes of scalp psoriasis range from thick adherent micaceous scale which demonstrates Auspitz's sign on manipulation to fine furfuraceous scale (Fig. 8.1). Scalp psoriasis may extend beyond the hairline onto the forehead (Fig. 8.2). This finding may be useful in differentiating scalp psoriasis from severe seborrheic dermatitis which is typically limited by the hairline. The scale of psoriasis often has a powdery consistency and silvery sheen whereas the scale of seborrheic dermatitis typically appears yellow and greasy. Involvement of the posterior auricular crease with

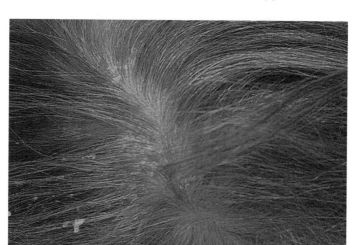

Figure 8.1 Psoriasis of the scalp demonstrating fine furfuraceous scale.

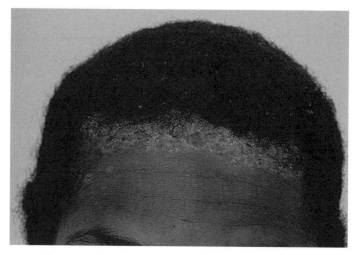

Figure 8.2 Psoriasis may extend beyond the hairline onto the forehead.

scaling and fissuring is common in psoriasis (see Plate 11, facing p. 34), although involvement in this location may also occur in other dermatoses, especially seborrheic dermatitis. The morphologic entity known as pityriasis (tinea) amiantacea consists of asbestos-like scales adhering to the scalp and hair shafts and may be an early manifestation of psoriasis (see Plate 12, facing p. 34).

The differential diagnosis of scaling plaques on the scalp includes:
1 Papulosquamous disorders such as lichen planus, allergic or irritant eczema, and atopic dermatitis.
2 Infectious or granulomatous causes such as tinea capitis, tertiary syphilis, deep fungal diseases, and sarcoidosis.
3 Neoplastic diseases such as mycosis fungoides, B-cell lymphoma, and histiocytosis-X.
4 Connective tissue diseases such as dermatomyositis and lupus erythematosus.

Usually, associated cutaneous findings or a history of prior skin disease allow for ready differentiation among these entities. Scalp psoriasis may be accompanied by nail pitting or onycholysis which are valuable clues to the correct diagnosis. If scaling of the scalp is diffuse, seborrheic dermatitis is more likely. Microscopic examination of scale digested by 10% potassium hydroxide is useful to exclude dermatophyte infection, and culture for fungal organisms, and serological testing for syphilis may also be useful adjunctive tests in certain situations. Psoriasis of the scalp is frequently accompanied by pruritus, but this is true for most of the other disorders which may mimic psoriasis. Occasionally, a biopsy must be performed to confirm the diagnosis of scalp psoriasis, especially in cases where there is significant hair loss, scarring, or when malignant infiltrations are diagnostic possibilities.

Biopsy of the scalp is readily achieved by the punch biopsy technique. A 4 mm specimen will usually suffice, so long as care has been taken to orient the punch parallel to the hairs exiting the scalp. Although epidermal changes are diagnostic for psoriasis, excision of the biopsy material with iris scissors at the level of the deep subcutaneous fat underneath the hair bulbs will ensure that an adequate specimen has been obtained so that other possible entities can be ruled out. Although psoriasis does not usually cause alopecia, scarring alopecia has been associated with familial and sporadic psoriasis and in the setting of the acquired immunodeficiency syndrome (AIDS).

Etiology

The etiology of scalp psoriasis is unknown, although it seems to be aggravated by some microbial organisms. *Pityrosporum ovale* and *Streptococcus pyogenes* have been implicated as organisms that might trigger the alternate complement pathway and stimulate the development of psoriatic plaques. As in the other forms of psoriasis, HLA antigens Cw6, HLA B16, B18, and B27 are found in a higher percentage than in the population at large. It is unclear whether these HLA antigens are associated with genes that produce an excessive inflammatory response to infectious organisms or are merely incidental findings.

Studies of follicular kinetics in psoriatic scalp have demonstrated unaltered hair growth in unaffected versus lesional skin. The percentage of cells in the S-phase in nonlesional follicular infundibulum of psoriatic scalp is increased compared to normal controls. This is in keeping with cutaneous psoriasis in which the epidermal turnover time is sharply reduced. Compulsive and subconscious scratching or rubbing of scalp psoriasis may induce the isomorphic response and perpetuation of lesions.

Treatment

A variety of treatments may prove helpful in controlling scalp psoriasis, but no single treatment is consistently effective. The most commonly used treatments include shampoos, keratolytics, tar derivatives, antibiotics and antifungal agents, corticosteroid preparations, Grenz ray therapy, softening agents such as mineral oil, and systemic medications such as methotrexate, cyclosporine, PUVA, biologic response modifiers, and retinoids. These agents will be reviewed in a sequential manner with reference to commonly available products. The subsections are arranged in order of decreasing popularity.

Mechanical debridement

Shampoos are substances used to wash the hair. These liquid formulations are usually sodium or potassium salts of fatty acids which act as anionic surfactants. Although simple soaps and mild detergents with surfactants may be used alone in the treatment of mild scalp psoriasis, formulations with additives like selenium sulfide, zinc pyrithione, chloroxine, sulfur, or salicylic acid often help speed clinical improvement (Table 8.1). Agents such as menthol may be added to combat pruritus. Coal tars are useful additives in disorders of keratinization because epidermal proliferation is inhibited and because of their antipruritic effects. Selenium sulfide has substantivity, meaning it remains on the skin and hair after shampooing.

Table 8.1 Common anti-psoriatic shampoos.

Capitrol 2% chloroxine 4-oz bottle

Danex 1% pyrithione zinc 4-oz bottle

Denorex (Regular and mountain fresh herbal) coal tar solution 9% and 1.5% menthol; (extra strength and extra strength with conditioners) 12.55 coal tar and 1.5% menthol 4-, 8-, and 12-oz bottles

Dermazinc soap bar zinc pyrithione

DHS tar shampoo 0.5% coal tar 4-, 8-, and 16-oz bottles

DHS zinc Dandruff Shampoo 2% pyrithione zinc 6- and 12-oz bottles

Doak 3% coal tar

Doctar Shampoo coal tar

Exsel 2.5% Selenium Sulfide Lotion 120 ml

Head and Shoulders 1% pyrithione zinc lotion 4-, 7-, 11-, and 15-oz bottles "Normal to Dry Scalp" 7-, 11-, 15-oz

Head and Shoulders Intensive Treatment 1% selenium sulfide in surfactant base 4-, 7-, 11-oz bottles

Ionil T Coal Tar Solution, salicylic acid; Ionil T Plus 2% Crude Coal Tar (Owentar II)

Iosel 250 selenium sulfide 2.5% lotion 240-ml bottle

Lavatar shampoo

Metec 5% sulfur 3% salicylic acid 120 ml

Neutrogena T/gel 2% coal tar 4.4, 8.5 16 oz

Neutrogena T/gel 3% sal acid 4.5 oz

Nizoral Shampoo 2% ketoconazole

Nizoral Shampoo 1% ketoconazole

P&S liquid mineral oil, glycerin, and phenol 4- and 8-oz bottles

P&S Plus Tar Gel 8% coal tar solution (1.6% crude coal tar, 6.4% ethyl alcohol), 2% salicylic acid 3.5-oz tube

Packer's pine tar 0.82% pine tar 180 ml

Pentrax tar 4.3% crude coal tar 120, 240 ml

Polytar 1% mixture of tars 180, 360 ml

Psorigel

Sebulex 2% sulfur 2% salicylic acid 4 and 8 oz

Sebutone coal tar 0.5%, salicylic acid 2%, and sulfur 2% 4- and 8-oz bottles

Selsun 2.5% selenium sulfide 120 ml

Selsun Blue selenium sulfide 1% (Dry, Oily, Normal, Extra Conditioning); extra medicated also contains 0.5% menthol 4-, 7-, and 11-oz bottles

Sebulon Shampoo

Sulfoam 2% sulfur 4, 8, 16 oz

Tarsum shampoo/gel 4, 8 oz

T/Gel 2% coal tar solution

Tegrin 5% coal tar solution, concentrated gel 2.5-oz tube, lotion 3.75- and 6.6-oz bottles

Table 8.1 (*cont'd*)

Theraplex Z 2% zinc pyrithione 8 oz bottle

Theraplex T shampoo 1% coal tar 8 oz

Vanseb salicylic acid 1%, sulfur 2% 3-oz tube or 4-oz bottle

Vanseb-T salicylic acid 1%, sulfur 2%, coal tar solution USP 5% 3-oz tube or 4-oz bottle

X-seb shampoo 4% salicylic acid 4-oz bottle

X-seb Plus 1% pyrithione zinc, 2% salicylic acid 4-oz bottle X-seb T 10% coal tar solution (2% crude coal tar, 8% ethyl alcohol) 4% salicylic acid, X-seb T Plus 10% coal tar solution (2% crude coal tar, 3% salicylic acid, 1% menthol) 4-oz bottle

Zetar shampoo

Zincon 1% pyrithione zinc 4- and 8-oz bottles

ZNP Bar Shampoo 2% zinc pyrithione

Selenium sulfide inhibits mitosis of keratinocytes, thereby controlling hyperproliferation. It also inhibits the growth of pityrosporum spores. Ketoconazole shampoo 2% also inhibits growth of pityrosporum and has proven useful in the treatment of scalp psoriasis as well as seborrheic dermatitis. Pyrithione zinc shampoos have substantivity and inhibit proliferation of keratinocytes, but have the advantage of causing less irritation of the skin than tar or selenium sulfide products. Therapeutic shampoos are usually lathered into the scalp and left in place for 5–10 minutes before thorough rinsing. Tar shampoos may discolor light or gray hair.

Adjunctive treatment, with a scalp debridement and shampoo machine may lead to rapid improvement of scalp psoriasis in the hospital or psoriasis day care setting, while freeing up nursing time. The machine consists of a chamber that encloses the scalp which is then exposed to a high-pressure liquid jet that contains water plus the therapeutic shampoo. It may be valuable for scale reduction.

Keratolytics

Many topical agents influence the production of scale. The most widely used keratolytic agents in dermatology include urea, propylene glycol, resorcinol, and salicylic acid. Salicylic acid is added to shampoo and lotion products to help control flaking of the scalp, but may also be applied directly to the scalp. If widespread areas are treated, salicylism may result. Tinnitus is the premonitory symptom. This may occur because salicylic acid is well absorbed through the skin, but renal secretion is slow.

Epilyt^R has been recommended for scalp psoriasis, and leads to improvement within 2 weeks when applied under a shower cap overnight. Baker's P&S liquid is also quite effective when used in a similar fashion. The full regimen consists of a morning shampoo followed by the application of a corticosteroid lotion which helps to reduce inflammation and control pruritus.

For recalcitrant heavy crusts in the scalp, Mayo Clinic dermatologists advocate a preparation consisting of 20% oil of Cade (juniper wood tar), 10% sulfur, and 5% salicylic acid in a water-soluble base, thoroughly rubbing it into the scalp. Some patients find the odor of oil of Cade offensive, but the product is beneficial.

Topical tar

The efficacy of tar products in psoriasis (Table 8.2) has been recognized for many years. The mechanism by which tar products work is not well understood. Antibacterial, antifungal, vasoconstrictive, and keratolytic effects as well as suppression of epidermal DNA synthesis have all been claimed. Use of these products may lead to folliculitis, and the odor of crude coal tar is unmistakable, making compliance with tar therapy in some patients difficult.

Table 8.2 Commonly used tar formulations.

Liquid formulations
Alphosyl Lotion 1% crude coal tar 1.7% allantoin
Doak Tar Lotion 5% tar distillate
Eltatar 10% coal tar solution
MG 217 5% coal tar solution
Oxipor Lotion 48.5% tar, benzocaine, salicylic acid,
    30 and 60 ml
P&S Plus 8% coal tar solution, 2% salicylic acid 3.5 oz
T/Derm Lotion 5% crude coal tar 120 ml
Tegrin Lotion 5% crude coal tar
Zetar Emulsion 300 mg coal tar/ml 6 oz

Gel formulations
Aquatar 0.5% crude coal tar 90-g tube
Estar Gel 5% crude coal tar 90-g tube
P&S Plus 1.6% crude coal tar, 2% salicylic acid 105 g
Psorigel 1.5% crude coal tar 120 g

In one study, topical tar products alone led to improvement in up to 75% of patients within 6 weeks of beginning treatment. Coal tar solution in gel form (Psorigel) was applied to plaques for five days of the week, with only mineral oil application on the sixth day and no treatment on the seventh day. Use of a tar shampoo (Ionil T) increased the time interval between relapses.

Tar oils are also used in the Goeckerman regimen. A combination of Nivea Oil, 3% salicylic acid, and 20% liquor carbonis detergens was popular in the past, but now because of a change in Nivea Oil formulation, the mixture will not support the addition of salicylic acid. An alternative solution can be made by adding 4 ml of polysorbate 80 and 13 ml coal tar emulsion (Zetar) to each 100 ml of New Improved Nivea Oil. Applied nightly under a shower cap, this product loosens scale and controls psoriatic plaques. The mixture is massaged into the scalp by parting the hair every 1 cm until the entire scalp is covered. A separate dose of UVB can be delivered to the scalp with a hot quartz lamp while shielding the face from secondary exposure.

Anthralin

Anthralin is a derivative of the South American araroba tree. It has antimitotic activity but frequently causes irritation when used in concentrations higher than 0.1%. Anthralin also causes a brown–red discoloration of the skin and scalp, and may cause a yellow discoloration of hair. Application to chronic scalp plaques for 8–12 hours may prove very helpful, but application to acute, exudative, or highly inflamed plaques should generally be avoided.

Anthralin pomade consisting of anthralin 0.4%, salicylic acid 0.4%, mineral oil 76%, cetyl alcohol 21.1% and sodium lauryl sulfate 2.1% left on overnight and then shampooed out clears patients' scalps quickly (Table 8.3). Anthralin is now not widely used, mainly because of irritation and discoloration of skin and light hair.

Corticosteroid preparations

Because they are effective, cosmetically elegant, and generally odorless, topical corticosteroid products have overtaken tar products in the treatment of scalp psoriasis. If corticosteroids are used for extended periods of time in an uninterrupted fashion, tachyphylaxis may occur, although this is controversial. Tachyphylaxis implies

Table 8.3 Anthralin preparations.

Anthra-Derma Ointment 0.1%, 0.25%, 0.5%, 1%
 (42.5-g tube)
Anthranol 0.1%, 0.2%, 0.4% (Canada)
Anthraforte 1%, 2%, 3% (Canada)
Drithocreme 0.1%, 0.25%, 0.5%, 1% 50 g
Dritho Scalp 0.25% and 0.5% 50 g
Micanol cream 1% 50 g
Psoriatec 1% anthralin cream 50 g

that a decreased therapeutic response is observed with the same dose of medication that was previously effective. The newer high potency products may potentially cause hypothalamic-pituitary-adrenal suppression, even if used on only a limited part of the body. Notwithstanding, if used prudently, these products can bring most cases of severe scalp psoriasis under control quickly (Table 8.4).

Corticosteroid sprays have been popular for many years. Spray delivery of corticosteroids minimizes the greasy feel to the hair that

Table 8.4 Corticosteroid scalp solutions and sprays.

Aeroseb-Dex 0.01% dexamethasone (alcohol 59%)
Barseb-HC 1% hydrocortisone, 0.5% salicylic acid 52-ml bottle
Cortaid/Rhulicort 0.5% hydrocortisone acetate lotion
Cyclocort Lotion amcinonide 0.1% 20 and 60 ml
Decaspray (dexamethasone spray) 25-g pressurized container
Dermazinc Spray
Dermovate 0.05% clobetasol propionate (Canada)
Diprolene Lotion betamethasone dipropionate 0.05%
Elocon Lotion mometasone furoate 0.1% 30- and 60-ml bottles
Emo-Cort Scalp Solution 2.5% hydrocortisone
Kenalog Lotion/Spray 0.025% triamcinolone acetonide 60-ml bottle, 23 g- and
 63 g-cans
Lidex fluocinonide 0.05% solution 20- and 60-ml bottles
Luxiq spray foam 0.12% betamethasone valerate
Maxivate betamethasone dipropionate 0.05% 60-ml bottle
Olux spray foam 0.05% clobetasol proprionate
Penecort alcohol 57%, hydrocortisone 1%
Synalar, Fluonid Solution fluocinolone acetonide 0.01% 20- and 60-ml bottles
Temovate Solution clobetasol propionate 0.05% 25- and 50-ml bottles
Texacort Scalp Solution alcohol 33%, hydrocortisone 1%
Uticort 0.025% betamethasone benzoate

Table 8.5 Commonly used salicylic acid products.

DHS Sal shampoo 3% salicylic acid
Hydrisalic Gel 6% salicylic acid 30 g
Ionil Plus Shampoo 2% salicylic acid
MG 217 Sal-Acid ointment 3% salicylic acid 60 g
Keralyt Gel 6% salicylic acid, 60% propylene glycol 30 g
Sal-Clens Shampoo 4% salicylic acid
Saligel 5% salicylic acid
T Sal shampoo 3% salicylic acid

may result from topical lotions. Clobetasol foam has been shown to be more cosmetically acceptable than cream and ointment vehicles when used as a twice-daily scalp application. Betamethasone valerate foam has been shown to decrease plaque thickness, scaling, and erythema when used either once or twice daily. The foams are readily accepted by patients because of their ease of use and absence of residue.

High potency corticosteroids may not always offer much more clinical benefit when compared to less potent products in the Stoughton classification. When desoximetasone gel 0.05% was compared to fluocinonide gel 0.05% for the treatment of scalp psoriasis, comparable improvement was seen in both groups. One cannot always predict the degree of improvement in scalp psoriasis by a corticosteroid product merely by knowing its potency rating. The vehicle and delivery mechanism probably cause changes in effectiveness and type of side-effects.

We recommend beginning therapy with a midpotency topical corticosteroid product. Patients should be advised to shampoo the hair and then apply the corticosteroid solution while the scalp is still damp, thereby enhancing absorption. Shower cap occlusion may be useful in selected cases, but is generally not necessary. Once daily application suffices in most cases. More extensive cases may require twice daily application, or application of a keratolytic gel containing salicylic acid to remove scales and improve absorption (Table 8.5).

If psoriasis is severe, many patients benefit from a regimen in which topical corticosteroids are used nightly for 1–2 weeks, and tar solutions are used on alternate weeks. One popular regimen is to use a keratolytic product (e.g. Epilyt or Baker's P&S) overnight with corticosteroid lotion in the morning until thick scale has been debrided. A combination product, such as Derma-Smoothe-

FS which contains peanut oil, isopropyl alcohol, and fluocinolone acetonide 0.01%, can then be used nightly as needed thereafter.

In selected resistant cases where only a few, small, discrete plaques remain on the scalp, intralesional injections of triamcinolone acetonide suspension (5 mg/ml) may be extremely helpful in temporarily clearing psoriasis locally, sometimes for many months.

Topical calcipotriene

Topical calcipotriene solution (50 µg/ml) is helpful in clearing scalp psoriasis. More than half of patients had marked improvement in one large study, but three-quarters of individuals treated with betamethasone had marked improvement. Irritation of perilesional skin was more common in calcipotriene treated patients. Topical treatment with calcipotriene does not alter the anagen/telogen ratio and is presumed not to alter hair growth. It has been used safely twice daily (maximum 50 ml/week) for 1 year with optimal response seen after 6 months and sustained. Tacalcitol cream twice daily may be effective for sebopsoriasis of the face and scalp.

Antibiotics and antifungal agents

The role of microbial agents in psoriasis is uncertain. *Pityrosporum ovale* has been implicated in the etiology of scalp psoriasis, and oral ketoconazole appears to be of benefit. Whether the effect of ketoconazole is due to its antifungal properties or its effect on follicular keratinization remains to be shown. Ketoconazole (1% and 2%) shampoo is available and effective but appears to have a similar efficacy to 1% selenium sulfide shampoos. Hepatotoxicity is not a concern with the topical formulations of ketaconazole. A pilot study showed effectiveness of a regimen consisting of 40% urea plus 1% bifonazole ointment and 1% bifonazole shampoo.

Grenz ray therapy

Grenz ray therapy is a very effective way to control scalp psoriasis. The addition of topical corticosteroids offers little additional benefit. Grenz ray treatment with 10 kV, 10 mA, and a half value layer of 0.3 mm aluminum, with a target skin distance of 10 cm and a half value depth of 0.5 mm, is an effective setting. Four hundred rads are given weekly for 6 weeks. When given by experienced clinicians and recommended total doses of 1000 rads are not exceeded, this is a safe and effective alternative to cumbersome topical treatments. Carcinogenesis becomes a serious concern only at higher doses of radiation. Rare disorders, such as the nevoid basal cell carcinoma syndrome or xeroderma pigmentosum, are obviously contraindications to radiation therapy.

Systemic therapy

Treatment with the systemic agents such as methotrexate, retinoids, cyclosporine, and vitamin D_3, covered in separate chapters, all lead to improvement in scalp psoriasis. Transient alopecia may, however, result from some of these medications, particularly the retinoids. The new biologic agents (Chapter 22), such as efalizumab, etanercept, infliximab, and alefacept, all help scalp psoriasis when used to treat widespread psoriatic involvement.

Phototherapy

Ultraviolet B phototherapy can control scalp psoriasis advancing beyond the frontal hairline if the hair is held or tied back during phototherapy. If the scalp hair is fine-textured and of decreased density as in androgenetic alopecia, either ultraviolet B or PUVA phototherapy may be of benefit in clearing scalp psoriasis. Some hand-held UVA/UVB irradiation sources that are commercially available have a removable comb for parting the hair. A unique broadband UVB fiberoptic comb with peak emission of 311–315 nm has shown benefit in scalp psoriasis when used at 72-hour intervals. The 308 nm excimer laser may also be used to treat localized plaques directly with the small hand piece.

Summary

Scalp involvement is a very common problem which can be extremely troubling to patients with psoriasis because it is usually symptomatic and difficult to hide. Although the etiology of scalp psoriasis is unclear, many effective treatments are available for its control. Judicious use of these agents can lead to remission of scalp disease with a minimum of side-effects.

Selected references

Anderson R. R. (2000) Lasers in dermatology—a critical update. *J Dermatol* **27**, 700–705.

Baden H. P. (1991) Epilyt for scalp psoriasis (letter). *Arch Dermatol* **127**, 274.

Barnes L., Altmeyer P., Forstrom L. *et al.* (2000) Long-term treatment of psoriasis with calcitriol scalp solution and cream. *Eur J Dermatol* **10**, 199–204.

Cockayne S. E., Messenger A. G. (2001) Familial scarring alopecia associated with scalp psoriasis. *Br J Dermatol* **144**, 425–427.

DuVivier A., Stoughton R. B. (1982) Tachyphylaxis to the action of topically applied corticosteroids. *Arch Dermatol* **111**, 581–583.

Duweb G. A., Abuzariba O., Rahim M. *et al.* (2001) Scalp psoriasis: topical calcipotriol 50 micrograms/g/ml solution vs. betamethasone valerate 1% lotion. *Int J Clin Pharmacol Res* **20**, 65–68.

Feldman S. R., Ravis S. M., Fleischer A. B. *et al.* (2001) Betamethasone valerate in foam vehicle is effective with both daily and twice a day dosing: a single-blind open-label study in the treatment of scalp psoriasis. *J Cut Med Surg* **5**, 386–389.

Gibson L. E., Perry H. O. (1991) Goeckerman therapy. In: Roenigk H. H. Jr, Maibach H. I. (eds) *Psoriasis*, 2nd edn. Marcel Dekker, New York, p. 537.

Helm T. N., Ferrara R. J., Dijkstra J., Soukup J. (1989) New improved Nivea Oil cannot be used alone as vehicle for salicylic acid. *J Am Acad Dermatol* **21**, 814.

Katz H. I., Lindholm J. S., Weiss J. S. *et al.* (1995) Efficacy and safety of twice-daily augmented betamethasone diproprionate lotion versus clobetasol propionate solution in patients with moderate to severe scalp psoriasis. *Clinical Therapeutics* **17**, 390–401.

King L. Jr, Webb B., Zanolli M. (1999) Experience in treating recalcitrant scalp psoriasis with automated shampooing and debridement. *J Am Acad Dermatol* **41**, 638–640.

Klaber M. R., Hutchinson P. E., Pedvis-Leftick A. *et al.* (1994) Comparative effects of calcipotriol solution (50 micrograms/ml) and betamethasone 17-valerate solution (1 mg/ml) in the treatment of scalp psoriasis. *Br J Dermatol* **131**, 678–683.

Kuijpers A. L., van Baar H. M., van Gasselt M. W., van de Kerkhof P. C. (1995) The hair root pattern after calcipitriol treatment for psoriasis. *Acta Dermato-Venereol* **75**, 388–390.

Lowe N. J. (1984) Therapy of scalp psoriasis. *Dermatol Clin* **2**, 471–476.

Lowe N. J., Breeding J. (1981) Anthralin: different concentration effects on epidermal DNA synthesis rates in mice and clinical responses in human psoriasis. *Arch Dermatol* **117**, 698–700.

Lowe N. J., Breeding J. H., Wortzman M. S. (1982) New coal tar extract and coal tar shampoos: evaluation by epidermal DNA synthesis suppression assay. *Arch Dermatol* **118**, 487–489.

Melian E. B., Specer C. M., Jarvis B. (2001) Clobetasol propionate foam, 0.05%. *Am J Clin Dermatol* **2**, 89–93.

Schon M. P., Reifenberger J., Gantke B. *et al.* (2000) Progressive cicatricial psoriatic alopecia in AIDS (German). *Hautarzt* **51**, 935–938.

Thaci D., Daiber W., Boehncke W. H., Kaufmann R. (2001) Calcipotriol solution for the treatment of scalp psoriasis: evaluation of efficacy, safety and acceptance in 3,396 patients. *Dermatology* **203**, 153–156.

van der Vleuten C. J., van der Kerkhof P.C. (2001) Management of scalp psoriasis: guidelines for corticosteroid use in combination treatment. *Drugs* **61**, 1593–1598.

van de Kerkhof P. C., Franssen M. E. (2001) Psoriasis of the scalp. Diagnosis and management. *Am J Clin Dermatol* **2**, 159–165.

9   Nail psoriasis

Charles Camisa

Psoriasis affecting the nails is very common, being found in up to 50% of patients. The prevalence of nail psoriasis is much higher in patients with psoriatic arthritis, occurring in over 80% of such patients. The fingernails seem to be affected more often than the toenails. In most patients, the changes are easier to identify in the fingernails because they are more accessible to examination, and patients are more likely to complain about changes visible to the public eye. Many of the alterations of toenails associated with aging can be confused with psoriasis: thickening and yellowing of the nail plate, longitudinal ridges, and dystrophies. Onycholysis may be secondary to trauma, ill-fitting shoes, bone deformities, vascular insufficiency, and dermatophytosis. The conventional wisdom is that dermatophytes are infrequently found in association with psoriatic nails, but it is advisable to examine the scales of the palms, soles, and subungual debris with potassium hydroxide and culture whenever the diagnosis is in doubt. In one study, the prevalence of cultures positive for dermatophyte from toenails of psoriatic patients was 8% compared to 4% of dermatologic patients who were not referred for nail problems. Treatment of a fungal component of skin and nail disease could provide some symptomatic and cosmetic relief to the patient.

The morphologic alterations seen in the nail unit are, by themselves, not specific or diagnostic of the disease unless there is associated cutaneous psoriasis of the proximal and lateral nailfolds or the volar finger pad (see Plate 13, facing p. 34); present in only about one-third of cases. The constellation of nail changes taken together, however, is strongly *suggestive* of psoriasis, even in the absence of any obvious cutaneous lesions. The latter scenario occurs in less than 5% of patients with psoriasis and may be seen in association with arthropathy as a precursor to the development of

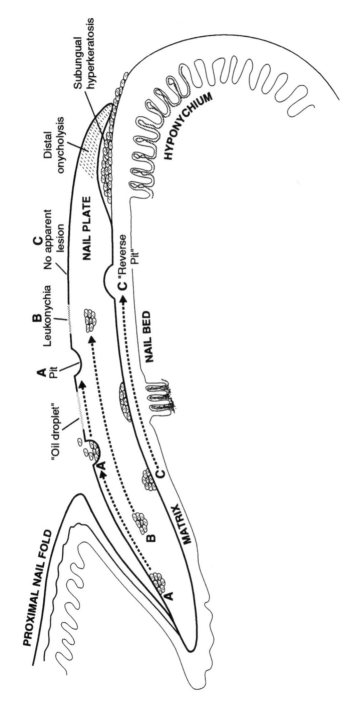

Figure 9.1 Correlation of psoriasis of the nail unit with morphologic changes.

skin lesions, or as the only manifestation of psoriasis an individual ever develops.

The end-result of psoriasis involving the cells of the nail matrix is usually but not always, manifested in the surface texture of the nail plate, while lesions in the nail bed are generally transmitted through the plate as color changes or onycholysis. Thickening or lifting of the nail and subungual hyperkeratosis, result from accumulation of scales in psoriatic lesions of the nail bed and hyponychium (Fig. 9.1).

There is a direct link between the linear growth rate of nails and nail matrix kinetics, consistent with in vivo thymidine-labeling studies of psoriatic epidermis. The growth rate of psoriatic nails with pitting was significantly greater than normal-appearing psoriatic nails (125 vs. 109 µm/day). Both rates were significantly greater than the rate in pooled normal controls (98 µm/day). Systemic cytotoxic drugs, such as methotrexate and azathioprine, markedly reduced the growth rate of nails while corticosteroids did not. Etretinate has the effect of increasing the rate of fingernail growth in psoriasis. The nail growth rate in palmoplantar pustulosis is not significantly different from that in normal control subjects.

Pitting of the nail plate is the most commonly recognized nail sign of psoriasis (Table 9.1). The pits are usually larger, deeper, and more randomly dispersed on the nail plate than those observed in alopecia areata. They are believed to be secondary to parakeratosis of the

Table 9.1 Clinicopathologic correlation of nail changes in psoriasis.

Clinical finding	Pathologic correlate
Pitting	Psoriasis in proximal matrix
Red spots in lunula	Active psoriasis in distal matrix
Transverse ridges (Beau's lines) or horizontal line of pits	Transient growth arrest of matrix or confluence of parakeratosis in proximal matrix
Thickening of nail	Hyperkeratosis of nail bed and adherence to nail plate
Lifting of distal end of nail plate, onycholysis	Hyperkeratosis of distal nail bed and hyponychium with separation of nail plate from nail bed
Yellow-brown spot ("oil droplet" sign)	Guttate psoriasis of nail bed with serum glycoprotein deposits
Splinter hemorrhages	Bleeding of superficial dilated capillaries in nail bed due to trauma

proximal matrix resulting in nucleated cells in the upper plate that eventually desquamate (Fig. 9.1). Similarly, parakeratosis in an intermediate portion of the matrix may result in leukonychia. Parakeratosis in the distal matrix or lunula results in no discernible change in the plate or focal onycholysis. Small red spots in the lunula may indicate active distal matrix psoriasis, another change that is very similar to that seen in alopecia areata. Transverse ridges may represent transient matrix arrest (Beau's lines) or a confluence of parakeratosis in the proximal matrix, thereby connecting the pits. Longitudinal ridges, elevations resembling drops of melted wax, result from alternating thinning and thickening of the nail plate and may correspond to psoriatic involvement focally or at regular intervals in the intermediate and distal matrix.

Splinter hemorrhages, longitudinal collections of extravasated blood under the nail plate, are very common after trauma of normal nails. Psoriatic nails with involvement of the nail bed are especially prone to these if psoriasis involves the nail bed because of the superficial location of dilated tortuous capillaries. The oil droplet appearance of the nail bed corresponds to an early guttate lesion of psoriasis. There is a yellowish-brown spot surrounded by erythema (see Plate 14, facing p. 34). The yellow greasy look is due to a serum glycoprotein, which accumulates in and under the abnormal nail. Large amounts of this material may be inhibitory for dermatophytes but not to yeasts. While the oil droplet sign is very suggestive of the diagnosis of psoriasis, almost identical lesions have been noted in onychomycosis (candidiasis) and tinea unguium (dermatophytosis). Complete crumbling of the nail plate is the result of extensive involvement of the matrix forming a nail plate of varying thicknesses, with deep pits and ridging dispersed throughout. In such an extensive case, there is likely to be psoriasis of the distal nail bed and hyponychium as well, which further elevates the nail plate to reveal accumulated keratinaceous debris.

In patients with psoriatic arthritis, the severity of skin and nail involvement does not correlate with severity of the joint disease. However, there is a significant association between psoriatic involvement of a fingernail and arthropathy of the adjacent distal interphalangeal joint. Whereas the most frequent fingernail change is pitting, subungual hyperkeratosis is the most common toenail alteration in psoriatic arthritis.

While it is true that one or more of the features listed for psoriatic nails can be seen in the nails of patients with alopecia areata, lichen planus, or eczema, these diseases can usually be diagnosed readily by their distinctive cutaneous lesions. There are two uncommon entities with papulosquamous skin lesions and nail changes that may be referred to a dermatologic consultant. In the classic adult-onset type (Type I) of *pityriasis rubra pilaris* (PRP), papulosquamous lesions spread from the head down to the feet, evolving into an erythroderma with islands of sparing. The skin may have a salmon or orange hue with palmoplantar keratoderma. When fully developed, the nails are thickened with subungual hyperkeratosis, distal yellow–brown discoloration, longitudinal ridges, and splinter hemorrhages. These changes are very similar to those seen in patients with erythrodermic forms of cutaneous T-cell lymphoma (CTCL) including Sézary syndrome. Another diagnostic challenge is *paraneoplastic acrokeratosis of Bazex* which typically occurs in middle-aged men in association with a squamous cell carcinoma of the upper aerodigestive tract. Psoriasiform lesions affect the ears, nose, hands, and feet. The nail changes may be the first clue to the diagnosis of the underlying neoplasm. They become thin, soft, fragile, and crumble. Subungual hyperkeratosis develops, and the nail plate may be lost. The skin and nail changes are reversible if the malignancy is cured. The skin biopsy findings of acrokeratosis of Bazex and PRP are fairly nonspecific, but the diagnosis of CTCL can usually be confirmed by skin biopsy or by peripheral blood smear if greater than 5% circulating Sézary cells are found.

Even the most severe changes of the nail in psoriasis are reversible because they are due to aberrations in epidermal cell kinetics and differentiation, which usually do not result in scarring or permanent nail loss. Therefore, it is reasonable to expect therapy will reverse the changes and induce remission if it can do so for the rest of the integument. This is only partially true and difficult to obtain for several reasons. Over time, the chronic inflammatory and reparative processes may effect subtle changes in the matrix or nail bed that do not allow a new nail plate to regrow and adhere normally to the nail bed, even after the most aggressive treatments.

I consider acrodermatitis continua of Hallopeau (ACH) to be a localized variant of pustular psoriasis or subcorneal pustular dermatosis. Histopathologic findings (Munro microabscesses or spongiform pustules of Kogoj) and responsiveness to methotrexate tend to support this position, but the same type of lesion can also be

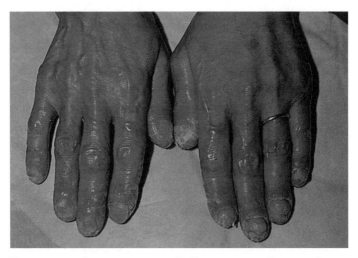

Figure 9.2 Acrodermatitis continua of Hallopeau causes yellowing and crumbling of nail plates.

seen in Reiter's syndrome. Perhaps it is best to lump ACH, Reiter's syndrome, and palmoplantar pustulosis (PPP) under the rubric of "acropustulosis." In both acrodermatitis continua of Hallopeau and PPP, sterile pustules arise beneath the nail plate in the nail bed and matrix, coalescing and reforming, producing necrosis of tissue, thinning and crumbling of the nail plate, scaling and crusting of nailfold skin, and eventually shedding of the nail (Fig. 9.2). Permanent nail loss, scarring, and bone resorption with tapering of the digit may occur after years of unchecked disease. Acropustulosis may affect one or several digits.

Nail biopsy

It is usually not necessary to perform a biopsy on the nail unit of psoriasis patients because the diagnosis can be reliably made based on the morphologic changes in the nail plate or the surrounding skin. In the patients with unexplained nail dystrophy without skin lesions or with seronegative arthritis, particularly when there is suppurative inflammation of the nail bed, it is important to perform a biopsy through the nail plate and nail bed or matrix. Psoriasis of the skin and nail bed have many histopathologic features in common.

Technique

Modern textbooks on nail surgery refer to the: (1) longitudinal biopsy which includes the proximal nailfold, matrix, nail bed and hyponychium; (2) longitudinal incision of the nail bed after nail avulsion; and (3) punch biopsy of the nail bed through the nail plate. To confirm the diagnosis of psoriasis, it is rarely ever necessary to perform a longitudinal biopsy because most of the diagnostic changes are in the nail bed and hyponychium. It is preferable to avoid the matrix, including the lunula, when one is performing biopsies of small areas that will not require suturing, because they can produce a permanent defect. I recommend a punch biopsy of the nail bed through the nail plate followed by incisional biopsy of the nail bed to the hyponychium.

After providing digital block or a thorough ring block with local infiltration of 1% lidocaine, select for biopsy a red spot or "oil droplet" between the lunula and hyponychium. Punch out a 4-mm cap of the nail plate; remove it and place it in formalin. Next, perform a 3-mm punch biopsy through the exposed nail bed (see Fig. 9.3A). Because it is still often difficult to remove the cylinder of tissue without crushing or macerating it, cut away a residual triangle of distal nail plate with cuticle scissors (see Fig. 9.3B). This specimen may now be submitted for fungal culture. Detach the punch biopsy specimen with gradle scissors and place in the formalin bottle containing the nail plate cap. Both specimens will be stained for organisms and with hematoxylin-eosin. If a second specimen is desired, using a scalpel, describe a small ellipse extending from the punch defect in the nail bed to the hyponychium (see Fig. 9.3C). One or more 6–0 sutures may be placed here for hemostasis and to expedite healing (see Fig. 9.3D). This technique is particularly useful in the diagnosis of acropustulosis. If a vesicle or pustule is accidentally

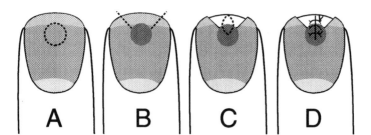

Figure 9.3 Biopsy of the nail bed and hyponychium. (See text for details.)

ruptured during the first procedure, thereby destroying the characteristic architecture, the second biopsy with the scalpel includes some hyponychium and volar skin where there is likely to be an extension of the primary disease.

Treatment

Topical corticosteroids

If topical therapy is selected, the first obstacle is reaching the diseased area. As Fig. 9.1 shows, the proximal matrix is obscured by the proximal nail fold and the nail plate while the distal matrix and bed are blocked by the nail plate. The hyponychium may be covered with scales, dirt, and contaminating microorganisms. A topical corticosteroid may improve psoriasis of the surrounding skin but has little to no effect on the appearance of the nail. Superpotent steroids under occlusion for two consecutive weeks may give further benefit but the need for repetitive use risks tachyphylaxis and atrophy of the nail fold skin.

Getting directly at the nail bed and exposed matrix by avulsion of the nail plate may be indicated in those patients with thick, crumbling nails. This may be accomplished atraumatically with an extemporaneously compounded formulation—urea 40%, white beeswax or paraffin 5%, anhydrous lanolin 20%, white petrolatum 35%—applied under plastic occlusion for seven days. After removing the dystrophic nail, apply a potent corticosteroid impregnated tape (flurandrenolide) or ointment to the denuded nail bed and proximal nail fold. A 50% success rate in regrowing "normal nails" has been reported. Atrophic nails treated in this manner will not respond as well.

A double-blind randomized study compared twice daily application of calcipotriene ointment and a combination of betamethasone dipropionate and salicylic acid and measured nail thickness as the end-point. Both treatments reduced nail thickness by about 50% after 5 months.

Intralesional corticosteroid

Another method of delivering medication directly to the area is by intralesional injection of corticosteroid. It is usually possible to deduce the location of active psoriasis in the nail unit with accuracy.

With highly motivated patients and skillful operators, the results can be most satisfying. The disadvantages of the procedure are that it is painful for the patient and tedious time-consuming work for the operator. It must be repeated at one- to two-monthly intervals until the desired result is obtained, and then at some less-frequent interval to treat new lesions as they arise. In a study of injecting 4 mg triamcinolone acetonide (TAC) suspension into nail units, subungual hyperkeratosis, ridging and thickening responded well, but pitting and onycholysis did not.

I routinely use TAC suspension 10 mg/ml diluted 1 : 1 with 1% lidocaine yielding a final concentration of 5 mg/ml. The patient scrubs his or her hands with chlorhexidine cleanser. Prior to injection the area is sprayed with a refrigerant such as Flurethyl (Fig. 9.4A). To treat pitting, injections are given into the proximal and lateral nail fold skin extending into the proximal lunula (Fig. 9.4B). When there are oil spots, onycholysis, or subungual hyperkeratosis, the 30 gauge needle is directed under the nail plate right to the affected areas. A total dose of less than 1.0–1.5 mg of TAC is deposited under or around a given nail unit. I have not observed atrophy of the nail fold, skin or nail plate with this dose. Subungual hematomas and increased numbers of splinter hemorrhages do occur, however, and patients should be forewarned and reassured that they are harmless. Infections have not occurred.

Chemotherapy

Topical nitrogen mustard (mechlorethamine), well known to dermatologists as the treatment of choice for certain forms of cutaneous T-cell lymphoma, is also very effective at clearing psoriasis. In aqueous solution, the rate of inducing delayed hypersensitivity reactions was unacceptably high. It was later recognized to be a carcinogen for the skin in patients with CTCL, an acceptable risk for treating a malignancy but not for psoriasis. There are no systemic effects of topical nitrogen mustard. In the setting of acropustulosis, it would be appropriate to try nitrogen mustard, compounded in an ointment base (10 mg mechlorethamine [Mustargen] dissolved in 95% ethyl alcohol and mixed into 100 g Aquaphor), applied daily to the affected digits and covered for up to 6 months, the shelf-life of the compound. Another topical chemotherapeutic agent for nails with pitting and hypertrophy is 1% 5-fluorouracil (5-FU). Applied to nail fold areas twice daily, it produces local inflammatory reactions and hyperpigmentation and may exacerbate onycholysis. Five per-

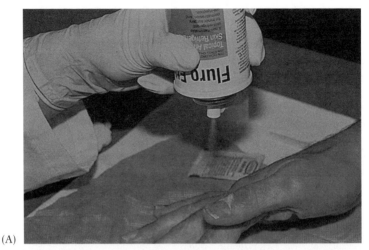

(A)

(B)

Figure 9.4 Intralesional injection of triamcinolone acetonide for psoriasis of the nail unit. (A) Spray nail fold with refrigerent. (B) Inject triamcinolone acetonide into the lateral and proximal nail folds.

cent 5-FU cream applied 1–3 times per week and washed off after 20 minutes was effective in a case report.

Miscellaneous

Tazarotene 0.1% gel applied once daily under occlusion for 24 weeks provided significantly more reduction of onycholysis and pitting then vehicle gel. Local irritation occurred in about one-fourth of cases. In an open study, anthralin ointment 0.4–2% was applied to nails daily for 30 minutes followed by 10% triethanolamine cream to prevent discoloration. Twelve of 20 patients (60%) showed moderate improvement in thickness, onycholysis and pitting after 5 months. Topical cyclosporine 70% dissolved in corn oil produced substantial improvement in 8/8 patients treated for 12 weeks.

Systemic

The best systemic medication for psoriasis of the nails appears to be methotrexate, but most clinicians would not use it exclusively for nail disease unless it was disabling or destructive as in acropustulosis. In the latter case, doses of 15 mg weekly are usually sufficient. When methotrexate is used to treat severe or extensive skin involvement or arthropathy, the nails benefit incidentally.

The synthetic retinoids, etretinate and acitretin, like methotrexate, are not used specifically to treat psoriatic nails although patients with prominent nail involvement may experience significant improvement in crumbling of the nail plate, oil droplets, onycholysis, and subungual hyperkeratosis. These beneficial changes may outweigh the unwanted effects of retinoids on nails, such as thinning and fragility, onychorrhexis, onychoschizia, onychomadesis, and paronychia, with granulation tissue. The nail changes of patients with HIV-associated psoriasis respond to zidovudine along with the skin changes. Oral cyclosporine 3.3 mg/kg/day combined with a superpotent topical corticosteroid has been used to control acrodermatitis continua associated with plaque psoriasis after the failure of methotrexate, retinoids, and localized superficial radiotherapy.

Radiation therapy

In a double-blind study, superficial radiotherapy given as three fractionated doses of 150 cGy (90 kV, 5 mA, 1.00 mm aluminum filter) significantly improved psoriatic fingernails compared to sham-treated nails. The improvement lasted for 10–15 weeks after treatment.

Phototherapy

Marx and Scher closely followed nail signs in 10 patients with generalized psoriasis receiving PUVA. They found that most changes showed 50% or more improvement after therapy (crumbling of nail plate, onycholysis, oil droplet) but that pitting was unchanged by this treatment. They hypothesized that, while the 8-MOP reached the entire nail matrix via the circulation, only limited UVA radiation could penetrate the nail plate to reach the distal matrix (lunula) and nail bed to improve abnormalities there, but the proximal matrix was not penetrable. It was later shown that only about 20% of the peak emission of conventional UVA lamps was transmitted through a nail 0.5 mm thick. For 330 nm, an order of magnitude more effective at clearing cutaneous psoriasis than 360 nm, the percent transmission drops to 10% and approaches zero for thicker nails (0.8–1.0 mm). It is possible to treat psoriatic nails with either systemic or bath PUVA delivering 2.5–5.0 times the therapeutic dose of UVA needed to induce resolution of psoriasis of the surrounding glabrous skin. Shielding of this skin while delivering the higher energy to the nail surface is necessary with the concomitant risk of PUVA-induced photo-onycholysis or photohemolysis (hemorrhage followed by onycholysis).

UVB therapy is unlikely to help psoriatic nails because the nail, like window glass, filters out much of it, and there is very low transmission of UVB (290–320 nm) to the nail bed.

Selected references

Baran R., Dawber R. P. R. (1994) *Diseases of the Nails and their Management*, 2nd edn. Blackwell Scientific Publications, Oxford.

Burden A. D., Kemmett D. (1996) The spectrum of nail involvement in palmo-plantar pustulosis. *Br J Dermatol* **134**, 1079–1082.

Cannavo S. P., Guarneri F., Vaccaro M. *et al.* (2003) Treatment of psoriatic nails with topical cyclosporin: a prospective randomized placebo-controlled study. *Dermatol* **206**, 153–156.

de Berker D. A. (2002) Diagnosis and management of nail psoriasis. *Dermatologic Therapy* **15**, 165–172.

de Berker D. A., Lawrence C. M. (1998) A simplified protocol of steroid injection for psoriatic nail dystrophy. *Br J Dermatol* **138**, 90–95.

de Jong E. M., Menke H. E., van Praag M. C. *et al.* (1999) Dystrophic psoriatic fingernails treated with 1% 5-Fluorouracil in a nail penetration-enhancing vehicle: a double-blind study. *Dermatol* **199**, 313–318.

Farber E. M., Nall L. (1992) Nail psoriasis. *Cutis* **50**, 174–178.

Gupta A. K., Lynde C. W., Jain H. C. *et al.* (1997) A higher prevalence of onychomycosis in psoriatics compared with non-psoriatics: a multicentre study. *Br J Dermatol* **136**, 786–789.

Harland C. C., Kilby P. E., Dalziel K. L. (1992) Acrodermatitis continua responding to cycolsporin therapy. *Clin Exp Dermatol* **17**, 376–378.

Jones S. M., Armas J. B., Cohen M. G. *et al.* (1994) Psoriatic arthritis: outcome of disease subsets and relationship of joint disease to nail and skin disease. *Br J Rheumatol* **33**, 834–839.

Kaur I., Saraswat A., Kumar B. (2001) Nail changes in psoriasis: a study of 167 patients. *Int J Dermatol* **40**, 601–603.

Lavaroni G., Kokelj F., Pauluzzi P., Trevisan G. (1994) The nails in psoriatic arthritis. *Acta Dermato-Venereol* (Suppl) **186**, 113.

Marx J.L., Scher R.K. (1980) Response of psoriatic nails to oral chemotherapy. *Arch Dermatol* **116**, 1023–1024.

Rich P. (1992) Nail biopsy. Indications and methods. *J Dermatol Surg Oncol* **18**, 673–682.

Scher R. K., Stiller M., Zhu Y. I. (2001) Tazarotene 0.1% gel in the treatment of fingernail psoriasis: a double-blind, randomized vehicle-controlled study. *Cutis* **68**, 355–358.

Schissel D. J., Elston D. M. (1998) Topical 5-fluorouracil treatment for psoriatic trachyonychia. *Cutis* **62**, 27–28.

Tosti A., Piraccini B. M., Cameli N. *et al.* (1998) Calcipotriol ointment in nail psoriasis: a controlled double-blind comparison with betamethasone dipropionate and salicylic acid. *Br J Dermatol* **139**, 655–659.

Yamamoto T., Katayama I., Nishioka K. (1998) Topical anthralin therapy for refractory nail psoriasis. *J Dermatol* **25**, 231–233.

Yu R. C., King C. M. (1992) A double-blind study of superficial radiotherapy in psoriatic nail dystrophy. *Acta Dermatol Venereol* **72**, 134–136.

10 Childhood psoriasis

Allison L. Holm
Thomas N. Helm

The onset of psoriasis during childhood is relatively common: 30% of all new cases of psoriasis start before the age of 15 years, 10% before 10 years, and 2% before 2 years. The incidence has been estimated at 3.1 new cases per year per 1000 children. Although the diagnosis may be straightforward in some cases, differentiation from other disorders including pityriasis rosea, lichen planus, atopic dermatitis, lupus erythematosus, seborrheic dermatitis, and dermatophyte infection may be difficult. Family history helps to clarify the diagnosis in some cases. Widespread and extensive involvement in childhood is uncommon but may occur at birth. Treatment options are limited by the desire to avoid toxicity and long-term health consequences. In this chapter, we review the presentation, precipitating factors, and important treatment options for clinicians in the diagnosis and treatment of psoriasis in children.

Epidemiology

Childhood psoriasis has an average age of onset between 7 and 8 years of age. One in 25 children under the age of 16 seeking medical attention for a dermatosis has psoriasis. Two-thirds of all children with psoriasis give a family history of psoriasis. Girls outnumber boys by two to one. Psoriasis in children is often associated with preceding infection, emotional distress, or trauma. Plaque-type psoriasis is the most common form noted and occurs in about 80% of children. The scalp is the most frequent site of involvement. The face and ears are often involved in children, and psoriasis may present as a single plaque on the eyelid. Guttate psoriasis is the second most common variant in children. Nail pitting is seen in one-third of children.

Presentation and precipitating factors

Psoriasis often develops in areas of irritation and may exhibit an isomorphic (Koebner) response. In infants, psoriasis develops in an area of diaper dermatitis. Psoriasis in the diaper area may present as "diaper rash" with sharp margination and bright, "glazed" erythema. The diagnosis of psoriasis later becomes clear after a primary irritant or diaper dermatitis fails to respond to treatment in a typical manner. Some authorities believe that psoriasis in the diaper area is the precursor of classic psoriasis in later life. Children with infantile psoriasis often have a mild course. In children and young adults, preceding streptococcal infections such as pharyngitis or perianal dermatitis with beta-hemolytic streptococci of the Lansfield Group A may be associated with a guttate flare of psoriasis. Widespread 3–6 mm papules on the trunk and extremities typically develop shortly after the infection. Psoriasis may be aggravated directly by streptococcal superantigens activating CD4+ T-cells or by T-cells reacting to streptococcal M protein, which exhibits similarity to keratin 14. Individuals with the Cw0602 allele are particularly subject to guttate flares. Psoriasiform eruptions have been noted in the setting of Kawasaki's disease and chronic recurrent multifocal osteomyelitis.

Classic plaque-type psoriasis may affect knees, elbows, buttocks, and scalp with erythematous scaly plaques. It may also involve intertriginous sites. Pustular and erythrodermic forms of psoriasis comprise only 1% of cases. The morphology and systemic signs in children are the same as those seen in widespread psoriasis of adults. The skin becomes diffusely erythematous and scaly in erythrodermic psoriasis. Small pinpoint pustules become confluent in pustular psoriasis and are often associated with fever and arthropathy. Underlying infections are thought to be culprits in some cases. Exposure to irritants such as coal tar or excessive sun exposure also may be associated with a psoriatic flare. Pustular and erythrodermic psoriasis may occur at any age, but congenital psoriasis is rare. Annular pustular psoriasis may be a fairly common and under-recognized variant of childhood psoriasis.

Another rare presentation of psoriasis is micropapular psoriasis. The form presents as 1–2 mm papules in dark-skinned individuals. The individual papules show scale after they have been scratched. Psoriatic arthritis is relatively rare in children and can occur with either plaque or guttate psoriasis.

Treatments

Many treatments commonly used in adults are not approved for use in children. Nonetheless, small studies or anecdotal reports indicate that many of the therapies used in older individuals are also effective in children. Clinicians must weigh the risks and benefits of treatment and carefully document discussions showing that adequate informed consent was given by guardians. We approach therapy in an organized therapeutic ladder in which emollients, topical immunomodulating agents, and topical steroids are tried prior to systemic agents such as phototherapy, retinoids, and immunosuppressive agents.

Topical therapy

Topical emollients

Emollient creams and lotions are helpful in controlling scale and relieving pruritus. Bland emollients are preferred, and we often prescribe a regimen that includes warm baths with colloidal oatmeal additive (Aveeno) followed by the application of emollient cream. We recommend products that are free of common sensitizers such as diazolidinyl urea, Quaternium 15, lanolin, or fragrance. Whereas ammonium lactate containing products can be very helpful in adults, the prescription ammonium lactate products equivalent to 12% lactic acid are not recommended in children less than two years of age because of irritation of the eyes, lids and mucous membranes with stinging and burning sensation. Older children often complain of irritation when such products are used on broken skin. Emollients made for sensitive skin, containing ingredients such as mineral oil, dimethicone, petrolatum, and glycerin, are particularly helpful at relieving dryness without causing irritation.

Topical steroids

Topical steroids are useful in the pediatric population. Topical steroids are recommended to be applied two to three times daily as a thin film to psoriatic plaques. The product is used for 2–3 weeks and then tapered in favor of emollient creams. After 1–2 weeks, topical calcipotriene or coal tar may be added in combination with topical corticosteroids. Some fluorinated steroids, such as fluocinonide

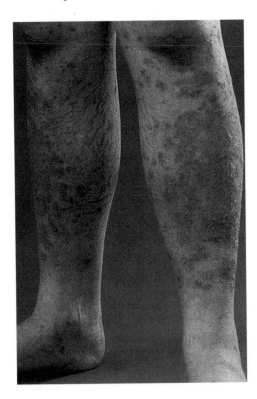

Figure 10.1 Striae distensae developed on the legs of a young girl with psoriasis where a medium potency corticosteroid was applied under plastic wrap occlusion.

0.05% gel, cream, ointment and solution, may be used in children. The risk of hypothalamic-pituitary-adrenal axis suppression must be considered whenever fluorinated steroids are used in the pediatric population. Striae distensae, telangiectasias, atrophy, and folliculitis are all possible complications of topical steroid use (Fig. 10.1). Careful attention must be taken to avoid long-term use and abuse.

Calcipotriene (0.005% ointment)

Calcipotriene is used for plaque-type psoriasis. It is not currently recommended for children, although many practitioners have used calcipotriene in the pediatric population in an "off label" fashion. Hypercalcemia and vitamin D toxicity are potential risks, although this occurrence is rare. Calcipotriene ointment is not recommended for use on the face as it may cause discomfort, although the cream formulation may be well tolerated on the face and intertriginous areas. Calcipotriene is rated as pregnancy category C and has not been shown to be safe during pregnancy.

Studies have shown topical calcipotriene to be a safe and effective treatment for chronic plaque psoriasis, with 60% of pediatric patients judged as "cleared" or "markedly improved" at the end of a study that involved an 8-week, twice daily application of medication. There have been case reports of the use of calcipotriene in infantile psoriasis.

Immunomodulating agents

Tacrolimus ointment and pimecrolimus 1% cream are valuable additions to the therapeutic armamentarium. Although not recommended for children under two years of age, both work well for atopic dermatitis and less so for psoriasis. These products should not be applied to areas that appear to be secondarily infected. Burning and stinging as well as pyrexia and headache may rarely occur. Plaques may become less red and inflamed as patients notice less pruritus. These products may be especially helpful for psoriasis if used on the face or in intertriginous areas.

Coal tar

Coal tar preparations can be effective for long-term management of psoriasis, with less side effects and rebound upon cessation than topical steroids. For plaque-type psoriasis in children under 12, coal tar can be used in combination with moderate natural sun exposure or UVB phototherapy. The gel formulations are more cosmetically acceptable to children than creams, ointments, and oils.

Systemic therapy

Cyclosporine

Cyclosporine has not been recommended for children less than 18 years of age. The risk of renal impairment, uncontrolled hypertension, and drug interactions with many medicines such as trimethoprim-sulfamethoxazole, cimetidine and ranitidine causes concern. There are case reports of the use of low-dose cyclosporine (1–2 mg/kg/day) being used effectively in limited courses for the treatment of episodes of severe pustular psoriasis.

Methotrexate

Methotrexate is not recommended for children but is often used in the pediatric setting. Baseline complete blood cell count, platelet, chest x-ray, liver and kidney function tests, and pulmonary function tests are recommended. The hematologic count parameters are usually monitored on a monthly basis, and the liver and kidney function tests are monitored every 1–2 months. When methotrexate is prescribed to the pediatric population, it is important to avoid other hepatotoxic drugs as well as live virus vaccines. Toxicity is increased by nonsteroidal anti-inflammatory agents, salicylates, phenytoin, sulfonyurea, sulfonamides, penicillins, and tetracyclines. Nausea, vomiting, stomatitis, pruritus as well as thrombocytopenia and elevated liver enzymes may all occur.

When methotrexate is used in children, most clinicians still opt to perform a pretreatment liver biopsy. Weekly oral doses range from 3.75 to 25 mg with an average dose of 16.6 mg. The lowest possible dose should be prescribed, usually in the range of 0.2–0.7 mg/kg/week.

PUVA

Psoralen ultraviolet A phototherapy is potentially useful in children but poses a difficulty because children may behave unpredictably while in the phototherapy cabinet. There are anecdotal reports of children taking off their goggles or leaning too close to a light source. For this reason, we do not advocate the use of PUVA in the pediatric population under age 12 years. Both PUVA and UVB may be associated with an increased risk of photoaging and skin cancer.

Retinoids

The retinoids have been reported to be effective in resistant severe erythrodermic or pustular psoriasis in children. Etretinate has been used in doses ranging from 0.25 to 0.6 mg/kg/day with improvement noted within one month of therapy. While etretinate and acitretin are not approved for use in children, they can be considered in exceptionally severe cases of psoriasis. The risks to monitor include premature epiphyseal closure, spinal hyperostosis, pseudotumor cerebri, and elevated liver function tests. Monitoring with a bone scan every 12–18 months has been recommended for children on long-term therapy with retinoids.

Antibiotics

Infection is one of the most important triggers of psoriasis in children. Guttate psoriasis or a guttate flare in a patient with stable plaque-type psoriasis often improves after a 10-day course of penicillin V or erythromycin on the presumption that a streptococcal infection may have induced the flare. Documentation by throat culture or rectal culture (in the case of perianal streptococcal dermatitis) or anti-streptococcal serology can be helpful to confirm the association of a streptococcal etiology with the flare.

In conclusion, psoriasis may present at an early age in genetically predisposed individuals and may be aggravated by an underlying infection. Although physicians must be wary about using therapies not approved for use in children, the accurate diagnosis of psoriasis and the judicious use of the therapeutic agents discussed, can dramatically relieve the suffering of affected children and their parents.

Selected references

Beretta-Piccoli B. C., Sauvain M. J., Gal I. *et al.* (2000) Synovitis, acne, pustulosis, hyperostosis, osteitis (SAPHO) syndrome in childhood: a report of ten cases and a review of the literature. *Eur J Pediatr* **159**, 594–601.

Burden A. D. (1999) Management of psoriasis in childhood. *Clin Exp Dermatol* **24**, 341–345.

Camisa C. (1998) Childhood Psoriasis. In: Camisa C. (ed.) *Handbook of Psoriasis*. Blackwell Science, Malden, MA, 114–118.

Choi Y. J., Hann S. K., Chang S.-N., Park W. H. (2000) Infantile Psoriasis: successful treatment with topical calcipotriol. *Pediatr Dermatol* **17**, 242–244.

Cofey J., Landells I. (2002) Topical treatment of psoriasis in children. *Skin Therapy* **7**, 4–7 (Letter).

Eberhard B. A., Sundel R. P., Newburger J. W. *et al.* (2000) Psoriatic eruption in Kawasaki disease. *J Pediatr* **137**, 578–580.

Farber E. M., Mullen R. H., Jacobs A. H., Nall L. (1986) Infantile psoriasis; a follow up study. *Pediatr Dermatol* **3**, 237–243.

Farber E. M., Nall L. (1999) Childhood psoriasis. *Cutis* **64**, 309–314.

Fond L., Michel J. L., Gentil-Perret A. *et al.* (1999) Psoriasis in childhood [French]. *Arch Pediatr* **6**, 669–674.

Freeman A. K., Linowski G. J., Brady C. *et al.* (2003) Tacrolimus ointment for the treatment of psoriasis on the face and intertriginous areas. *J Am Acad Dermatol* **48**, 564–568.

Ham M.-H., Jang K.-J., Moon K.-C. *et al.* (2000) A case of guttate psoriasis following Kawasaki disease. *Br J Dermatol* **142**, 548–550.

Herbst R. A., Hoch O., Kapp A. *et al.* (2000) Guttate psoriasis triggered by perianal streptococcal dermatitis in a four year old boy. *J Am Acad Dermatol* **42**, 885–887.

Honig P. J. (1988) Guttate psoriasis associated with perianal streptococcal disease. *J Pediatr* **113**, 1037–1039.

Judge M. R., McDonald A., Black M. M. (1993) Pustular Psoriasis in Childhood. *Clin Exp Dermatol* **18**, 97–99.

Khoo B. P., Giam Y. C. (2000) A pilot study on the role of intralesional triamcinolone acetonide in the treatment of pitted nails in children. *Singapore Med J* **41**, 66–68.

Kilic S. S., Hacimustafaoglu M., Celebi S. *et al.* (2001) Low dose cyclosporin A treatment in generalized pustular psoriasis. *Pediatr Dermatol* **18**, 246–248.

Kumar B., Dhar S., Handa S., Kaur I. (1994) Methotrexate in childhood psoriasis. *Pediatr Dermatol* **11**, 271–273.

Mahe E., Bodemer C., Pruszkowski A., Teillac-Hamel D., de Prost Y. (2001) Cyclosporine in childhood psoriasis. *Arch Dermatol* **137**, 1532–1533.

Mallon E., Bunce M., Savoie H. *et al.* (2000) HLA and guttate psoriasis. *Br J Dermatol* **143**, 1177–1182.

Morris A., Rogers M., Fischer G. *et al.* (2001) Childhood psoriasis: a clinical review of 1262 cases. *Pediatr Dermatol* **18**, 188–198.

Oranje A. P., Marcoux D., Svensson A. *et al.* (1997) Topical calcipotriol in childhood psoriasis. *J Am Acad Dermatol* **36**, 203–208.

Rasmussen J. E. (2000) The relationship between infection with Group A beta hemolytic streptococci and the development of psoriasis. *Pediatr Infect Disease J* **19**, 153–154.

Rattet J., Headley J., Barr R. (1981) Diaper dermatitis with psoriasiform id eruption. *Int J Dermatol* **20**, 122–125.

Raychaudhuri S. P., Gross J. (2000) A comparative study of pediatric onset psoriasis with adult onset psoriasis. *Pediatr Dermatol* **17**, 174–148.

Rogers M. (2002) Childhood psoriasis. *Curr Opin Pediatr* **14**, 404–409.

Rotstein H. (1996) Psoriasis: Changing clinical patterns. *Aust J Dermatol* **37** (Suppl. 1), 27–29.

Travis L. B., Silverberg N. B. (2001) Psoriasis in infancy: therapy with calcipotriene ointment. *Cutis* **68**, 341–344.

Weigl B. A. (1998) Immunoregulatory mechanisms and stress hormones in psoriasis (Part 1). *Int J Dermatol* **37**, 350–357.

Yamamoto T., Nishioka K. (2000) Topical tacrolimus is effective for facial lesions of psoriasis. *Acta Dermatol Venereol* **80**, 451.

11   Corticosteroids

Charles Camisa

Introduction

The first successful use of topical hydrocortisone for skin disease was described in 1952. Synthetic alteration of the parent compound has allowed for the proliferation of molecules that express potent glucocorticoid activity. Although their long-term efficacy is questionable, topical corticosteroids have been prescribed for the majority of patients with localized psoriasis for the past three decades in the United States. Recent surveys of visits by psoriasis patients to all physicians and to dermatologists revealed that topical corticosteroids were prescribed at 70% and 85%, respectively. The dermatologists estimated that, in 30% of patients with mild psoriasis, the lesions would clear with the most potent topical agents, but that satisfactory improvement was maintained in only 40% and 7% 1 month or 12 months, respectively, after stopping therapy. The mid- and low-potency preparations were rated considerably lower in effectiveness. Overall, topical corticosteroids were considered to be less effective than either phototherapy or systemic therapy.

What are the reasons for the popularity of topical corticosteroids in the treatment of localized psoriasis? The drugs are small molecules that penetrate the stratum corneum and bind to steroid receptors in the cytosol of living keratinocytes, ultimately altering DNA synthesis and gene transcription. The potency of the drug correlates with the affinity of the receptor for it. Glucocorticoids exert both receptor-mediated and direct inhibitory effects on the inflammatory cells seen in biopsies of psoriasis. They also inhibit mediators of inflammation such as phospholipase A2, the enzyme that initiates the arachidonic acid cascade.

Topical corticosteroids

Potency

The ideal topical corticosteroid would embody all of the following characteristics: penetration, clinical efficacy, no tachyphylaxis, no side-effects, cosmetic elegance, and low cost. Increasing potency correlates with increasing local and systemic toxicity. The super-potent corticosteroids are the newest and the most expensive compounds. Penetration is enhanced in thinner skin. Thus, penetration through eyelid skin is 36–40 times that of the palms or soles. Increased hydration and temperature increase penetration, factors that are exploited with application after a warm bath or occlusion of the corticosteroid with plastic wrap or tape. Increasing the concentration of drug does not necessarily result in greater penetration or potency.

Potency and therefore clinical efficacy are increased by molecular modification of the parent compound such as by halogenation, or by producing acetonide or valerate analogues which both increase the tightness of binding to glucocorticoid receptor, or by changing the vehicle by adding high concentrations of the solvent propylene glycol which enhances percutaneous absorption.

The vasoconstrictor assay was introduced by McKenzie and Stoughton in 1962 and has been used ever since for screening new corticosteroids and as an indirect bioassay of clinical effectiveness. In its current modification, the formulation is applied to the volar surface of the forearms of normal volunteers, covered with an elevated perforated guard for 16 hours, washed off, and "read" two hours later in a blind manner by an experienced investigator. Readings of vasoconstriction are graded qualitatively from 0 to 3, and the results are analyzed statistically by nonparametric tests.

In 1985, Cornell and Stoughton demonstrated an excellent correlation between the results of the vasoconstrictor assay and the results of bilateral symmetric paired comparisons of psoriatic target lesions treated 1–3 times daily for 2–3 weeks, for 30 of 32 different compounds. Alclometasone ointment 0.05% and hydrocortisone valerate cream 0.2% were the exceptions, resulting in greater vasoconstriction than clinical effectiveness. The most precise method of evaluating the potency of a topical steroid is by well-controlled clinical studies comparing one drug with another or its vehicle (placebo). Psoriasis is particularly well suited for study early in the course of treatment because lesions tend to be bilateral, symmetric, and of equal severity on either side. The literature abounds with this type of study. After the vasoconstriction classification for a drug has been determined, the manufacturers typically sponsor studies comparing their drug to others in the same potency group. Any edge in clinical efficacy, rapidity of onset of action, patient acceptance, side effect profile, or relapse rate is then marketed.

Superpotent topical corticosteroids

A study comparing diflorasone diacetate ointment 0.05% and clobetasol propionate ointment 0.05% confirmed that reductions in severity scores were greater on the clobetasol side but emphasized that "preatrophy" was also more evident. Applied twice weekly for 2 weeks, diflorasone ointment was as effective as betamethasone dipropionate in optimized vehicle (OV). Two double-blind multicenter studies compared halobetasol propionate ointment 0.05% to clobetasol ointment 0.05% or betamethasone dipropionate OV ointment 0.05%. After 28 days of twice daily application, marked improvement or clearing occurred in 96% of subjects treated with halobetasol and 91% of those treated with clobetasol.

Potency in the vasoconstrictor assay is generally correlated with clinical efficacy in psoriasis. Potency is also correlated with bioavailability and adverse effects, both local and systemic. Therefore, the advent of superpotent group I steroids opens new vistas for dermatologists. On the one hand, plaques of psoriasis may be completely cleared after 2–4 weeks of twice daily application, but more importantly, maintenance of remission by intermittent pulsing of topical therapy becomes possible. Unfortunately, serious unwanted effects such as striae and hypothalamic-pituitary-adrenal (HPA) axis suppression can occur, and there is potential for abuse of these agents. Abusive or inappropriate use includes more than twice-daily application (wasteful), use under occlusion, and use in children under 12 years (more atrophogenic and increased systemic absorption), use on the face or intertriginous areas (more risk of steroid-induced rosacea and atrophy with telangiectasia or striae), use for more than 2 consecutive weeks, or more than 50 g per week.

Gammon *et al.* used successive courses of clobetasol ointment 0.05% (twice daily for 14 days) separated by one or more weeks determined by the rate of relapse. The treatment was effective, but

Table 11.1 Recommended guidelines for the use of superpotent topical corticosteroids.

---

1 Do not use more than 50 g per week
2 Do not use under occlusion
3 Do not use on the face, axillae, submammary area, and groin
4 Do not use in children under 12 years of age
5 Allow a 1–2 week "drug holiday" between successive full courses of therapy (as is done in intermittent pulsing for maintenance)
6 If using for more than two consecutive weeks, consider measuring morning plasma cortisol; reduce or stop daily dosing if it is below normal
7 If the morning plasma cortisol level is considered borderline or unreliable, order corticotropin releasing hormone stimulation test

---

mild local adverse effects and transient low morning plasma cortisol levels were found in 20% and 12% of patients, respectively.

Katz *et al.* studied the effects of two superpotent steroids, 3.5 g applied twice daily for 3 weeks, on the HPA axis. They showed that both clobetasol and betamethasone dipropionate in OV dramatically suppress morning plasma cortisol (<5 µg/dl) and urinary free cortisol levels (<35 µg/dl) in 20% of patients. None of the patients manifested any classic signs of adrenal insufficiency. Clinical effectiveness with the superpotent topical steroids parallels suppression of the HPA axis. A ranking of clinical effectiveness among the superpotent agents in descending order would be clobetasol, halobetasol, betamethasone dipropionate in OV, and diflorasone diacetate.

Patients whose plasma morning cortisol value drops below 5 µg/dl could conceivably develop clinically significant adverse effects if they sustained coincident serious trauma, or infection, or underwent major surgery with general anesthesia. Therefore, certain guidelines for the use of the superpotent agents have been suggested (Table 11.1).

Generic formulations of topical corticosteroids

As the patents on brand-name corticosteroids expire, generic formulations will proliferate and be marketed for the same indications as the innovator product without the benefit of clinical efficacy studies. The bioavailability and rate of release of the corticosteroid is dependent not only on the concentration of corticosteroid in the vehicle but also on the composition of the vehicle itself. The design of the vehicle and manufacturing methodology of the final product are not likely to be identical for most proprietary and generic topical corticosteroids.

There is political and economic pressure on physicians to prescribe generic medicines. Patients want the best drug that gives the fastest relief from suffering, preferably at low cost or gratis. Physicians prescribe what they think will work the best with the least toxicity in a given situation, without regard to rapidity in a chronic incurable condition such as psoriasis and often without regard to price. Pharmacists want to fill prescriptions correctly and legally while realizing a reasonable profit. Some physicians dispense their own prescriptions. Governments, institutions, and prescription insurance plans usually include the drugs on their formularies that can be obtained at the lowest wholesale price, regardless of generic or brand-name status.

Some popular brand-name topical corticosteroids have been compared to themselves and their generic equivalents by the vasoconstrictor assay. Valisone® 0.1% (Schering Corp., Kenilworth, NJ), Kenalog® 0.1% (Bristol-Myers Squibb Co, Princeton, NJ), and Synalar® 0.025% (Medicis, Phoenix, AZ) creams were significantly more potent than some generic formulations. However, generic triamcinolone acetonide creams 0.025% and 0.05% (E. Fougera & Co, Melville, NY) were more potent than the corresponding Aristocort® creams (Fugisawa USA, Inc., Deerfield, IL). In addition, higher concentrations of the same corticosteroid in the same vehicle made by the same manufacturer do not necessarily predict higher activity or bioavailability. In most cases, no differences in activity were found for Kenalog® ointment 0.025, 0.1, 0.5%; Aristocort® ointment and creams 0.1, 0.5%; Topicort® 0.05, 0.25%; and Hytone cream 1.0, 2.5%. The Fougera generic triamcinolone acetonide creams 0.025 and 0.5% were also equivalent. Because the topical corticosteroids are so widely used in the treatment of psoriasis, it should be pointed out that:

1 Brand-name topical corticosteroids are priced according to concentration. If the lower concentration is equipotent, it should be prescribed preferentially.

2 Where generic formulations are equivalent in potency to brand-name formulations, the former should be prescribed for the cost savings. The physician would have to know which generic manufacturer the pharmacist dispenses, however, since the generics are

not all the same. For example, Fougera betamethasone valerate 0.1% ointment is equivalent to Valisone ointment.

3 Until comparative potency labeling of all generic topical corticosteroids is required, it is not feasible to prescribe the most cost-effective generic drug in all cases. As a general rule, generic ointment formulations are closer to brand names in vasoconstriction assays. The physician should prescribe generic ointments or specify brand-name creams if that vehicle is desired.

Adverse effects

While the effects of systemic absorption, HPA-axis suppression, and iatrogenic Cushing's syndrome are serious concerns with conservative use of the superpotent topical steroids, they may occur with the intermediate- to high-potency compounds as well (Table 11.2). Fortunately, such reports are rare and usually implicate grossly inappropriate or unsupervised use of the medication. While the potential hazards of superpotent steroids are greater, the tendency for abuse of the former is more likely because there are no limitations on quantities dispensed, recommendations for daily dosage and rest periods, prohibitions against occlusive dressings and use in children. Notwithstanding, in practice, it is the local unwanted effects of topical corticosteroids that give the most frequent cause for concern.

Atrophy

The most common adverse effect of topical corticosteroid use is cutaneous atrophy. This atrophy involves both the epidermis with thinning secondary to decreased mitotic activity and DNA synthesis as well as the dermis with decreased fibroblast synthesis of collagen and ground substance. The clinical counterpart to steroid-induced atrophy is increased transparency, shininess of the skin with loss of skin markings, and telangiectasia.

Atrophy is most commonly detected on the face as telangiectasias, but these may represent normal or preexisting dilated capillaries in the papillary dermis made more obvious by thinning of the epidermis. Moreover, patients with solar elastosis or rosacea may already have preexisting telangiectasia. For this reason, low potency nonfluorinated topical steroids are recommended for psoriatic lesions on the central face (e.g. hydrocortisone, desonide,

Table 11.2 Potency ranking of some commonly used topical corticosteroids based on vasoconstrictor assay and clinical studies in psoriasis.

Potency group	Concentration	Generic name	*Brand name (U.S.)
I Super-High	0.05%	Clobetasol propionate	Temovate
	0.05%	Halobetasol propionate	Ultravate
	0.05%	Betamethasone dipropionate (in optimized vehicle)	Diprolene
	0.05%	Diflorasone diacetate (in optimized vehicle)	Psorcon
II High	0.1%	+Amcinonide	Cyclocort oint
	0.05%	Betamethasone dipropionate	Diprosone oint
	0.25%	Desoximetasone	Topicort***
	0.05%	Diflorasone diacetate	Fluorone+Maxiflor oint
	0.05%	Fluocinonide	Lidex
	0.1%	Halcinonide	Halog cream
III Intermediate	0.05%	Betamethasone dipropionate	Diprosone cream
	0.1%	Betamethasone-17-valerate	Valisone oint
	0.05%	Diflorasone diacetate	Maxiflor+Florone cream
	+++0.005%	Fluticasone propionate	Cutivate oint
	0.1%	Triamcinolone acetonide	Aristocort A oint***
	0.1%	Mometasone furoate	Elocon oint
IV Intermediate	0.025%	Fluocinolone acetonide	Synalar oint
	0.05%	Flurandrenolide	Cordran oint/tape
	0.1%	Triamcinolone acetonide	Kenalog cream
	0.1%	Mometasone furoate	Elocon cream
	0.2%	Hydrocortisone 17-valerate	Westcort oint
V	0.1%	++Betamethasone-17-valerate	Valisone cream
	0.1%	Prednicarbate	Dermatop cream
	0.025%	Fluocinolone acetonide	Synalar cream
	0.05%	Fluticasone propionate	Cutivate cream
	0.1%	Hydrocortisone butyrate	Locoid cream
	0.2%	Hydrocortisone-17-valerate	Westcort cream
VI Low	0.05%	++Aclometasone dipropionate	Aclovate cream + oint
	0.01%	Betamethasone-17-valerate	Valisone cream
	0.05%	Desonide	Tridesilon and DesOwen creams
	0.1%	Triamcinolone acetonide	Aristocort cream
	0.01%	Fluocinolone acetonide	Synalar cream
VII Very low	0.1%	Dexamethasone	Decadron cream
	**1%,2.5%	Hydrocortisone	Hytone***
	0.25%	Methylprednisone	Medrol cream

*Product refers to both cream and ointment vehicle unless specified.

**Also available without prescription.

***A dose–response curve has not been demonstrated in either vasoconstriction assay or clinical activity for the same formulations of these brands.

+With few exceptions, the ointment formulation of the same concentration of corticosteroid is one class higher in potency than the cream formulation.

++Potency rating based on clinical activity in psoriasis, not vasoconstriction assay.

+++Note that concentrations of ointment and cream formulations are different.

Table 11.3 Strategies to avoid tachyphylaxis.

---

1 Apply steroid only once daily or on alternate days
2 Combine steroid treatment with coal tar, anthralin, calcipotriene, or tazarotene
3 Use intermittent courses of therapy (e.g. 2 weeks on, 1 week off) or apply superpotent steroid three times in 36 hours each week
4 Alternate among different steroids within the same potency class at periodic intervals

---

and hydrocortisone-17-valerate). More potent steroids should not be used on the eyelid skin because of the risk of increasing intraocular pressure (glaucoma). Fluticasone propionate 0.005%, a group V fluorinated steroid, was applied to the face and the intertriginous areas twice daily for 2 weeks, then once daily for two consecutive days each week for 8 more weeks. Clearance was maintained in 85% of patients without causing atrophy. It is often necessary and appropriate to apply intermediate- to high-potency steroids to psoriasis of the ears and scalp. Thorough washing of hands or covering with gloves if they are also under treatment cannot be overemphasized. Shower caps worn over anointed scalps at bedtime are also helpful.

Steroid-induced rosacea (Table 11.3)

Another common adverse effect occurring on the face is a papulopustular reaction, usually in a perioral or periocular distribution, particularly in acne- or rosacea-prone individuals. This may have resulted after intentional treatment of facial psoriasis or inadvertent contact. In some instances, patients may have learned by trial and error that the steroid helps incidental acneiform lesions and use it on their own.

Striae distensae

While preatrophy and atrophy of the skin are reversible, striae caused by rupture of connective tissue and stretching of the epidermis are permanent. They may result from the application of medium- to high-potency steroids to flexural or intertriginous areas such as the axillae and groin which are naturally moist and partially occluded.

Purpura

In mature patients with age-related atrophy and solar elastosis, purpura occurs frequently on the backs of the arms and hands after minor or imperceptible trauma, even with use of low- to intermediate-potency steroids. Many patients find these annoying and complain about them. Stellate pseudoscars may develop, particularly if shearing of the epidermis occurs.

Infections

Long-term use of topical steroids can mask cutaneous infections with scabies or dermatophytes because of the blunted inflammatory response and slowed rate of epidermal turnover. Fungal infections of the groin, buttocks, and feet that are inappropriately treated as psoriasis will be aggravated. Bacterial folliculitis may develop in a hairy area related to occlusive ointments.

Tachyphylaxis

Tachyphylaxis is defined as the diminishing effect of a pharmacologic agent as it is repeatedly used to achieve a clinical response. This was described for potent steroids when no further vasoconstriction could be elicited after 96 hours. Recovery generally occurred after a 4-day rest period. The pathomechanisms of tachyphylaxis are unknown. Loss of clinical effect is a common problem with chronic application of higher potency steroids, but tachyphylaxis is difficult to demonstrate in the clinical setting. The perception of tachyphylaxis may be related to failure of therapeutic efficacy, noncompliance, or a flare of psoriasis unrelated to therapy. Strategies to avoid tachyphylaxis are listed in Table 11.3.

Rebound and pustular flares

After abrupt withdrawal of a potent topical steroid, a rebound flare of psoriasis may ensue. Rapid proliferation of the epidermis and stoking of the synthetic machinery of the dermis occur within days after the steroid is stopped. Since both mechanisms may be involved in the pathogenesis of psoriasis, it is easier to understand why an incompletely treated psoriatic lesion may rebound. It is not uncommon to observe sterile pustules developing within a plaque during therapy. A full generalized pustular flare rarely occurs upon withdrawal of therapy. For this reason, it is advisable to utilize intermittent therapy with potent steroids or continuous therapy with the weakest steroid that is effective, at the same time taking care to alternate chemical structures periodically to avoid tachyphylaxis.

Systemic corticosteroids

To the extent that one can say "never" in medicine, systemic corticosteroids should probably never be prescribed for psoriasis. However, physicians must deal with their complications when they are prescribed by other physicians for psoriasis or when they are used appropriately for concomitant conditions that may overshadow psoriasis in terms of severity and disability, for example, Crohn's disease, rheumatoid arthritis, systemic lupus erythematosus, and renal allograft transplantation.

A 1992 survey of 225 dermatologists revealed that 11% still used systemic steroids to treat some of their patients with severe psoriasis. Studies and experience have shown that it is not systemic steroid treatment per se that aggravates psoriasis, but rather the tapering or withdrawal of the drugs. Most patients with psoriasis are initially quite responsive to systemic steroids, as judged by clearing of the skin during treatment. It is during the taper that the skin disease becomes labile and more inflammatory, spreads, and develops pustulation. In the past, dermatologists who treated psoriasis with prednisone noted that the dose needed to maintain the disease spiraled upward until reaching an uncomfortably high dose that eventually became ineffective. Upon subsequent tapering and withdrawal of the steroid, a rebound flare, exacerbation, and pustular or erythrodermic psoriasis may occur unless there is intervention with systemic anti-psoriatic treatment or hospitalization. Consultation at a tertiary care center is indicated prior to the desperate use of systemic steroids for a patient with severe psoriasis.

For patients with psoriasis and serious concomitant systemic diseases, it is imperative to collaborate with colleagues in the selection of adjunctive therapy that will help psoriasis but not aggravate the underlying disease and vice versa (Table 11.4).

Allergic contact dermatitis

Hypersensitivity to a topical corticosteroid should be suspected when the skin disease not only fails to respond but worsens during

Table 11.4 Treatment of disease concomitant with psoriasis.

Concomitant disease	Treatment with beneficial effect on psoriasis
Crohn's disease	Sulfasalazine, cyclosporine, infliximab
Rheumatoid arthritis	Sulfasalazine, methotrexate, azathioprine, infliximab, etanercept
Systemic lupus erythematosus	MTX, azathioprine, retinoids (cutaneous signs)
Allograft transplant rejection	Azathioprine, cyclosporine, tacrolimus, mycophenolate mofetil

treatment. Patients may become sensitized to ingredients in the vehicle or to the active corticosteroid itself. They may become sensitized to steroids, such as triamcinolone, mometasone, and budesonide, which are found in nasal sprays and inhalers. Allergic contact dermatitis to corticosteroids is believed to be uncommon in psoriasis because almost all of the published reports involved patients with underlying chronic eczematous conditions or venous stasis ulceration. However, when hospitalized psoriatics were subjected to allergy patch testing, 4/140 (2.9%) patients gave positive results to topical steroids. Coal and wood tars and anthralin are more important allergens, however. Tixocortol pivolate, hydrocortisone-17-butyrate, and budesonide are excellent steroid screening compounds, but most patch-test experts use a larger topical medicament allergen series.

Occlusive dressings

The use of impermeable polyethylene wraps and plastic sauna suits has declined in popularity with the development of potent and superpotent topical corticosteroids and the trend toward outpatient therapy, home UVB units, and psoriasis day treatment centers. The group I and II steroids are powerful enough without occlusion. Moreover, occlusion may enhance local side-effects such as atrophy and increase systemic absorption. Occlusive dressings are uncomfortable for some patients and may be complicated by sweating, miliaria, and folliculitis. Because of the thickness of volar skin and reduced absorption of steroids, and relatively resistant psoriasis there, occlusion of a superpotent steroid on the palms or soles is tolerable and acceptable using vinyl medical examining gloves or plastic wrap (Saran wrap).

An alternative occlusive dressing that is elegant and well tolerated is flurandrenolide impregnated tape (4 $\mu g/cm^2$) which is only practical for relatively small lesions and may be left in place for a full day. Flurandrenolide tape applied once daily for up to 16 hours produced consistently greater clearing than diflorasone acetate ointment applied twice daily for 4 weeks.

A modification of the hydrocolloid patches developed for wound healing have been marketed for occlusion of localized psoriatic plaques over an intermediate- or high-potency steroid for 48 hours. The patches (DuoDERM Extra Thin, Convatec, Montreal, Canada) are small, self-adhesive, and waterproof. They absorb transepidermal water, keeping the stratum corneum well hydrated and optimal for topical steroid delivery. Maceration and bacterial overgrowth are significantly less with hydrocolloid patches compared to plastic-film occlusion. Mild folliculitis occurs infrequently. Epilation typically occurs upon removal of the dressing.

David and Lowe showed that improvement of chronic plaque psoriasis was most rapid and persistent with triamcinolone acetonide (TAC) 0.1% under occlusion with a hydrocolloid dressing compared to TAC and plastic-film occlusion or TAC alone. This technique used every third day for palmoplantar pustulosis was more effective than clobetasol propionate cream 0.05% applied twice daily. Four weeks after stopping both treatments, the lesions returned to their pre-treatment status. Clobetasol lotion 0.05% applied once weekly under a hydrocolloid dressing gave more rapid clearance than the same steroid ointment applied twice daily without occlusion. The rate of relapse was comparable for both treatments, and atrophy was not observed.

Hydrocolloid patches may be ideal as primary therapy for limited plaques of psoriasis on the palms, soles, elbows, knees, and sacrum, for localized pustular psoriasis, and for patients with residual lesions after UVL or systemic therapy. The hydrocolloid patches are expensive but can be obtained without a prescription and can be cut to the desired size. An inexpensive generic ointment such as TAC 0.1% or betamethasone-17-valerate 0.1% can be used with it every 5–7 days. In frequently traumatized areas, the patches may afford a level of protection (from picking and scratching) that prevents the isomorphic response and allows healing to occur.

An alternative technique for treating limited or residual psoriasis is intralesional injection of triamcinolone acetonide, 5 mg/ml. The suspension must be well mixed and the material must be injected in the dermis so that an immediate blanch is seen. There will be a response unless the drug is diluted improperly or injected too deeply. I inject a maximum of 4 ml (20 mg) per month. Atrophy, which is unlikely to occur at this concentration, is reversible. Healing of plaques may persist for 3 months or longer. This treatment is ideal for the scalp and is preferred by patients who are noncompliant with the applications of lotions, ointments, and dressings and who can tolerate the slight discomfort of intradermal injections.

A new hydro-ethanolic foam vehicle has been developed which incorporates betamethasone valerate 0.12% or clobetasol propionate 0.05%. The steroid foams are significantly more effective at treating psoriasis of the scalp and other body areas than the foam vehicle. The foam may enhance bioavailability of the steroids without increasing toxicity. Although the steroid foams are more expensive than their conventional cream or lotion counterparts, patient acceptance and possibly compliance is higher.

Compounding

It is risky business to compound chemicals with proprietary formulations without knowing the effects on physicochemical stability and skin penetration rate. Krochmal *et al.* showed that urea 10% caused significant chemical degradation of the active steroid in Westcort, Topicort, and Kenalog creams. On the other hand, such frequently used additives as 0.25% camphor, 0.25% menthol, 0.25% phenol, 2% salicylic acid, or 5% LCD solution caused no degradation. Salicylic acid 2% enhanced the penetration rate 2–3-fold while the others did not. A proprietary combination ointment of mometasone furoate 0.1% and salicylic acid 5% was significantly more effective than the steroid ointment alone in the treatment of target lesions twice daily for 3 weeks. We recommend that extemporaneous compounding be performed by an experienced pharmacist using USP chemicals and petrolatum, Aquaphor or Eucerin, as a vehicle. We frequently compound triamcinolone acetonide USP and hydrocortisone USP with some of the additives listed above excluding urea.

Combination therapy

Topical corticosteroids are most useful for patients with limited psoriasis (<10%). Therefore, in patients with more extensive disease, the role of steroids as adjunctive therapy with ultraviolet light has been explored and reviewed. Combining UVB phototherapy and topical steroids confers little advantage in treating psoriasis compared to UVB alone. Most studies showed a more rapid early, but not final, clearing. Two of seven reports noted a shorter remission time when UVB was combined with clobetasol ointment or hydrocortisone valerate cream, respectively. In only one study was the remission time longer when UVB was combined with a topical steroid (fluocinonide cream 0.05%), but the results did not attain statistical significance.

In conclusion, the combination of topical steroids with UVB phototherapy appears to have no substantial effect on the time to clearing or the proportion of responders. The long-term effects on remission are inconclusive and may be detrimental. Therefore, because of potential toxicity discussed previously and the increased cost, high-potency topical corticosteroids should not be used in combination with UVB therapy. However, low-potency steroids for light-protected areas and mid-potency lotions for the scalp are probably still warranted.

At least five studies compared PUVA photochemotherapy with and without various topical corticosteroids. All studies showed more rapid clearing rates of psoriasis with the combination of PUVA plus corticosteroid compared to PUVA alone. There were no differences in the percentage of patients cleared in each group, and only one study reported a higher relapse rate in the patients who received fluocinolone acetonide cream or ointment 0.025% under plastic-film occlusion until clearing was achieved. The psoriasis in patients who had a relapse progressed to a more aggressive form. In the two studies where it was reported, the cumulative UVA dose required for clearing on the corticosteroid side was approximately half that required on the placebo-treated side.

In conclusion, an intermediate- to high-potency topical steroid may be used concurrently during PUVA photochemotherapy in order to achieve faster clearing and a lower cumulative UVA dose at clearing. With weaning of the topical steroid (decrease frequency of application or decrease potency) and continuous maintenance PUVA, higher relapse rates are unlikely to occur.

In one study, combining triamcinolone cream 0.1% with 5% salicylic acid (which probably increases the penetration rate of the steroid) allowed low-dose oral etretinate to be as effective as higher doses. This helped decrease retinoid-related side-effects and reduced the cost of therapy.

In a bilateral paired comparison, combining fluocinonide 0.01% with increasing concentrations of anthralin did not change the final time to clearance. The sides receiving the steroid showed less burning and more staining from the anthralin but unfortunately a significantly more rapid relapse of psoriasis. It may be advisable to reserve topical steroids for brief stints as a "fireman" if intolerable anthralin-related irritation occurs while reducing the working concentration of anthralin for further treatment. Because their main side-effects consist of erythema and skin irritation, the response to vitamin D analogues (calcipotriene and tacalcitol) and acetylenic retinoid (tazarotene) are improved by combinations with topical corticosteroids.

Many studies have shown that various topical steroids used in combination with calcipotriene work synergistically to improve the efficacy and reduce the side-effects of either treatment used alone. The two drugs have been used in different sequences: (1) two weeks' treatment with twice daily application of clobetasol ointment 0.05%, followed by 4 weeks of calcipotriene, was superior to 6 weeks' treatment with calcipotriene alone; (2) betamethasone dipropionate OV cream 0.05% once daily for the first and third weeks and calcipotriene ointment twice daily for the second and fourth weeks was more effective than the steroid cream alone once daily for 4 weeks; (3) calcipotriene ointment in the morning and halobetasol ointment 0.05% in the evening for 2 weeks. Three-quarters of patients maintained remission for 6 months with application of halobetasol twice daily on weekends and calcipotriene twice daily on weekdays. A proprietary ointment formulation of calcipotriene 0.005% and betamethasone dipropionate 0.05% has been developed. After 4 weeks' twice daily application, the combined formulation was significantly more effective and produced less local adverse reactions than either calcipotriene or the vehicle ointment.

The adjunctive use of mid- and high-potency topical creams (but not low-potency) improved the therapeutic efficacy and tolerability of tazarotene gel 0.1%. With tazarotene applied in the evening and the steroid in the morning, the best-performing steroid was betamethasone dipropionate cream 0.05%, followed by mometasone furoate ointment 0.1%, and diflorasone diacetate ointment 0.05%.

How much to use

It is only necessary to apply a quantity of cream or ointment sufficient to cover the lesion site with a thin, uniform, barely perceptible

Table 11.5 Amount of ointment required to treat anatomic areas for 1 and 7 days.

Anatomic area	No. of FTUs required to cover	Quantity (g) required for twice-daily application	Quantity (g) required for one week of twice-daily treatment
Face and neck	2.5	2.5	17.5
Anterior trunk	7	7.0	49
Posterior trunk	7	7.0	49
Arm	3	3.0	21
Hand (two sides)	1	1.0	7
Leg	6	6.0	42
Foot	2	2.0	14

FTU, fingertip unit.

layer. Previous estimations of body surface area have used a "hand" as representing approximately 1%. Long *et al.* have calculated one flat closed hand to represent about 0.75% of the body surface area. They further determined that one fingertip unit or FTU (the amount of ointment applied from the distal skin crease to the tip of the palmar aspect of the index finger) of ointment weighs about 0.5 g. One FTU of ointment covers about two hand areas. The amount of ointment required to treat each anatomic area twice daily can be estimated (Table 11.5). The entire body skin treated twice daily requires 28.5 g for one day and 200 g of medicine for one week. The concept of the FTU helps provide a more convenient means for the physician to estimate the quantities to dispense and for the patient to translate lesion size (one hand) into a quantity of medication (0.5 FTU or 0.25 g) to apply with less wastage.

Summary

Although topical steroids are important in the treatment of psoriasis because of their sheer volume and relative ease of use and cosmetic elegance, their long-term efficacy and safety have not been established. While a few new compounds were approved in existing potency groups, and a novel foam vehicle was developed for delivery of conventional steroids, it would be desirable if future steroid uses were developed to exploit the synergism found with popular anti-psoriatic treatments such as calcioptriene and tazarotene. As the patents of the brand-name innovators expire, there will be a proliferation of generically equivalent steroids. Paired comparisons of the brand-name and generic formulations on psoriatic subjects should be performed prior to marketing, and the package labeling should include the vasoconstrictor potency rating.

Selected references

Abma E. M., Blanken R., de Heide L. J. (2002) Cushing's syndrome caused by topical steroid for psoriasis. *Neth J Med* **60**, 148–150.

Austad J., Bjerke J. R., Gjertsen B. T. *et al.* (1998) Clobetasol propionate followed by calcipotriol is superior to calcipotriol alone in topical treatment of psoriasis. *J Eur Acad Dermatol Venereol* **11**, 19–24.

Cornell R. C., Stoughton R. B. (1985) Correlations of the vasoconstriction assay and clinical activity in psoriasis. *Arch Dermatol* **121**, 63–67.

David M., Lowe N. J. (1989) Psoriasis therapy: comparative studies with a hydrocolloid dressing, plastic film occlusion, and triamcinolone acetonide cream. *J Am Acad Dermatol* **21**, 511–514.

Franz T. J., Parsell D. A., Halualani R. M. *et al.* (1999) Betamethasone valerae foam 0.12%: a novel vehicle with enhanced delivery and efficacy. *Int J Dermatol* **38**, 628–632.

Gammon W. R., Krueger G. G., Van Scott E. J., Kamm A. (1987) Intermittent short courses of clobetasol propionate ointment 0.05% in the treatment of psoriasis. *Curr Ther Res* **42**, 419–427.

Green L., Sadoff W. (2002) A clinical evaluation of tazarotene 0.1% gel, with and without a high- or mid-high-potency corticosteroid, in patients with stable plaque psoriasis. *J Cut Med Surg* **6**, 95–102.

Griffiths C. E. M., Tranfaglia M. G., Kang S. (1995) Prolonged occlusion in the treatment of psoriasis: A clinical and immunohistologic study. *J Am Acad Dermatol* **32**, 618–622.

Guenther L., van de Kerkhof P. C., Snellman E. *et al.* (2002) Efficacy and safety of a new combination of calcipotriol and betamethasone dipropionate (once or twice daily) compared to calcipotriol (twice daily) in the treatment of psoriasis vulgaris: a randomized, double-blind, vehicle-controlled clinical trial. *Br J Dermatol* **147**, 316–323.

Hepburn D. J., Aeling J. L., Weston W. L. (1996) A reappraisal of topical steroid potency. *Pediatr Dermatol* **13**, 239–245.

Heule F., Tahapary G. J. M., Bello C. R., van Joost T. (1998) Delayed-type hypersensitivity to contact allergens in psoriasis. A clinical evaluation. *Contact Dermatitis* **38**, 78–82.

Jackson D. B., Thompson C., McCormack J. R., Guin J. D. (1989) Bioequivalence (bioavailability) of generic topical corticosteroids. *J Am Acad Dermatol* **20**, 791–796.

Katz H. I., Hien N. T., Prawer S. E. *et al.* (1987) Betamethasone dipropionate in optimized vehicle. *Arch Dermatol* **123**, 1308–1311.

Katz H. I., Hien N. T., Prawer S. E. *et al.* (1987) Superpotent topical steroid treatment of psoriasis vulgaris—clinical efficacy and adrenal function. *J Am Acad Dermatol* **16**, 804–811.

Koo J., Cuffie C. A., Tanner D. J. *et al.* (1998) Mometasone furoate 0.1% or salicylic acid 5% ointment versus mometasone furoate 0.1% ointment in the treatment of moderate-to-severe psoriasis: a multicenter study. *Clin Therapeutics* **20**, 283–291.

Krochmal L., Wnag J. C. T., Patel B., Rodgers J. (1989) Topical corticosteroid compounding: effects on physicochemical stability and skin penetration rate. *J Am Acad Dermatol* **21**, 979–984.

Krueger G. G., O'Reily M. A., Weidner M. *et al.* (1998) Comparative efficacy of once-daily flurandrenolide tape versus twice-daily diflorasone diacetate ointment in the treatment of psoriasis. *J Am Acad Dermatol* **38**, 186–190.

Lebwohl M. G., Tan M. H., Meador S. L., Singer G. (2001) Limited application of fluticasone propionate ointment, 0.005% in patients with psoriasis of the face and intertriginous areas. *J Am Acad Dermatol* **44**, 77–82.

Lebwohl M. G., Breneman D. L., Goffe B. S. *et al.* (1998) Tazarotene 0.1% gel plus corticosteroid cream in the treatment of plaque psoriasis. *J Am Acad Dermatol* **39**, 590–596.

Lebwohl M., Yoles A., Lombardi K., Lou W. (1998) Calcipotriene ointment and halobetasol ointment in the long-term treatment of psoriasis: effects on the duration of improvement. *J Am Acad Dermatol* **39**, 447–450.

Lebwohl M., Sherer D., Washenik K. *et al.* (2002) A randomized, double-blind, placebo-controlled study of clobetasol propionate 0.05% foam in the treatment of nonscalp psoriasis. *Int J Dermatol* **41**, 269–274.

Long C. C., Finlay A. Y., Averill R. W. (1992) The rule of hand: 4 hand areas = 2 FTU = 1 g. *Arch Dermatol* **128**, 1129–1130.

McCullough J. L., Weinstein G. D. (1995) Topical therapy for psoriasis: results of national survey. *Cutis* **55**, 306–310.

McKenzie A.W., Stoughton R.B. (1962) Method for comparing percutaneous absorption of steroids. *Arch Dermatol* **86**, 608–610.

Malhotra V., Kaur I., Saraswat A., Kumar B. (2002) Frequency of patch-test positivity in patients with psoriasis: a prospective controlled study. *Acta Derm Venereol* **82**, 432–435.

Miller J. J., Roling D., Margolis D., Guzzo C. (1999) Failure to demonstrate therapeutic tachyphylaxis to topically applied steroids in patients with psoriasis. *J Am Acad Dermatol* **41**, 546–549.

Olsen E. A. (1991) A double-blind controlled comparison of generic and trade-name topical steroids using the vasoconstriction assay. *Arch Dermatol* **127**, 197–201.

Singh S., Reddy D. C., Pandey S. S. (2000) Topical therapy for psoriasis with the use of augmented betamethasone and calcipotriene on alternate weeks. *J Am Acad Dermatol* **43**, 61–65.

Stinco G., Frattasio A., de Francesco V. *et al.* (1999) Frequency of delayed-type hypersensitivity to contact allergens in psoriatic patients. *Contact Dermatitis* **40**, 323–329.

Stroughton R. B., Cornell R. C. (1987) Review of super-potent topical corticosteroids. *Semin Dermatol* **6**, 72–76.

Stoughton R. B. (1987) Are generic formulations equivalent to trade name topical glucocorticoids? *Arch Dermatol* **123**, 1312–1314.

Theeuwes M., Bright R. (1996) Use of a hydrocolloid dressing in combination with a topical steroid in plaque psoriasis. *Cutis* **57**, 48–50.

Volden G., Kragballe K., van de Kerkhof P. C. *et al.* (2001) Remission and relapse of chronic plaque psoriasis treated once a week with clobetasol propionate occluded with a hydrocolloid dressing versus twice daily treatment with clobetasol propionate alone. *J Dermatology Treat* **12**, 141–144.

Warner M., Camisa C. (2001) Topical corticosteroids. In: Wolverton S. E. (ed.) *Comprehensive Dermatologic Drug Therapy.* WB Saunders, Philadelphia, 548–577.

Yohn J. J., Weston W. L. (1990) Topical glucocorticosteroids. *Curr Probl Dermatol* **2**, 31–63.

12   Anthralin

Charles Camisa

The active ingredient in Goa powder extracted from the bark of the Brazilian araroba tree is called *chrysarobin* and has a therapeutic effect in psoriasis. A substitute was synthesized during World War I, 1, 8-dihydroxy-9-anthrone, called anthralin or dithranol.

Mechanism of action

In the hairless mouse, a single topical application of anthralin results in depression of the mitotic index and DNA synthesis. Repeated application to the mouse tail results in a significant decrease in DNA synthesis, global reduction in protein synthesis, epidermal hyperplasia, and the presence of a continual granular layer. Anthralin and its dimer completely inhibit cell growth and thymidine incorporation in cultured human fibroblasts at concentrations ranging from 0.1 to 1.0 μM. Moreover, in a rapidly multiplying human keratinocyte line (HaCaT cells), anthralin inhibits DNA synthesis by 50% at 0.2 μM. The antiproliferative effects of anthralin are distinct from its inhibitory effects on the cytosolic enzyme glucose-6-phosphate dehydrogenase.

The effects of pharmacologic concentrations of anthralin on normal human keratinocytes (KC) in culture have been studied. Keratinocyte proliferation was inhibited by 98% at an anthralin concentration of 10 ng/ml, compared to only 9% inhibition of lymphocyte proliferation. Cell viability was not affected. Anthralin prolongs the prophase of mitotic KC about seven-fold at subtoxic doses. Transforming growth factor (TFG)-alpha expression and binding to its receptor, epidermal growth factor (EFG) receptor, were significantly downregulated.

In the concentration range expected with topical application, anthralin inhibits the secretion in vitro of IL-6, IL-8 and TNFα (but not IL-1) by activated monocytes. This may be clinically significant because circulating proliferating monocytes and lymphoid cells are increased in psoriasis and increase in step with disease activity. In KC culture, anthralin induces lipid peroxidation, which mediates the stress-activated protein kinase cascade. Peripheral blood mononuclear cells are significantly more sensitive to these effects than KC.

In cell culture, mitochondrial respiration is sensitive to anthralin. The mitochondria of keratinocytes increase in size and the cristae become less well defined. Ultrastructural changes in the mitochondria of the cells in psoriatic skin treated with anthralin are followed by inhibition of cell respiration. Langerhans' cells are more sensitive to these changes than keratinocytes. In summary, anthralin is probably an inhibitor of cell respiration, and the mitochondrial membrane is the primary site of action. During the oxidation reaction, anthralin is irreversibly degraded and the mitochondrion is inactivated.

Polymorphonuclear leukocyte (PML) but not monocyte chemotaxis in vitro is inhibited by concentrations of anthralin likely to be encountered in skin. Superoxide anion production of both cell types is inhibited by anthralin, but monocytes appear to be 100 times more sensitive to this effect. The increased chemotactic activities of both monocytes and PMLs in psoriatics is normalized after 3–4 weeks of anthralin therapy. The chemotaxis enhancing effects of plasma from psoriatic patients return to normal after 2 weeks of treatment.

During treatment of psoriasis, anthralin shows a rapid effect on the normalization of epidermal differentiation, with an increase in differentiation-associated keratins K1, K2 and K10 and reappearance of filaggrin. There is a concomitant reduction of proliferation-associated keratins K6, K16, K17, and minimal effect on transglutaminase and involucrin positive-cell layers.

Wang *et al.* found that anthralin penetrated faster through involved than uninvolved psoriatic skin in vitro, with large individual variations. They concluded that the stratum corneum is the rate-limiting step in normal skin but that in diseased skin the rate of release of drug from vehicle is rate limiting.

Clinical use of anthralin

Anthralin USP is available as a yellow powder, soluble in organic solvents. Anthralin may be dissolved in chloroform and added to petrolatum. The chloroform is allowed to evaporate off, leaving the suspension in petrolatum. Anthralin soft paste contains varying concentrations of anthralin (0.1–5%) in Lassar's paste, which contains zinc oxide 25%, starch 25%, and salicylic acid 2% in petrolatum. Paraffin 5–10% may be added to make a hard anthralin paste. Anthralin sticks (suspended in beeswax) for directed application to limited lesions are available in the U.K. Anthralin ointments, creams, and scalp solutions are commercially available in concentrations ranging from 0.1 to 1.0%.

Ingram method

The traditional use of anthralin was developed by Ingram in 1953. The use of anthralin paste was combined with the Goeckerman regimen. The current Ingram method consists of a bath for 15–30 minutes with a coal tar solution (e.g. Balnetar, Polytar, Zetar) followed by suberythemogenic doses of UVB irradiation starting with 1/3 or 1/2 minimal erythema dose (MED) exposure, which increases by this amount each treatment, provided no burning occurs. The anthralin paste is then applied with a spatula or tongue depressor to psoriatic plaques sparing normal surrounding skin, at an initial concentration of 0.1%. This can be increased every 2–3 days until irritation occurs. The paste is powdered with talc conveniently dabbed onto the treated area with a ball made from a cheesecloth filled with talcum powder. This procedure absorbs moisture from the paste and prevents staining of clothing. The whole body may be covered with a stocking net and worn for 6–24 hours. This type of treatment is most suitable for an outpatient psoriasis daycare situation or for a hospital inpatient.

Prior to repeating the cycle of tar bath and UVB exposure, the hardened paste must be removed by rubbing light mineral oil or baby oil onto it. Adherent scales are removed along with the paste. The rate of increase of UVB dose and anthralin paste concentration is flexible, based on therapeutic response and whether burning or irritation occurs. Some patients improve dramatically with low concentrations while others need concentrations of 4% or higher to achieve excellent responses. The therapy may be simplified by omitting the tar bath and suberythemogenic UVB. Alternatively, lower nonirritating concentrations of anthralin (0.01–0.05%) may be combined with suberythemogenic UVB irradiation.

Combination therapy

Because anthralin shows an absorption maximum at 350–360 nm, UVA irradiation may give additional benefit. The combination of PUVA with anthralin gives better results than either regimen alone. The combination of crude coal tar (CCT) 2% for 30–60 minutes, anthralin 1–10% for 15–60 minutes, followed by phototherapy from high-pressure metal halide lamps (consisting of UVA and UVB) 3–4 times weekly is as efficacious as PUVA or conventional psoriasis day care therapy for moderate to severe disease. The additional phototherapy may not be necessary when CCT and anthralin are combined. Clearance of psoriasis by the Ingram method allows maintenance of the remission by PUVA given once weekly for 4–5 months, then every other week for 4–5 months, then every third week for a mean dose rate of 28.6 J/cm^2 per month.

The combination of twice daily calcipotriene and 30 minutes' short contact anthralin therapy (SCAT) using 2% anthralin and 3% salicylic acid gave significantly better and faster improvement than the vehicle ointment plus SCAT. In a randomized open study of anthralin 0.1–2% SCAT compared to calcipotriene ointment twice daily for 3 months, 50% and 60% showed marked improvement, respectively (difference not significant). SCAT as first-line therapy is more cost-effective than calcipotriene, but more patients preferred calcipotriene. Calcitriol 3 µg/g ointment applied twice daily for 8 weeks and SCAT (0.25–2%) for 30 minutes are comparably efficacious; however, skin irritation occurred in 5% and 72% respectively.

The addition of clobetasol ointment 5 days per week to SCAT enhanced the clearing capability of SCAT without shortening remission duration. In biopsies of sites treated with both anthralin and clobetasol, there was a decrease in the number of cycling epidermal cells and in the number of perivascular T-lymphocytes.

Adverse reactions

The most important side effects of anthralin are staining and irritation of uninvolved skin (see Plate 15, facing p. 34). The reaction peaks three days after the first application and subsides after 4–5 days, even if one continues to apply the same anthralin concentration.

Topical application of 1% indomethacin gel, a prostaglandin-synthetase inhibitor, has no effect on irritancy due to anthralin. The standard dose of oral indomethacin, 25 mg three times daily has no significant harmful effects on patients receiving the Ingram regime, but it does not improve their tolerance to anthralin. The combination of 5% crude coal tar with anthralin 1–3% significantly reduces the irritancy of anthralin alone without decreasing its anti-psoriatic efficacy as long as the compound is kept refrigerated and used within 3 weeks.

The erythema reaction is not related to skin type. Westerhof *et al.* showed that there was no statistically significant difference in anthralin-induced irritation in vitiligo and normally pigmented skin. Moreover, there is less anthralin-induced inflammation in the skin of a psoriatic plaque than in surrounding uninvolved skin. The purplish-brown discoloration of uninvolved skin is caused by uncharacterized anthralin metabolites arising from extensive oxdation and melanin pigmentation. It is dose dependent and fades a few weeks after treatment is stopped. Other acute side-effects include itching, stinging, burning, folliculitis, and rarely conjunctivitis. A few cases of contact allergy to anthralin have been reported. No systemic toxicity due to anthralin has been reported in humans.

Short contact anthralin (SCAT)

It is possible to reduce the side-effects of anthralin while maintaining efficacy. It is not necessary to produce irritation or erythema in order to obtain the beneficial therapeutic effects of anthralin. Clinical studies indicate that short-contact anthralin (1–3%) therapy (SCAT) for 10–30 minutes is equivalent or superior to standard overnight anthralin therapy (Fig. 12.1). Contact times of 5–20 minutes daily are sufficient to clear psoriatic plaques in 22 days (2% anthralin, 0.5% salicylic acid). Short contact with hard anthralin paste for 2 hours in the Ingram regime is more effective than 30 minutes and equal to the standard 24-hour application. The overall shorter times needed for application and cleansing of anthralin in petrolatum or Lassar's paste are more acceptable and practical for patients and nursing staff. Physicians and patients should be aware that irritation and staining of skin and clothing can still occur with SCAT. Short-contact treatment with 1% anthralin microencapsulated in crystalline monoglycerides did not improve psoriasis as rapidly as anthralin in petrolatum but did produce less erythema, burning, and staining of skin and clothing. The manufacturer

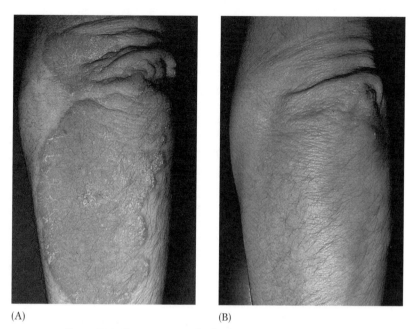

(A)   (B)

Figure 12.1 Short contact anthralin therapy (SCAT). Psoriasis of the arm before (A) and 2 weeks after (B) treatment with SCAT.

emphasizes rinsing the skin thoroughly with cool to lukewarm water before washing with soap.

Washing off anthralin with aqueous 1% potassium hydroxide folowing application periods of 40 minutes significantly reduced inflammation without sacrificing therapeutic efficacy. The peri-lesional inflammation induced by anthralin can be significantly reduced while maintaining clinical efficacy of SCAT by applying a cream containing 10% triethanolamine to the skin after the anthralin is applied (Cura Stain Spray, Young Pharmaceutical Inc., Wethersfield, CT 06109. Tel: (800) 874-9686). It is believed that KOH enhances the oxidation of anthralin to inactive products and that triethanolamine increases the solubility and removal of anthralin.

Although anthralin is still not well accepted by patients and is not widely used in the U.S., SCAT and new cream formulations have allowed use of this important topical agent at home in selected patients with plaque-type psoriasis. The search continues for a new anthralin analogue or formulation, e.g. in liposomes, with a more favorable benefit to side-effect ratio .

How to use anthralin at home

1 Patients start with a 0.1% or 0.25% concentration and increase it to 1.0% as tolerated. Most of my compliant patients settle on the 0.5% ointment. If required, concentrations higher than 1.0% must be compounded by the pharmacist.

2 Anthralin cream or ointment is applied daily to lesions and left on for 5 minutes, gradually increasing the contact time to 60 minutes as tolerated. Optional application of petrolatum or zinc oxide ointment to perilesional skin helps to prevent irritation. Because of staining, no clothing or loose-fitting old garments should be worn during treatment.

3 Scalp skin can be treated similarly with solution or cream. Face and body folds are usually avoided because of their increased irritation potential.

4 The anthralin is then washed off with liquid soap in the bath or shower.

5 Anthralin stains of white fabrics can be removed by a 10 minute soak in full-strength chlorine bleach followed by a water rinse and air drying. Color fabrics should be bleach-safe. A white plastic shower curtain should be cleaned within 5 minutes with 95% ethyl alcohol followed by a water rinse.

Selected references

Agarwal R., Saraswat A., Kaur I. *et al.* (2002) A novel liposomal formulation of dithranol for psoriasis: preliminary results. *J Dermatol* **29**, 529–532.

Ashcroft D. M., LiWan Po A., Williams H. C., Griffiths C. E. (2000) Cost-effectiveness analysis of topical calcipotriol versus short-contact dithranol. In the treatment of mild to moderate plaque psoriasis. *Pharmacoeconomics* **18**, 469–476.

Coaish S. (1965) Ingram method of treatment psoriasis. *Arch Dermatol* **92**, 56–58.

Hutchinson P. E., Marks R., White J. (2000) The efficacy, safety and tolerance of calcitriol 3 mcg/g ointment in the treatment of plaque psoriasis: a comparison with short-contact dithranol. *Dermatol* **201**, 139–145.

Mahrle G., Bonnekoh B., Wevers A., Hegemann L. (1994) Anthralin: How does it act and are there more favorable derivatives? *Acta Dermato Venereol Suppl (Stockh)* **186**, 83–84.

Monastirli A., Georgiou S., Pasmatzi E. *et al.* (2002) Calcipotriol plus short-contact dithranol: a novel topical combination therapy for chronic plaque psoriasis. *Skin Pharmacol Appl Skin Physiol* **15**, 246–251.

Mrowietz U., Jessat H., Schwarz A., Schwarz T. (1997) Anthralin (dithranol) in vitro inhibits human monocytes to secrete IL-6, IL-8 and TNF-α, but not IL-1. *Br J Dermatol* **136**, 542–547.

Muller K. (2000) Current status and recent developments in anthracenone antipsoriatics. *Curr Pharmaceutical Design* **6**, 901–918.

Peus D., Beyerle A., Rittner H. L. *et al.* (2000) Anti-psoriatic drug anthralin activates JNK via lipid peroxidation: mononuclear cells are more sensitive than keratinocytes. *J Invest Dermatol* **114**, 688–692.

Poyner T. F., Menday A. P., Williams Z. V. (2000) Patient attitudes to topical antipsoriatic treatment with calcipotriol and dithranol. *J Eur Acad Dermatol Venereol* **143**, 154–158.

Swinkels O. Q., Prins M., Kucharekova M. *et al.* (2002) Combining lesional short-contact dithranol therapy of psoriasis with a potent topical corticosteroid. *Br J Dermatol* **146**, 621–626.

Swinkels O. Q., Prins M., Tosserams E. F. *et al.* (2001) The influence of a topical corticosteroid on short-contact high-dose dithranol therapy. *Br J Dermatol* **145**, 63–69.

van der Vleuten C. J., de Jong E. M., van de Kerkhof P. C. (1996) Epidermal differentiation characteristics of the psoriatic plaque during short contact treatment with dithranol cream. *Clin Exp Dermatol* **21**, 409–414.

Wall A. R., Poyner T. F., Menday A. P. (1998) A comparison of treatment with dithranol and calcipotriol on the clinical severity and quality of life in patients with psoriasis. *Br J Dermatol* **139**, 1005–1011.

Wang J. C. T., Patel B. G., Ehmann C. W., Lowe N. (1987) The release and percutaneous permeation of anthralin products, using clinically involved and uninvolved psoriatic skin. *J Am Acad Dermatol* **16**, 812–821.

Westerhof W., Buehre Y., Pavel S. *et al.* (1989) Increased anthralin irritation response in vitiliginous skin. *Arch Dermatol Res* **281**, 52–56.

13 UVB phototherapy and coal tar

Charles Camisa

UVB phototherapy

The earliest experimentation with ultraviolet light and psoriasis was reported in the 1920s. Elucidation of the erythema action spectrum and the therapeutic action spectrum of psoriasis in 1981 made possible the development of modern bulbs which emit light capable of clearing psoriasis with less risk of burning. Short-wave ultraviolet B (broad-band UVB = 290–320 nm) light is now widely used in the treatment of psoriasis as monotherapy, with emollients, or with crude coal tar (the Goeckerman regimen). The treatments can be delivered in the office, hospital, day treatment center, or at home (by the patient).

There are basically three types of UVB sources that are practical for the office: the hot quartz Alpine lamp, high pressure metal halide lamps, and fluorescent sunlamps (UVB bulbs).

The hot quartz or high-pressure mercury vapor lamps (available from KBD, Inc., see Table 13.9) were used by the pioneers in phototherapy. The spectral power distribution (SPD) is discontinuous with wavelength peaks of emission including 254, 263, 297, 303, and 366 nm. The advantages and disadvantages of the hot quartz lamp are shown in Table 13.1.

The high-pressure mercury halide lamp system consists of five lamps stacked in columns that deliver a continuous spectrum of UV wavelengths (Dermalight Systems) (Table 13.2). The selection of UVA or UVB is effected by opening and closing filter doors.

The work horse in most offices for UVB phototherapy is the fluorescent sunlamp manufactured by Westinghouse (FS series, available as 2, 4, and 6 foot tubes) and Philips (TL-12) (Table 13.3). The glass tube is coated on the inside with a phosphor that emits a continuous spectrum primarily from 280 to 350 nm. About 60% of

Table 13.1 Hot quartz lamp.

Advantages	Disadvantages
Inexpensive	Ozone production when first
Small size needs less storage space	ignited causing 10–15 min
Mounted on pole with wheels allows	delay in treating first patient
portability to bedside	Heat production during treatment
Ideal for treating limited areas of	Adequate ventilation required
involvement such as palms, soles, elbows,	Small field size requires up to six
knees, scalp	exposures to treat entire body
Can be used for photopatch testing	skin

Table 13.2 High-pressure mercury halide lamp.

Advantages	Disadvantages
May be used for UVB, PUVA or	Very expensive
UVA + B	Three columns needed to give a
Potentially shorter treatment times	single even exposure
No claustrophobia from enclosed cabinets	Excessive heat production
Five stacked lamps needs only 12 × 16 inches'	Possibility of wavelength selection
floor space	errors if both filter doors left
Lamps have longer useful life with less	open
output degradation than fluorescent lamps	

Table 13.3 Fluorescent lamp (enclosed cabinet system with 12 or more tubes).

Advantages	Disadvantages
Highly effective UVB phototherapy	Expensive
Generalized exposure in relatively	Possible need for special ventilation and
short period of time	power sources
Inexpensive lamps	Heat production
No warm-up time	Risk of claustrophobia and falling in cabinet

the radiant energy is emitted at wavelengths below 320 nm (Fig. 13.1), falling into the therapeutic action spectrum for psoriasis, which peaks at 300–305 nm. The therapeutic and erythema action spectra parallel each other from 290 to 365 nm, but wavelengths shorter than 290 nm are far more erythemogenic than therapeutic. The sunlamps can be mounted in open banks or in enclosed cabinets

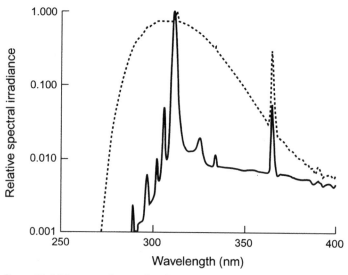

Figure 13.1 The spectral power distribution for TL-01 (narrow-band UVB) and TL-12 (broad-band UVB) lamps. *Solid line*, TL-01; *dashed line*, TL-12. (From Das *et al.*, Fig. 1, courtesy of Dr Farr.)

(Fig. 13.2). The output decreases to 70–80% of the original output after about 500 hours of use. The lamps should be replaced after 1000 hours of use.

A flat open bank of 4–6 lamps obviates some of the disadvantages of the enclosed cabinet (Table 13.3), but it does increase the treatment time because four exposures are necessary to treat generalized psoriasis (front, back, both sides).

All of the systems have problems delivering a uniform dose of irradiation to the skin surface. The irradiance from the ends of the tubes may be 10–30% less than the central portion. Photodosimeters applied to multiple anatomic sites of patients undergoing UVB phototherapy with a cabinet or flat bank revealed "cold" areas (receiving <50% of stated dose) and "hot" areas (receiving >100% of stated dose). The implications for under treatment and burning are obvious.

The lower parts of the legs and feet are "cold" areas in both open banks and enclosed cabinets, and psoriasis is ordinarily more resistant to phototherapy in these areas. Standing on a slightly raised platform may help, but it increases the risk of falling. Additional exposures to the legs and feet with shielding elsewhere is the solu-

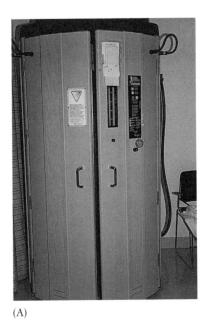 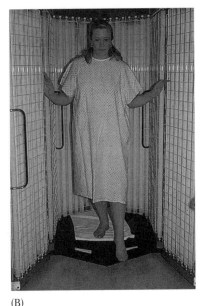

(A)   (B)

Figure 13.2 Narrow-band ultraviolet B phototherapy unit with doors closed (A) and with model shown exiting the unit (B) after removing goggles.

tion. Because the scalp receives very little exposure and the soles none, if psoriasis is active there, it may be necessary to shave and bow the head during treatment and purchase a UVB hand/foot unit.

In a practice with only a few patients eligible for UVB phototherapy, an open system with wheels is recommended. The cost is modest, but it requires more time for the treatment than the cabinet, and privacy screens are needed. The panel of lamps can be stored in one examination room, and the room can be dedicated to other purposes when the unit is not in use. A practice which intends to treat 10 or more psoriatic patients per week with a range of severity should invest about $15,000 in a combined UVA/B cabinet system (see Table 14.2 in Chapter 14 for sources) with safety features such as timer and automatic shutoff, handrails, protection from bulb breakage, and a window for direct visualization of the patient. In regions that are distant from referral centers, it is advisable for physicians in the community to encourage their local hospital's physical therapy department to purchase the necessary equipment and provide treatments based on the doctor's orders who continues to follow the patient in the office on a regular basis. In this way, there is a win-win situation: patients receive the best modality for their psoriasis at a centralized facility with expert follow-up care and the hospital recovers expenses by collecting the revenue for treatments.

Nurses and technicians should receive formal training in the operation of equipment such as offered by the National Psoriasis Foundation and be supervised by the physician. Even with the safety feature of automatic shutoff, a mishap could occur; for example, if the correct UVA time is keyed in, but the technician turns on the UVB lamp. Requesting dosimetry in terms of radiant energy per unit surface area helps to avoid errors because the typical UVB dose is measured in millijoules per square centimeter compared to UVA in Joules/cm^2. Errors could still occur if UVB dosing is not based on radiometric readings but rather in terms of seconds and minutes estimated on the basis of skin type or other factors. Separate cabinets for UVA and UVB avoids the issue of confounding the two wavebands but are only warranted for larger centers where 20 or more patients are treated, and the proper amount of space, ventilation, and air conditioning is available. Hand and foot units for UVA or UVB can be added one at a time to a practice at a cost of about $1500 each as the need arises for giving extra doses to palmoplantar psoriasis or as the primary treatment for palmoplantar pustulosis.

Phototherapy should probably be reserved as second-line treatment for those patients with extensive (defined as 10% or more involvement of body surface area) or disabling (defined as involving the face, hands, and feet) psoriasis who have had an insufficient response to aggressive topical regimens.

The physician who has a source of ultraviolet light in the office now prepares the patient for phototherapy. Those who do not have the equipment should refer to a facility that does rather than bypass UVB phototherapy and risk potentially more toxic systemic therapies that are more appropriately reserved for third- and fourth-line treatment.

There are many reputable suppliers of UV equipment and radiometers (see Table 14.2, Chapter 14). The selection should be based on the company's accessibility to your office, whether installation and service are provided, the frequency and cost of service and regular maintenance calls, space needs and availability of special power lines, ventilation, and air-conditioning.

I recommend that the unit be metered on a weekly basis so that dosages may be calculated in millijoules. This is important not only for standardization of dosages between different centers and different units in the same center but also so that modifications and improvements of protocols published in the medical literature can be immediately duplicated in practice. Metering helps to compensate for the declining output of bulbs. The clinician should be aware that great variability between specifications and quality control exists among manufacturers. One should purchase the UVB radiometer recommended by the manufacturer of the system. The radiometers themselves must be recalibrated at least once per year. Use the formula to calculate the time needed to administer a given dose in mJ/cm^2:

Dose desired (mJ/cm^2) ÷ output measured (mW/cm^2)
= time (seconds)

For a specific measured output, conversion tables can be derived in increments of 5 mJ/cm^2 for quick reference. Some manufacturers supply conversion tables with the unit. Newer UVB cabinets have a built-in panel with a calculator. The UVB output is measured with a UVB light meter and punched into the calculator. Next, the desired UVB dose in (mJ/cm^2) is punched into the calculator, which then computes and displays the treatment time (in minutes and seconds), thus eliminating the need for conversion tables. Some UVB units have a built-in UVB light meter that continuously monitors UVB output while light is being administered. After the desired UVB treatment dose (mJ/cm^2) is entered into the control panel, the treatment time is automatically calculated and delivered.

Another decision to be made is whether the patient should be treated as an outpatient, in a psoriasis day treatment center, in the hospital, or at home by the patient himself or herself. The final recommendation is usually based on the availability of facilities, the physician's philosophy, and patient's (or third-party payer's) preference.

During the last twenty years in the United States, there has been a precipitous decline in the number of patients admitted to the hospital as well as their length of stay for the treatment of dermatologic diseases. This change has occurred in part because of the federal government's insurance program for elders, which allows only 8.3 days of hospitalization for patients with major skin diseases. Most private third-party insurers approve admission for only the most acute and severe forms of disease, such as exfoliative dermatitis and generalized pustular psoriasis. In addition, technological refinements in drug and physical therapies of psoriasis, particularly

Table 13.4 UVB dosimetry.

Skin type	Broad-band UVB dose (mJ/cm^2)	
	Start	Increase per treatment
I–Always burn, never tan	10	5
II–Always burn, sometimes tan	20	5–10
III–Sometimes burn, always tan	30	10
IV–Never burn, always tan	40	10–20
V–Moderately pigmented	50	20
VI–Black	60	20–30

Skin type	Narrow-band UVB dose (mJ/cm^2)	
	Start	Increase per treatment
I–Always burn, never tan	50	10
II–Always burn, sometimes tan	100	15
III–Sometimes burn, always tan	220	25
IV–Never burn, always tan	260	40
V–Moderately pigmented	330	45
VI–Black	350	60

retinoids, cyclosporine, and phototherapy, have made it possible to significantly improve the condition in almost every patient in an outpatient setting. This trend will most certainly continue in the twenty-first century as more biologic agents are approved.

Psoriasis day treatment costs about half as much as inpatient treatment but is very time-consuming for patients and labor-intensive for staff. The clinical improvement at the time of discharge is probably equivalent to that from hospitalization, but there are intangible benefits that the hospital setting does not provide; for example, daily education about disease and treatment from specialized staff, socialization with other patients in all stages of disease, and reinforcement of good self-treatment habits and the need for follow-up maintenance. Familiarity with the treatment site, facilities, and professional staff encourages follow-up treatment and assessment. (Details of the daily routine in a psoriasis day treatment center will be presented later in this chapter.)

The starting dose of UVB can be estimated based on the skin type and increased according to Table 13.4. However, it is preferable to give the first dose based on the results of minimal erythema dose (MED) testing upon which all subsequent doses are based. Photo-

Table 13.5 MED testing for UVB.

Skin type	mJ/cm²
I, II	10 15 20 25 30
III, IV	20 30 40 50 60
V, VI	40 50 60 70 80

therapists should understand, meter and maintain their equipment, keep complete and detailed records of exposures for each patient and be able to provide current and cumulative dosages of UVB received in mJ/cm² if the patient moves to another facility.

MED testing is somewhat tedious and time-consuming. It is performed using a piece of flexible plastic foam large enough to cover the patient's back. Five 1.5-cm squares are cut into the foam and the rest of the skin is shielded with drapes before exposing each test site to varying doses of UVB according to skin type (Table 13.5). After 24 hours, the reactions at each site are graded. The dose, which has resulted in a barely perceptible erythema or pinkness, is defined as the MED. Because the breasts and abdomen are more likely to burn than the back, I recommend starting with one UVB dose below the MED. The MED result is valid for future treatment courses without the need to reproduce it. An alternative method of determining the initial UVB dose is measurement of skin pigmentation by skin reflectance.

Studies have demonstrated that erythemogenic UVB given as an outpatient was effective in 90–100% of patients in clearing moderate to severe psoriasis completely. The only adjunctive treatment was the application of white petrolatum immediately prior to exposure and as needed for dryness at home. Two such treatment protocols gave treatments five times per week or three times per week. The average extent of involvement was 38%. In the first protocol the initial exposure was 80% of the MED and subsequent exposures were increased by 17% of the previous dose. The second protocol administered MED on the first day and increased dosages by 50%, 50%, 30%, and 20% on subsequent exposures. (The reader is referred to Tables 1 and 2 in the article by Adrian *et al.*) Patients who had tender erythema at the time of a scheduled treatment were not treated and subsequently received a dose one increment lower than the one that apparently caused the burn. The authors gave additional increments of UVB to the extremities such that by the fifth treatment the arms and legs received 50% more radiation than the trunk. Other investigators advised against giving extra UVB doses to resistant plaques on the lower legs because they yielded only slight additional improvement (5–10%).

In both protocols, the number of treatments needed for clearance ranged from 20 to 30. There is a strong linear correlation between an individual's MED and the corresponding total dose needed for lesions to clear. The total number of treatments needed did not differ significantly according to the MED.

One should not expect the psoriasis in 100% of patients to clear completely as was achieved in the ideal studies cited. Moreover, I found that increasing the UVB dose by a varying percentage of the previous dose increases the potential for calculation errors. Increasing the dose by a fixed amount at each treatment (Table 13.4) gives equally gratifying results. Outpatient UVB phototherapy, as opposed to day treatment or hospitalization, is an approach worthwhile attempting in stable patients because of the dramatic cost savings and avoidance of the generally objectionable appearance, odor, and staining of clothing caused by combining UVB with coal tar.

Maintenance phototherapy

Standard clinical practice includes additional biweekly UVB treatments for 2–3 weeks after clearing at the final clearance dose. Defined as complete resolution of at least 90% of psoriasis present prior to initiation of phototherapy, "clearing" was achieved in 76% of patients. A multicenter study designed to determine the time to flare compared a group of patients receiving maintenance UVB biweekly for 4–8 weeks followed by at least weekly treatments for a total of 4 months to a group receiving no maintenance. The protocol called for a maintenance dose equal to 90% of the patient's final clearance dose. The probability of remaining in remission as defined by this study was significantly higher for those patients receiving UVB phototherapy maintenance. Based on a life table analysis, the psoriasis in 60% of maintenance-therapy patients vs. 28% of no-maintenance-therapy patients would still be clear 6 months after the initial clearing. In another study, clearing was defined less stringently as "at least 80% improved" and this was achieved in 81% of patients with four-times-weekly treatment. Maintenance therapy consisted of an attempt to gradually reduce the frequency of treatments to three, two, then one or less times weekly if possible, with the UVB dose equal to the last clearing dose. The authors estimated that the probability of remaining in remission for at least one year after clearing was 58%. In conclusion, it is cost-effective to administer outpatient UVB maintenance phototherapy to patients with moderate to severe psoriasis to prevent a relapse in at least 50% of patients for 6 months or longer until the patient can benefit from the next season of ambient sunlight.

In 1984, the therapeutic action spectrum of psoriasis (between 300 and 315 nm) was exploited with the development of a fluorescent UVB lamp with a peak narrow band of emission at 311–313 nm and a minor peak at 305 nm (Fig. 13.1). Treatment with the Philips TL-01 is now referred to as *narrow-band UVB phototherapy* and represents a significant advance in the treatment of psoriasis. Thus, narrow-band UVB avoids completely the shorter, more erythemogenic and carcinogenic UVB and UVC wavelengths that are emitted by conventional sunlamps (Westinghouse FS and Philips TL-12). In bilateral paired comparison studies of widespread symmetrical psoriasis, sides treated with the TL-01 were significantly better than the sides treated with TL-12 sun lamp at the end of study using both erythemogenic and suberythemogenic protocols. The number of burning episodes was significantly less with the TL-01 lamps. The TL-01-treated side received twice as much cumulative UVB dose, owing to the ability to increase the time by 40% if the previous exposure induced no perceptible erythema. An open study of narrow-band UVB phototherapy suggested that the 40% increment is too aggressive and recommended increments of 20% for no erythema and 10% for slight transient erythema. However, no difference was found in burning potential for the two lamps in in vivo experiments.

After considering all the published data, I have settled on a protocol for narrow-band UVB phototherapy that employs a skin-type based initial dose and fixed-dose increments given three times weekly. This conservative regimen has minimized the risk of serious erythema or blisters. The protocol in Table 13.4 is modified from the article by Shelk and Morgan.

The action spectrum for 8-MOP phototoxic erythema parallels the anti-psoriatic effect at around 330 nm; therefore, it is surprising that psoralen-311 nm UVB is effective in psoriasis. TL-01 lamps do emit in the 330 nm range albeit at 1/100 of its peak irradiance (Fig. 13.1). Narrow-band TL-01 radiation was compared with and without oral psoralen. More erythema and pigmentation occurred and clinical improvement was more rapid with psoralen. A comparison of conventional PUVA and psoralen-311 nm UVB revealed no differences in proportion of patients cleared, number of exposures, or durability of response at 3 months post-treatment. Similar results were obtained by comparing PUVA to psoralen-broad-band UVB in patients with type IV skin. The cumulative UV doses were much smaller for the UVB groups compared to the UVA groups.

When treatments were given twice weekly, PUVA cleared a significantly higher proportion of patients than narrow-band UVB (84% vs. 63%) with fewer treatments (17 vs. 25) and a longer duration of remission. Subsequent trials have shown, however, that narrow-band UVB given three times weekly is equivalent to twice weekly PUVA in time to clearance and maintenance of remission.

The efficacy and time to relapse were compared among: (1) TL-01 phototherapy, (2) etretinate 1 mg/kg/day 2 weeks prior to TL-01, and (3) or etretinate prior to PUVA (re-PUVA). Only concomitant emollients were allowed. The clearance rate was 80%, 93%, and 100% for the three groups. At 6 months' follow-up, 50%, 33%, and 50% remained in remission, respectively. The cumulative UVB exposure dose was 1/3 less in the group receiving etretinate. These studies show that TL-01 phototherapy with or without etretinate is less efficacious than re-PUVA and that etretinate does not extend the remission time of TL-01. The effect of maintenance therapy was not investigated. The long-term safety of cumulative doses of narrow-band UVB is unknown.

Monochromatic 308-nm excimer laser

A xenon-chloride excimer laser (XTRAC, PhotoMedex, Inc.) delivers UVB energy at 308 nm, similar to narrow-band UVB phototherapy (311–313 nm). Dose-response studies have clearly shown that the rapidity of clearing and severity of side-effects are dose-related. Significant clearing was seen after a single high-dose exposure of 8 or 16 times the MED. Using medium doses three times weekly and a flexible escalation scheme, the mean number of treatments to achieve >95% clearance was 10.6. The mean remission time was 3.5 months.

The advantages of the 308-nm excimer laser are that it directs energy toward lesional skin and spares unnecessary radiation exposure to uninvolved skin, and improves psoriasis in fewer treatments than standard UVB-phototherapy. Common acute side-effects include erythema, blisters, hyperpigmentation and erosions.

Disadvantages with using this modality are that the aperture of the handpiece is 4 cm^2, limiting practical use to patients with less than 10% body surface area involvement; unproven efficacy in palmoplantar and scalp psoriasis; and unknown long-term side-effects.

Coal tar

Introduction

The combination of crude coal tar and ultraviolet light used in the treatment of psoriasis was published by Goeckerman in 1925. Wood tars have been used in medicine since antiquity, but coal tar was not available until the second half of the 19th century when coal gas production was developed. Coal tar is a by-product of the processing of coke and gas from bituminous coal. Coal tar is chemically complex, consisting of 10,000 different compounds, of which only about 400, constituting 55–60% of the tar by weight, have been identified. Some of the major compounds in coal tar include aromatic hydrocarbons such as anthracene, benzene, benzo[a]pyrene, and naphthalene. In therapy, either crude coal tar or coal tar extract dispersed in a suitable vehicle is used. The extracts are produced by extraction with ethanol or surfactants or by distillation.

Mechanism of action

In healthy subjects, crude coal tar 5% in hydrophilic ointment initially causes a transient hyperplasia, followed over time by a 20% reduction in epidermal thickness. Thickening of the epidermis including the granular layer due to coal tar has also been found in some animal models. Coal tar alone or followed by UVB irradiation suppresses epidermal DNA synthesis significantly in the hairless mouse.

Efficacy

No method of chemical or biological standardization of the potency of coal tar products has ever been established, rendering direct comparisons between different products difficult if not impossible. Variability in potency between different products with the same concentration of active ingredient as well as variation between batches of the same product is the rule.

Is crude coal tar (CCT) effective as monotherapy for psoriasis in hospitalized patients? Using 1% and 5% or higher concentrations of CCT in yellow soft paraffin, the median whole body PASI score fell by about 50% during a 10-day treatment period. Moreover, the authors (Williams *et al.*) determined that the dose-response curve for anti-psoriatic effects peaked between the concentration of 1 and 5% of CCT. The patient's skin was in contact with tar for 24 hours daily, and UVB was not used.

Coal tar solution (15% v/w) was not as effective as calcipotriene in a 6-week study. An open left-right comparison of calcipotriene and 5% CCT ointments combined with sun exposure showed comparable efficacy at 8 weeks. Palmoplantar plaque psoriasis was treated with 6% CCT ointment overnight with glove or sock occlusion, and 76% showed "good improvement." Combined treatment with coal tar and anthralin significantly inhibited the anthralin-induced erythema/irritation of normal-appearing skin. The mechanism for this may be induction of aryl-hydrocarbon hydroxylase by coal tar, which metabolizes anthralin or its irritant by-products.

Clinical studies

The use of coal tar for the treatment of psoriasis has been inextricably tied to ultraviolet light therapy ever since Goeckerman popularized this combination. He used the hot quartz (high-pressure mercury vapor) lamp that emits discontinuous UV light bands in the short wave (B) and long wave (A) ranges corresponding to the spectral emission peaks of mercury. It is uncertain whether erythemogenic dosages were used. As currently employed by the Mayo Clinic, the Goeckerman regimen consists of a 24-hour per day program of frequent applications of 3–5% crude coal tar in petrolatum or Lassar's paste to the entire body skin. Excess tar is then physically wiped away with the aid of cottonseed or corn oil and then erythemogenic dosages of UVB are given.

Tar is a photosensitizer with an action spectrum in the longwave ultraviolet region (UVA = 320–400 nm). Some of the constituents of crude coal tar that define the action spectrum for photosensitivity in the longwave UVA and visible range include anthracene, phenanthrene, pyrene, fluoranthrene and acridine.

The tar distillate liquor carbonis detergens (LCD) alone has only a weak effect on psoriasis. The clearing effect of light alone was obtained at a maximum of 313 nm, which was not enhanced by pretreatment with LCD. Distinctly better healing was seen at 365 nm after the pretreatment. However, a smarting sensation that was most pronounced at 405 nm was produced. Erythemogenic dosages of UVA plus tar gel can be as effective as UVB plus tar gel at healing psoriasis but the former combination is limited by the "smarting reaction." Phototoxicity from coal tar is probably not a therapeutic mechanism in the modern Goeckerman regimen.

Tar may have a "UVB-sparing" effect; that is, it may allow the therapeutic benefits of tar and lower, suberythemogenic dosages of UVB to be additive. Pretreatment with LCD produced a 30–50% higher UVB erythema threshold than did petrolatum. Tar gel (5% crude coal tar in a hydroalcoholic gel containing 29% alcohol) alone is equally as effective as suberythemogenic UVB at improving psoriatic plaques (about 50%). The combination was more effective than either one alone. Moreover, the suberythemogenic UVB + tar gel group received 59% less total cumulative UVB dose than the erythemogenic UVB + tar gel group. The efficacy of suberythemogenic UVB + tar oil was roughly equivalent to maximally aggressive UVB + emollients given on an outpatient basis. The cumulative dose of UVB at the time of clearing, however, was 44% less in the suberythemogenic UVB + tar oil group. CCT 2% ointment gave no therapeutic advantage to either daily suberythemogenic UVB or maximally aggressive UVB in the time to clear psoriasis in hospital patients, or the time to relapse, but 80% less UVB was used with suberythemogenic UVB.

Several studies questioned whether crude coal tar (CCT) adds much, if any, therapeutic benefit to UVB irradiation. UVB radiation alone was almost as effective as 1, 5, or 25% CCT + UVB. Bilateral comparison studies have consistently shown that daily erythemogenic UVB + white petrolatum or 5% CCT in petrolatum were equally effective. Immediate broad-spectrum decreases in spectral remittance (reflectance) of psoriatic stratum corneum occur after the application of white petrolatum. It is possible that this vehicle, which is also used to formulate the tar, increases UVB transmission. Apparently, some of the commonly used emollients, including petrolatum and hydrophilic ointment absorb UVB, thereby reducing the potential for erythema in uninvolved skin. Fortunately, the peak absorption spectrum for most of these agents is between 270 and 290 nm, which causes erythema but is below the therapeutic action spectrum for psoriasis. If combined with UVB

Table 13.6 Guidelines for admission to psoriasis day treatment center.

---

1 Psoriasis involves 20% or more of body surface area or is disabling by affecting the face, scalp, hands, and feet
2 Psoriasis is recalcitrant to all reasonable attempts at outpatient therapy for 4 weeks or longer
3 The patient is a candidate for coal tar and UVB phototherapy; PUVA and systemic therapy are not indicated or not desired by patient or physician at the present time
4 Complications of systemic therapy necessitate a change to safer yet effective therapeutic alternative
5 The patient is sufficiently medically or emotionally compromised to require assistance and monitoring, but not severe enough to warrant hospitalization

---

phototherapy, anthralin or calcipotriene should be applied after the light treatment.

Psoriasis day treatment centers

To be considered a psoriasis day treatment center, a facility must be equipped with all of the modern tools, pharmaceuticals, and an experienced nursing staff. Hospitalization is still indicated for patients with erythrodermic or pustular psoriasis, severe plaque-type psoriasis with arthropathy, complications of systemic therapy, or concomitant illnesses (e.g. diabetes, emphysema, cardiovascular disease) although lengths of stay are reduced. While the majority qualify for routine or office phototherapy, certain patients have disease significant enough to justify treatment in a psoriasis day center. Suggested guidelines for admission and requirements of the center are shown in Tables 13.6 and 13.7, and a schedule is shown in Table 13.8.

UVB treatment

On day 1, treatment is given according to skin type (Table 13.4), and MED testing is done (Table 13.5). On day 2, a suberythemogenic dose (the dose just below the determined MED) is given. Subsequent daily increases are usually $10-20$ mJ/cm^2, as tolerated. Half the daily dose is given in the morning and the other half in the afternoon. This allows for greater flexibility in proper dosing and helps to prevent burning.

Table 13.7 Requirements to qualify as a psoriasis day treatment center.

Space
- Exam rooms for consultation with physician
- Treatment room for application of medicaments
- Toilet facilities for men and women
- Phototherapy room for UVL cabinets
- Bathrooms for tub bath, whirlpool
- Recreation/dining room
- Quiet room

Equipment
- UVB cabinet
- UVA cabinet
- Hand and foot units
- Sink for hair washing (Scalp debridement unit)
- Tub for bath PUVA
- Whirlpool for debriding scales (and for relief of joint pain)

Pharmaceuticals
- Emollients (Aquaphor, Petrolatum, Eucerin, mineral oil, etc.)
- 3% Crude coal tar with and without salicylic acid 3–5%
- Anthralin ointments 0.1, 0.25, 0.5, 1.0%
- Liquor Carbonis Detergens 10 and 20% in petrolatum and Nivea oil with and without salicylic acid 3–5%
- Low and medium potency corticosteroid creams and ointments and scalp solutions

---

Table 13.8 Sample schedule of psoriasis day treatment center.

8:00–10:00 am
- Examination by physician
- Whirlpool bath as needed
- UVB treatment
- Shampoo
- Application of coal tar and other topicals

10:00 am–1:00 pm
- Relaxation/work/sleep
- Lectures
- Lunch

1:00–3:00 pm
- Tar removal/bath
- UVB treatment
- Shampoo
- Application of anthralin if needed and other topicals

Trunk and extremities

AM: 3% crude coal tar in petrolatum applied by nurse in direction of hair follicle growth. Salicylic acid 3–5% is added in patients with severe scaling.

PM: Emollients (Aquaphor, Eucerin, etc.) are applied, to be repeated by the patient at bedtime. Some patients are instructed in the proper use of anthralin (short contact therapy), to be applied either at the center or in the evening at home, gradually increasing to 1% concentration. Others apply calcipotriene in the afternoon after the light treatments and at bedtime.

Scalp

AM: Tar shampoo (Zetar, T-gel, Ionil-T, etc.), followed by tar oil (Doak or the formulation of Zetar emulsion 13%, salicylic acid 3%, Tween-80 4% in Nivea oil) under a shower cap.

PM: Repeat tar shampoo, followed by application of a fluorinated corticosteroid solution as needed (e.g. fluocinolone 0.01%, betamethasone valerate 0.1%).

Facial areas

Nonfluorinated corticosteroid cream (e.g. hydrocortisone 1% with or without iodoquinol, hydrocortisone valerate 0.2%, desonide 0.05%): for hairline, ears, face, skin-folds in morning and afternoon as needed.

Bath treatment

Whirlpool in morning as needed for debridement of severe scaling. This is very relaxing to patients and makes arthritis feel better; many patients prefer to continue even after scaling subsides. Tepid emollient bath in afternoon. Tar (Balnetar, Zetar emulsion) is added mostly for instructional purposes for eventual outpatient use.

Weekend treatment

This depends on patient's anticipated activities (family, social, work). It varies from simple lubrication, tar bath, and shampoo to a full topical psoriasis day-care regimen without the light or with natural sunlight or with a home UVB unit if available.

Treatment after discharge from the psoriasis day treatment center

Ultraviolet B

UVB treatment is given three times per week. If possible, decrease the number of treatments every four weeks to maintenance frequency of one or two times per week. The starting dose is 70% of the last total daily dose in the center and is increased by $10-20$ mJ/cm^2 per treatment. When the skin is cleared, the UVB dose is held at the last daily dose attained.

Trunk and extremities

Emollients, or anthralin at the highest tolerated concentration, 10% LCD in petrolatum, or 3% crude coal tar are applied to active areas for a few hours in the evening. Administration of calcipotriene twice a day is continued. Fluorinated corticosteroid ointments are rarely used because of possible shortened remission time. A tepid tar bath is given daily.

Scalp

Tar shampoo is used daily. When the patient has a flare, tar oil is applied and a shower cap worn for a few hours in the evening, followed by a shampoo and application of fluorinated corticosteroid oil (Dermasmoothe F/S) or solution at bedtime. The solution can be reapplied in the morning as needed. Low-potency corticosteroid cream is applied to the hairline, ears, face, and skin-folds twice daily as needed.

A review of 300 patients with severe psoriasis receiving all treatment in the Dallas and San Francisco psoriasis day-care centers showed an average time of 18 days to at least 90% clearing. In 90% of the patients, the psoriasis remained clear for a minimum of 8 months, and 73% of patients were in remission one year after discharge. Patients were encouraged to receive regular exposure to natural sunlight or artificial UVB for one month after discharge. These results compare favorably to those of 123 patients treated with the Goeckerman regimen as inpatients at the Mayo Clinic for whom a median remission time of 1–1.4 years was reported (range, 0.2–8.0 years). In 1997, at the Cleveland Clinic Psoriasis Day

Treatment Center (which has since closed), 90% of the last 103 consecutive patients achieved an excellent response defined as less than 5–10% body surface area of residual psoriasis. The median length of stay was 15 treatment days. Modest or poor responders were switched to alternative therapy, either PUVA or systemic medications.

Alternatives to office phototherapy

Home ultraviolet B therapy

Home UVB or Goeckerman therapy is effective when prescribed for selected compliant patients who are educated in the use of the topical medications and the lamps, and who receive adequate follow-up assessments in the office. There are several excellent units designed for home UVB (or Goeckerman) treatment that are relatively inexpensive and often covered in part or in full by third-party insurers (Table 13.9). One of these, the Jordan light, was used in a study of home Goeckerman treatment. About 80% maintained satisfactory results for over a year with continuous treatments, 1–3 times per week. Other home units are probably equally as effective. Handy individuals can construct their own wall units or cabinets, and purchase either broad-band or narrow-band UVB lamps separately.

Home UVB should probably only be prescribed to patients who have undergone similar treatments in hospital, day treatment center, or office settings and achieved a good result. They have presumably learned how their skin reacts to UVB light and the technique of safely increasing or decreasing the dose for themselves depending on the clearing response of the involved skin and the burning or tanning of uninvolved skin. This assumption may not always be valid, however.

Physicians have the choice whether to write a prescription for a home UVB unit but implicit in the choice to do so is the obligation to instruct the patient in its proper use and to monitor them at intervals for progress and safe operation. Some units limit the session to a maximum of 10 minutes, while others, which I advocate, allow the physician to prescribe a fixed number of exposures (75 or more) by preprogramming a code number at the factory. A follow-up visit is then required to reprogram the unit.

If patients are stable, I recommend follow-up visits at least annually to renew topical prescriptions and examine the body skin for

Table 13.9 UVB phototherapy units available for home use.

Recommended units	Supplier
Jordan Light Model 648-BD	Richmond Light Co. 2301 Falkirk Drive Richmond, VA 23236
Panasol II or Foldalite-B	National Biological Corporation 1532 Enterprise Parkway Twinsburg, OH 44087
Spectra 724	Daavlin P O Box 626 Bryan, OH 43506
Panelite	Ultralite Enterprises, Inc. 390 Farmer Ct. Lawrenceville, GA 30045
Model 800B	Phototherapeutix 1260 Palmetto Ave, Suite C Winter Park, FL 32789
Hot quartz Alpine lamp	KBD, Inc. 20 Kenton Lands Rd. Erlanger, KY 41018
Model 2400	Psoralite Corporation 2806 William Tuller Drive Columbia, SC 29205

cancer. The main pitfall of home UVB therapy is that patients rarely test the irradiance of their units or replace expired lamps.

In 1925, Goeckerman suggested using phototherapy at home: "In exceptional instances, indeed, there is no reason why the patient should not install a lamp for his own personal use, and manipulate it with all the skill required." While the risk of ultraviolet carcinogenesis was not known at that time, the incidence of skin cancer 25 years after receiving inpatient Goeckerman therapy for psoriasis or atopic dermatitis was not increased compared to the general population. Several large epidemiologic studies comparing thousands of unselected psoriatics treated with the full range of modalities to the general population of their respective countries revealed a relative risk of developing nonmelanoma skin cancer of 1.17–2.5. A meta-analysis of four articles yielded estimates varying from 0.6 to 2 excess nonmelanoma skin cancers per 100 patients per year who were treated with UVB phototherapy.

In the long-term U.S. PUVA prospective studies, patients who received >260 treatments had an 11-fold risk of squamous cell carcinoma (SCC) and a two-fold risk of basal cell carcinoma (BCC) compared to those receiving <160 treatments. The statistics were adjusted for exposure to a "high tar dose" and ionizing radiation, which independently increased the risk of SCC. Since 1989, the risk of invasive SCC of the penis and scrotum was found to be increased 52.6-fold for PUVA-treated men compared to the general white population. The highest genital tumor risk was found among men who received high-dose exposure to PUVA and topical tar/UVB. The data suggest that PUVA, UVB and coal tar may act together as cocarcinogens.

Tanning salons

The cosmetic tanning industry has enjoyed astounding growth and profitability in the U.S. and Europe. Most commercial salons employ lamps that emit predominantly UVA radiation. In a study of the spectral power distributions of six UVA bulbs or blacklights as they are called, 96–99% of the radiation was emitted in the UVA band, 320–400 nm. Stated another way, only 0.4–3.8% was emitted at wavelengths less than 320 nm, which might be expected to improve psoriasis. There are two ultraviolet fluorescent lamps that diverge from the group. The Metec Helarium bulb emits about 8% below 320 nm and 30% between 320 and 340 nm, the most effective UVA wavelengths for psoriasis when combined with psoralens. A high intensity lamp has been developed called "UVA-Sun" which emits only UVA wavelengths above 340 nm; all UVB is effectively filtered out.

It is common for patients with skin diseases to ask their physician about the merits of exposures in a tanning salon for its *therapeutic* value. In a questionnaire survey of tanning salon proprietors, 80% stated that "skin therapy" was an important reason for their clients to visit. A survey of 1252 Swedish teenagers revealed that 57% used tanning salons four or more times per year. Students with skin diseases were more likely to go to tanning salons, especially if the disease was perceived to be improved by natural sunlight: of the 25 students with psoriasis, 18 (72%) used the salons.

An open study showed that commercial tanning beds modestly improved mild psoriasis in the majority of patients. This finding was confirmed in a placebo-controlled study of a UVA sunbed in the treatment of psoriasis. After 12 exposures given over a 4-week period, the PASI score decreased about 10% on the UVA-treated side. The change was statistically significant ($p < 0.05$), and the majority of the subjects said that they would use a sunbed again to treat their psoriasis.

Because of the possibility of low emission of UVB between 300 and 320 nm that may benefit psoriasis, I would accept a trial of exposures in a tanning salon for use by patients who:

1 live too far away from a bona fide treatment center;

2 cannot take time off from other responsibilities to travel to the office or clinic;

3 have little or no health insurance and cannot afford to pay the fees for phototherapy;

4 are willing to accept the risks involved (see below) for potentially little or no improvement of skin disease and "cosmetic tanning" of uninvolved skin;

5 spend the relatively small sums of money to attend the tanning bed in their local community.

We do not recommend UVA tanning for cosmetic purposes only. The use of concomitant photosensitizing agents such as coal tar should be discouraged. Topical and oral psoralens should not be prescribed unless the UVA is going to be administered in the office and supervised by the physician.

The most important verifiable short-term risks of UVA exposure in a tanning salon include the following:

1 Cutaneous eruptions due to the concomitant ingestion of phototoxic drugs such as some antibiotics, diuretics, psychotropic medications or photosensitizers (psoralens) in food (celery, parsnip, etc.) or in illicit "tan accelerators."

2 The aggravation or unmasking of photosensitive diseases such as polymorphous light eruption, lupus erythematosus, dermatomyositis, and porphyria cutanea tarda.

3 Eye injury such as corneal burns if protective goggles are not provided, not worn, or removed prematurely.

4 Skin infections from improperly cleaned surfaces transferred to subsequent clients such as impetigo, folliculitis, lice, and herpes simplex.

5 Proprietor or client error leading to overexposure resulting in tender erythema ("sunburn"); it is conceivable that a UVA burn could result in the Koebner phenomenon or provoke an annular pustular flare of psoriasis.

Conclusion

Based upon the published information available and personal experience, I offer the following recommendations:

1 UVB alone, especially near 311 nm, can clear psoriasis.

2 Erythemogenic doses of UVB given 3–5 times weekly yields the most rapid clearance.

3 Coal tar is weakly active as monotherapy.

4 White petrolatum, mineral oil, or Aquaphor in combination with erythemogenic UVB is as effective as crude coal tar in the same vehicle plus UVB.

5 Coal tar improves the time to clearing in suberythemogenic UVB protocols and may lower the total accumulated UVB dose.

6 While certain constituents of coal tar used in industry are known to be potent carcinogens for human skin, e.g. benzo[a]pyrenes, there is no convincing evidence that coal tar as it is used in the treatment of psoriasis, with or without UVB, significantly increases the risk of skin cancer. It is prudent, however, not to apply coal tar to the genitalia, and to shield them during UV exposures.

7 The risk of developing cutaneous squamous cell carcinoma after UVB and tar therapy is enhanced by PUVA, ionizing radiation, and possibly arsenic ingestion.

8 Coal tar is most useful for:

(a) Patients receiving modified Goeckerman regimens in a hospital, in a day treatment center, or at home.

(b) Patients limited to using topical regimens at home such as tar baths, ointments, oils, gels, or shampoos combined with anthralin, calcipotriene, or corticosteroids.

(c) Patients using natural sunlight when that is the only source of UV radiation available.

9 Commercial UVA sunbeds are weakly effective for psoriasis and may be recommended to patients who are unable to avail themselves of medical-grade UVB or UVA in a physician's office.

Selected references

Adrian R. M., Parrish J. A., Momtaz -T. K., Karlin M. J. (1981) Outpatient phototherapy for psoriasis. *Arch Dermatol* 117, 623–626.

Alora M. B. T., Taylor C. R. (1997) Narrow-band (311 nm) UVB phototherapy: an audit of the first year's experience at the Massachusetts General Hospital. *Photodermatol Photimmunol Photomed* 13, 82–84.

Asawanonda P., Anderson R. R., Chang Y., Taylor C. R. (2000) 308-nm excimer laser for the treatment of psoriasis: a dose-response study. *Arch Dermatol* **136**, 619–624.

Bagel J. (2000) Establishing a practical and effective psoriasis treatment center. *Dermatol Clin* **18**, 349–357.

Boer J., Hermans J., Schothorst A. A., Suurmond D. (1984) Comparison of phototherapy (UV-B) and photochemotherapy (PUVA) for clearing and maintenance of psoriasis. *Arch Dermatol* **120**, 52–57.

Boldeman C., Beitner H., Jansson B. *et al.* (1996) Sunbed use in relation to phenotype, erythema, sunscreen use and skin diseases. A questionnaire survey among Swedish adolescents. *Br J Dermal* **135**, 712–716.

British Photodermatology Group (1997) An appraisal of narrowband (TL-01) UVB phototherapy. British Photodermatology workshop Report (April 1996). *Br J Dermatol* **137**, 327–330.

Cameron H., Darve R.S., Yule S. *et al.* (2002) A randomized, observer-blinded trial of twice vs. three times weekly narrowband ultraviolet B phototherapy for chronic plaque psoriasis. *Br J Dermatol* **147**, 973–978.

Coven T. R., Burack L. H., Gilleaudeau P. *et al.* (1997) Narrowband UV-B produces superior clinical and histopathological resolution of moderate-to-severe psoriasis patients compared with broad-band UV-B. *Arch Dermatol* **133**, 1514–1522.

Das S., Lloyd J. J., Farr P. M. (2001) Similar dose-response and persistence of erythema with broad-band and narrow-band ultraviolet B lamps. *J Invest Dermatol* **117**, 1318–1321.

De Berker D. A. R., Sakuntabhai A., Diffey B. L. *et al.* (1997) Comparison of psoralen-UVB and psoralen-UVA photochemotherapy in the treatment of psoriasis. *J Am Acad Dermatol* **36**, 577–581.

Feldman S. R., Clark A., Reboussin D. M., Fleischer A. B. (1996) An assessment of potential problems of home phototherapy treatment of psoriasis. *Cutis* **58**, 71–73.

Fleischer A. B., Clark A. R., Rapp S. R. *et al.* (1997) Commercial tanning bed treatment is an effective psoriasis treatment: Results from an uncontrolled clinical trial. *J Invest Dermatol* **109**, 170–174.

Goeckerman W. H. (1925) The treatment of psoriasis. *Northwest Med* **24**, 229–231.

Gordon P. M., Diffey B. L., Matthews J. N., Farr P. M. (1999) A randomized comparison of narrow-band TL-01 phototherapy and PUVA photochemotherapy for psoriasis. *J Am Acad Dermatol* **41**, 728–732.

Hudson-Peacock M. J., Diffey B. L., Farr P. M. (1994) Photoprotective action of emollients in ultraviolet therapy of psoriasis. *Br J Dermatol* **130**, 361–365.

Levine M. J., Parrish J. A. (1980) Outpatient phototherapy of psoriasis. *Arch Dermatol* **116**, 552–554.

Lowe N. J., Lowe P. S., Wasiowich E. (1991) Psoriasis ambulatory treatment centers: United States experience. In: Roenigk H. H. Jr, Maibach H. I. (eds) *Psoriasis*, 2nd edn. Marcel Dekker, Inc, New York, 547–552.

Markham T., Rogers S., Collins P. (2003) Narrowband UV-B (TL-01) phototherapy vs. oral 8-methoxypsoralen psoralen-UV-A for the treatment of chronic plaque psoriasis. *Arch Dermatol* **139**, 325–328.

Morison W. L., Pike R. A. (1984) Spectral power distributions of radiation sources used in phototherapy and photochemotherapy. *J Am Acad Dermatol* **10**, 64–68.

Pasker-de Jong P. C., Wielink G., van der Valk P.G., van der Wilt G. J. (1999) Treatment with UVB for psoriasis and nonmelanoma skin cancer: a systematic review of the literature. *Arch Dermatol* **135**, 834–840.

Sakuntabhai A., Diffey B. L., Farr P. M. (1993) Response of psoriasis to psoralen-UVB photochemotherapy. *Br J Dermatol* **128**, 296–300.

Selvaag E., Caspersen L., Bech-Thomsen N. *et al.* (2000) Optimized UVB treatment of psoriasis: a controlled left-right comparison trial. *J Eur Acad Dermatol Venereol* **14**, 19–21.

Shelk J., Morgan P. (2000) Narrow-band UVB: a practical approach. *Dermatol Nursing* **12**, 407–411.

Snow J. L., Muller S. A. (1996) Surface dosimetry in phototherapy: comparison of three ultraviolet B lamps used in the treatment of psoriasis. *Br J Dermatol* **135**, 949–954.

Stern R. S., Armstrong R. D., Anderson T. F. *et al.* (1986) Effect of continued ultraviolet B phototherapy on the duration of remission of psoriasis: a randomized study. *J Am Acad Dermatol* **15**, 546–552.

Stern R. S., Bagheri S., Nichols K. (2002) PUVA follow up study. The persistent risk of genital tumors among men treated with psoralen plus ultraviolet A (PUVA) for psoriasis. *J Am Acad Dermatol* **47**, 33–39.

Trehan M., Taylor C. R. (2002) Medium-dose 308-nm excimer laser for the treatment of psoriasis. *J Am Acad Dermatol* **47**, 701–708.

Turner R. J., Walshaw D., Diffey B. L., Farr P. M. (2000) A controlled study of ultraviolet A sunbed treatment of psoriasis. *Br J Dermatol* **143**, 957–963.

Walters I. B., Burack L. H., Coven T. R. *et al.* (1999) Suberythemogenic narrow-band UVB is markedly more effective than conventional UVB in treatment of psoriasis vulgaris. *J Am Acad Dermatol* **40**, 893–900.

Williams R. E. A., Tillman D. M., White S. I. *et al.* (1992) Re-examining crude coal tar treatment for psoriasis. *Br J Dermatol* **126**, 608–610.

14 Psoralens and photochemotherapy (PUVA)

Thomas N. Helm
Charles Camisa

Introduction

Psoralens are natural compounds that interact with sunlight to produce biological effects. Psoralens were initially used for the treatment of vitiligo in ancient times. In the 1940s, Egyptian scientists isolated the photoactive furocoumarin ingredients from *Ammi majus* plants. The active compounds are found in diverse plant families which include parsnip, celery, lemon, lime, fig, parsley, and bishop's weed.

In clinical trials, sunlamp irradiation or natural sunlight combined with oral 8-methoxypsoralen (8-MOP) was found to be an effective treatment for some cases of vitiligo. Oral 8-MOP given at doses corresponding to patients' weights, followed by high intensity ultraviolet A (UVA) irradiation in the 320–390 nanometer wavelength range was found to be effective for psoriasis and was well tolerated. This form of treatment has become widely known as "PUVA" therapy; the acronym stands for psoralen (P) and ultraviolet A (UVA) light. PUVA is much more effective than ultraviolet light therapy given with conventional fluorescent bulbs or a xenon source. Up to 85% of patients on outpatient maintenance treatments remain in remission for up to 400 days. Psoralen therapy has become a mainstay of treatment for psoriasis and has supplanted other modalities such as methotrexate and cytotoxic drug therapy.

The psoralens

The psoralens most widely used for psoriasis therapy are 8-methoxypsoralen (8-MOP), 4,5,8-trimethylpsoralen (TMP), and

191

5-methoxypsoralen (5-MOP). Each of these preparations has different photobiological effects. 8-Methoxypsoralen is the most widely used preparation. Dosages of 0.6 mg/kg are required in the average patient. 5-MOP produces less nausea and gastrointestinal upset than 8-MOP and also produces less photosensitivity when given at the same dosage as 8-MOP. 5-MOP, however, appears less effective in the treatment of psorasis. TMP stimulates melanocytes more than the other two commonly used preparations. TMP is most often used in the treatment of vitiligo or psoriasis which has not responded to 8-MOP or 5-MOP. The dosage of TMP is approximately 0.2–0.5 mg/kg.

Mechanisms of action

Psoralens belong to the group of compounds known as furocoumarins. Furocoumarins are formed by the combination of a furan ring with a coumarin ring. When the linear structure is formed, the product is known as a psoralen. If an angular structure is formed, it is known as an angelican. The tertiary structure of these compounds dictate how they will react with cellular constituents after photoactivation. The 3–4 bond of psoralen molecules interacts with the 5–6 bond of the thymidine constituents of deoxyribonucleic acid (DNA), even in the absence of light. This is known as a "dark complex." With activation by sunlight, some psoralens are capable of producing cross-linking of DNA strands known as "bifunctional adducts." Differing wavelengths of light change the type of complexes which form. At wavelengths below 250 nm, greater amounts of mono-adducts are formed than at higher wavelengths.

Initial research suggested that DNA cross-linking is responsible for the biological effect of PUVA therapy in diseases like psoriasis. Cross-linking of DNA leads to inhibition of DNA synthesis in epidermal basal cells and thereby creates a marked antiproliferative effect. It is not necessary for binding of DNA constituents to occur in order to produce phototoxicity. Recent studies suggest that cross-linking may not be necessary to have a biologic effect. The therapeutic effects of PUVA may be related to toxic effects on activated lymphocytes. Interaction with proteins, RNA, and cellular organelles may also be important to PUVA response.

The exact mechanism of psoralen therapy remains undetermined. Cell proliferation is inhibited by the production of monofunctional and bifunctional DNA adducts. High quantities of monofunctional adducts lead to cell death. Faulty repair of this type of adduct may give rise to some of the carcinogenic effects that have been attributed to PUVA therapy. It is also possible that the photosensitizing, Langerhans' cell-depleting, and anti-psoriatic effects of PUVA therapy are independent of one another.

Pharmacokinetics of specific psoralens

8-Methoxypsoralen

8-Methoxypsoralen gives maximum photosensitivity about 3.9–4.25 hours after ingestion. The 8-MOP binds reversibly to serum albumin and is distributed throughout the body by the circulatory system. Concomitant administration of food may also affect peak concentrations. The 8-MOP generally causes higher serum levels when taken while fasting rather than with meals. There is great variability from person to person. A significant proportion of patients receiving 8-MOP for the first time also have a "first-pass effect," a phenomenon in which the first administration of medication does not give rise to significant serum levels as expected. The "first-pass effect" is due to rapid metabolism by liver enzymes and diminishes upon further dosing with 8-MOP. New galenic formulations of 8-MOP with penetration enhancers have been developed for sublingual administration which bypasses hepatic first-pass metabolism.

Oral 8-MOP gives peak concentrations in 1.5 hours after administration, whereas soft gelatin oral preparation gives a peak level one hour after ingestion. Levels after ingesting hard gelatin 8-MOP capsules peak at 2–3 hours after ingestion. The skin concentration of 8-MOP seems to approximate one-third of the serum level. Plasma concentration of 8-MOP correlates with the intensity of an erythema response at a given wavelength but not with minimal phototoxic dose.

In the U.S., the original crystalline form of 8-MOP (Oxsoralen) has been widely replaced by a liquid preparation in a capsule which has a more rapid rate of absorption (Oxsoralen-Ultra). Oxsoralen-Ultra capsules lead to a faster clearing of psoriasis and may produce a more consistent clearing response, but the incidence of gastrointestinal side-effects is slightly increased . If severe, rectal suppositories of 8-MOP may be used instead and are not associated with nausea.

Trimethylpsoralen

TMP differs from 8-MOP in that it is more effective in stimulating pigmentation. TMP levels peak two hours after ingestion. Oral TMP is not as potent a photosensitizer as 8-MOP because of its poor solubility and quick metabolism to nonphotosensitizing compounds like 4,8 dimethyl, 5-carboxypsoralen (DMeCP). Topical application of TMP, a strong photosensitizer, may be helpful in treating psoriasis. TMP was found to be 10,000 times more active as a lymphotoxic agent compared to 8-MOP in an in vitro assay. Moreover, at concentrations achieved in vivo, lymphocytes were more sensitive to the toxic effects of TMP and UVA than keratinocytes.

5-Methoxypsoralen

5-Methoxypsoralen (5-MOP) is a psoralen with comparable efficacy to 8-MOP in treating psoriasis. The 5-MOP causes less phototoxicity than 8-MOP and has a lower incidence of acute cutaneous and gastrointestinal side-effects than 8-MOP. The serum half-life of 5-MOP is about one hour. The rapid rate of 5-MOP metabolism holds undesired photosensitivity after treatment to a minimum. This preparation is most useful for patients who do not tolerate 8-MOP. 5-Methoxypsoralen is available in Europe (Gerot Pharmazeutika Gmbh; Vienna, Austria) but not in the U.S.

Oral PUVA (photochemotherapy)

8-MOP is the most widely used psoralen for psoriasis treatment. When first-line therapies such as corticosteroid preparations, anthralin, or coal tar have not been effective at controlling psoriasis, and the Goeckerman regimen does not produce clearing of psoriasis after a 2–3-week period of intensive inpatient or outpatient day care treatment, PUVA therapy is usually the next alternative.

A careful history should be taken prior to starting therapy, with special emphasis on photosensitivity diseases. PUVA therapy should be avoided in patients with previous bronchiolar or hypersensitivity reactions to psoralens, systemic lupus erythematosus, some types of porphyria (such as porphyria cutanea tarda and variegate porphyria), and xeroderma pigmentosa (Table 14.1). Pregnant

Table 14.1 Considerations that may contraindicate PUVA therapy.

Ability to comply with eye protection and sunscreen use
Melanoma and nonmelanoma skin cancer
Cataracts
Medications (photosensitizers)
Photosensitivity disorders (e.g. albinism, lupus, porphyria, xeroderma pigmentosa, etc.)
Pregnancy

women or women planning pregnancy in the immediate future should also be excluded because PUVA is mutagenic and effects on pregnancy have not been adequately studied. PUVA does not seem to be a potent teratogen. However, PUVA exposure in women around the time of conception or pregnancy has been associated with a greater abortion rate. Since the lens of the eye shields the retina from incident ultraviolet A light, an aphakic patient has greater potential for retinal damage, and PUVA therapy should be reserved as a treatment of last resort. The effects of PUVA on children are not well studied, and the use of this modality in children is controversial, although some investigators report a favorable experience. Lasting eye disease attributable to PUVA therapy is very rare. Nevertheless, a baseline eye examination which measures not only visual acuity, but includes slit-lamp examination looking for lenticular opacities is recommended. In this way, lenticular abnormalities which antedate PUVA therapy can be clearly identified and later screening studies can better evaluate changes. If no abnormalities are detected on initial examination, follow-up examinations by the same ophthalmologist at intervals ranging from 6 to 12 months seem to help detect any changes early.

Because hepatic inactivation of psoralens is necessary for clearance, oral psoralen therapy should be used with caution in patients with active liver disease. Liver function tests should be screened prior to beginning PUVA therapy. Although some investigators perform antinuclear and Ro (SSA) antibody tests in addition to a urinary porphyrin screen and complete blood count to ensure that no photosensitive diseases have been overlooked, a careful history and examination usually render these tests unnecessary.

A cumulative dose of ultraviolet A light greater than 1000 J/cm^2, concomitant ingestion of photosensitizing drugs such as thiazide diuretics, tetracyclines, or nonsteroidal anti-inflammatory drugs (like piroxicam), previous skin cancer or exposure to cancer promoters such as x-ray or trivalent inorganic arsenic are relative contraindications to PUVA therapy. The use of concurrent topical photosensitizers such as tar preparations needs to be avoided.

Because PUVA therapy has been shown to depress the immune system, patients on other immunosuppressive medications such as azathioprine, cyclosporine, or cyclophosphamide should be treated with caution if PUVA is used at all. PUVA therapy seems to be safe in individuals with AIDS.

Another variable which must be assessed is whether or not a patient is able to cooperate with therapy, stand unassisted for several minutes in a light box, and withstand the cardiovascular stress caused by prolonged vasodilation in the phototherapy unit. (Lie-down units which help avoid some of these problems are available from some companies.) Patients must also be able to comply with the use of photoprotective lenses that need to be worn the remainder of the day of therapy.

Although some physicians have advocated the use of patient consent forms prior to starting PUVA therapy, a careful and fully documented discussion regarding the side-effects of PUVA therapy is essential before starting therapy and may obviate the need for standardized consent forms. No consent form can foresee all possible outcomes of therapy and an open discussion is most helpful. (ICN pharmaceuticals has prepared a patient instruction video on PUVA which serves as a good adjunct to the physician's discussion.)

Preparing for PUVA treatment

For suitable candidates, two or three treatments/week may be anticipated to control psoriasis and at least 20 treatments must be given before a maximal therapeutic effect can be expected (Fig. 14.1). PUVA erythema peaks at 48–96 hours compared to 8 hours for UVB erythema. Patients are issued wrap-around style glasses which can be either tinted or clear depending upon the patient's preference. Some dermatologists have recommended that more fashionable eye glasses with specially coated or treated lenses be worn instead of wrap-around glasses to increase compliance.

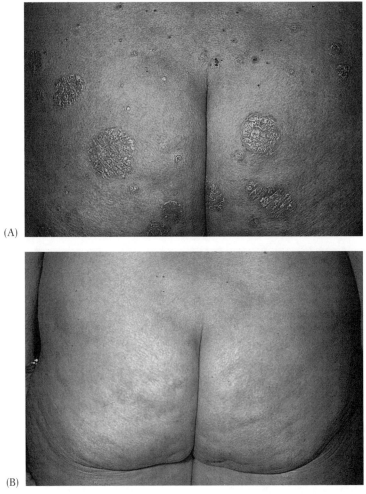

Figure 14.1 Psoriasis of buttocks before (A) and after (B) 12 weeks of PUVA.

Acceptable transmission of light has been reported to be less than 10% at 390 nanometers, less than 5% at 380 nanometers, less than 2% at 370 nanometers, and less than 1% at 360 nanometers. Table 14.2 lists some sources of acceptable UVA blocking optical equipment.

Use of skin type information obtained from patient history can give useful estimates of appropriate starting UVA dosing. A widely used regimen is shown in Table 14.3.

Table 14.2 Sources of phototherapy and protective optical equipment.

daavlin.com	Phototherapy units, protective equipment, meters
dioptics.com	UV protective glasses
homephototherapyexpert.com	Home UV units distributor
natbiocorp.com	Phototherapy units, protective equipment, meters
solarcsystems.com	UV phototherapy units
spectroline.com	Hand-held UV lamps
summertan.com	ph-36 Cooper Hewitt psoriasis UV lamp
trlc.com	Jordan light UV system
ultralite-uv.com	UV phototherapy units
uvbiotek.com	UV phototherapy units
uvp.com	UV meters, UV blocking eyewear

Table 14.3 Protocol for photochemotherapy based on skin type.

Skin type	History	Initial UVA dose	Subsequent UVA increases
I	Always burns, never tans	0.5 J/cm^2	0.5 J/cm^2
II	Always burns, sometimes tans	1.0 J/cm^2	1.0 J/cm^2
III	Sometimes burns, always tans	1.5 J/cm^2	1.0 J/cm^2
IV	Never burns, always tans	2.0 J/cm^2	1.0 J/cm^2
V	Darkly pigmented	2.5 J/cm^2	1.5 J/cm^2
VI	Black	3.0 J/cm^2	1.5 J/cm^2

Dosage of psoralen

For the initial dose of 8-MOP, patients bring their medication to the office and take their first dose under the supervision of the nurse. The time of taking the medication is recorded in the chart, and ultraviolet A light is adminstered $1\frac{1}{2}$ to 2 hours later. Although higher levels of psoralen in serum can be achieved when psoralen is taken on an empty stomach, the preparations are much better tolerated if they are taken with a small meal. A similar amount and type of food should be taken each time to help maintain relatively consistent serum levels. In this way, the desired response can be achieved by changing the UVA dosage. If patients do not respond to PUVA at all, it is reasonable to measure serum levels. A level of >50 ng/ml is considered to be therapeutic, and the dosage of 8-MOP can be increased until this level is reached.

Although skin type determined by history can be a rough starting point for UVA dosage, history may be an unreliable indicator of the minimal phototoxic dose (MPD). Minimal phototoxic dose testing gives an accurate estimate of optimal starting dose. To perform MPD testing, small squares on the back or buttock are irradiated with differing amounts of ultraviolet A light one to two hours after ingesting the appropriate dose of 8-MOP. An opaque plastic sheet with six 1.5 cm squares is used for this purpose. We usually test in a range of $1–10$ J/cm^2. Each square is irradiated with a different incremental amount of light and in 48–72 hours, the squares are evaluated to find the lowest dose that gives complete erythema of the irradiated area. Seventy to 100% of the MPD can then be given as the starting dose of irradiation and further treatments can be increased by $0.25–1.0$ J/cm^2 as tolerated. A half-body study of both regimens based on MPD and skin type gave equivalent clearing and remissions, but the cumulative UVA dose was higher with the MPD regimen. Patients with types I and II skin should be treated with the fixed starting dose to avoid the risk of burns. A suggested treatment protocol for inducing remission is shown in Table 14.3, but many variations are available.

After the psoriasis is almost clear or clear (90–100% improved), maintenance PUVA is begun by holding steady at the final dose and reducing the frequency of treatment by once per week, every 4 weeks. For example, if cleared at three times weekly, then treat twice weekly for 4 weeks, once weekly for 4 weeks, then stop and follow for relapse.

Less commonly used psoralens

5-Methoxypsoralen

5-Methoxypsoralen treatment is accomplished in an analogous fashion to 8-MOP treatment. After identical history and laboratory evaluations are performed, patients are begun on a 1.2 mg/kg dose. Unfortunately, 5-MOP is not available in the U.S. and must be obtained from Europe. It shows great promise in the therapy of psoriasis because of greater tolerance by patients and lower incidence of unwanted photosensitivity subsequent to therapy. Oral 5-MOP may also modify circadian rhythm regulation because it stimulates melatonin secretion.

Trimethylpsoralen (TMP)

Oral trimethylpsoralen has limited use in the treatment of common psoriasis. However, if patients fail to respond to 8-MOP or 5-MOP, this modality can be tried before advancing to therapies such as retinoids, methotrexate or cyclosporine. In the setting of photosensitive psoriasis, TMP PUVA has given excellent results and may be the treatment of choice.

Side-effects of oral PUVA

Acute side-effects

Side-effects of PUVA treatment can be divided into acute and chronic effects. **Acute reactions** include phototoxicity manifest by erythema (and possibly edema); nausea, which occurs in 20–30% of patients; pruritus; dizziness; flu-like symptoms; headache; and the isomorphic response of Koebner. Phototoxic reactions are more likely to occur with pustular or erythrodermic psoriasis, and dosages should be adjusted accordingly. Some individuals also may develop itching, pain, and tenderness while on maintenance therapy after psoriasis has cleared. Slight scaling and erythema may occur and be confused with a flare in psoriasis, but this eruption responds to a 2-week respite from phototherapy. **Chronic side-effects** include enhanced photoaging, pigmented macules known as "PUVA lentigines" (see Plate 16, facing p. 34), actinic keratoses, squamous cell carcinomas, and possibly anterior cortical cataracts. Development of fever and liver function test elevation has been reported during PUVA therapy. The liver function abnormalities returned to normal, but with the next PUVA treatment the same reaction occurred. No significant changes, however, have been demonstrated by liver biopsies done before and after PUVA therapy. It seems that psoralens have little or no lasting hepatotoxicity.

The prolonged exertion of standing and thermal exposure during PUVA therapy raises concerns about cardiovascular stress. PUVA must be used with caution in patients with unstable angina at risk for myocardial infarction. Several studies have not shown any substantial cardiovascular risk, however.

Chronic side-effects

PUVA therapy is associated with an increased incidence of skin cancer. Histologic changes such as hyperkeratosis, acanthosis, melanosis, and focal dysplasia in the epidermis occur after PUVA therapy. The presence of PUVA lentigines correlates with the risk of nonmelanoma skin cancer. An increased deposition of acid mucopolysaccharides and a decrease in elastic fibers in the dermis has been found. Most of these changes are irreversible. Unexpected findings include mutations in the tumor suppressor gene *p53* that consist predominantly of the cytosine to thymidine transitions typically encountered from UVB irradiation and relatively few of the thymidine to adenine transversions expected from PUVA therapy.

Melanoma

In the 1380 patients enrolled in the U.S. PUVA Follow-up Study (Stern, 2001), the incidence of melanoma was similar to that expected in the general population for the first 10 years, but was found to be increased in later years. The risk has been found to be most significant in individuals who have undergone more than 250 treatments more than 15 years previously and is increasing with the passage of time. However, in the Swedish PUVA cohort of 4799 patients followed for 16 years, there was no increased risk of melanoma. Taken together with the development of PUVA lentigines with cytologically atypical melanocytes, these findings indicate that photochemotherapy contributes to the induction of malignant melanoma and accounts for some of the diminution in the enthusiasm for PUVA therapy.

Squamous cell carcinoma

The incidence of squamous cell carcinomas is substantially increased by PUVA therapy. More than one-fourth of patients treated with high dose PUVA in some studies developed squamous cell carcinoma. A history of methotrexate or cyclosporine treatment further increases this risk. Human papillomavirus DNA can be isolated in many of these tumors, suggesting that PUVA treatment alters the extent and pathogenicity of papillomavirus infection. Genital cancers are more common in PUVA-treated men, possibly because of concomitant papillomavirus infection. For this reason, shielding the genital area during treatment is strongly recommended. Both men and women who have undergone extensive PUVA therapy may be at higher risk for respiratory cancer, and females may be at greater risk for colonic and renal cancer. The usual relative incidence of one squamous cell for every three basal cell carcinomas is reversed by PUVA therapy. The time interval over which UVA is given, not just the total UVA dose, may be important in carcinogenesis, with longer treatment periods correlating with increased tumor production. These observations, if confirmed, would make aggressive short-term treatment the method of choice for PUVA therapy. These observations may also, in part, explain the discrepancy between the European and American experience with PUVA carcinogenesis; the Europeans have noted a lower incidence of skin cancer and in general do treat their patients more aggressively. Most patients who develop SCC have PUVA lentigines, and one study suggests that absence of PUVA lentigines may be a useful indicator for a lower risk of malignancy.

Basal cell carcinoma

The incidence of basal cell carcinoma in PUVA patients without other predisposing risk factors is slightly increased over the normal population. The main carcinogenic effect of PUVA therapy is noted as an increased production of actinic keratoses and squamous cell carcinomas while the effect of PUVA on production of basal cell carcinoma appears to be relatively small. Basal cell carcinomas have occurred before age 21 in some individuals treated with PUVA.

Connective tissue disease

Because PUVA therapy amplifies the effects of sunlight on the skin, researchers have suspected that PUVA therapy could cause connective tissue diseases such as lupus erythematosus. PUVA therapy can lead to SSA (Ro) expression in fibroblasts. This may, in part, explain the phenomenon of antinuclear antibody (ANA) development during PUVA therapy. There might be a statistically significant correlation between the duration of PUVA therapy and conversion from a negative to positive ANA test. A large multicenter study did not, however, show a higher incidence of ANA in PUVA patients than the population at large. Other studies have suggested that the addition of etretinate could lower the expression of ANA. It is not clear if phototherapy can cause connective tissue disease, but if this occurs it must be uncommon. A greater concern is the exacerbation of unrecognized or misdiagnosed connective tissue disease. For example, dermatomyositis and the papulosquamous type of subacute cutaneous lupus erythematosus may closely mimic psoriasis and must be considered in any atypical response of "psoriasis" to PUVA.

Miscellaneous

Vitiligo, bullous pemphigoid, pemphigus, and lichen planus have been associated with PUVA therapy. Other conditions resulting from keratinocyte mutation, such as disseminated superficial actinic porokeratosis, and multiple keratoacanthomas, have been reported. The onset of neurofibromas, myelomonocytic leukemia, evolution of myelodysplasia to acute myeloid leukemia, melanonychia striata, zosteriform acantholytic dyskeratotic, epidermal nevus and photo-onycholysis have also been observed.

The eye

Ultraviolet radiation alone can damage the lens of the eye and 8-MOP seems to enhance these ultraviolet changes. 8-MOP could be detected in human lenses up to 12 hours after a dosage of 8-MOP. If 8-MOP is exposed to ultraviolet light, irreversible binding to the lens occurs. If no photoactivation of the 8-MOP occurs, diffusion from the lens without appreciable binding was noted. The importance of proper ultraviolet eye protection therefore becomes obvious.

Ordinary eyeglasses give little protection from incident ultraviolet radiation as compared to eyeglasses such as Noir, Blak-ray, and Polaroid. Table 14.2 shows some sources for UVA protective optical equipment. It is important to stress to patients that outdoor sunlight poses the greatest hazard for inducing lenticular changes during PUVA therapy. Indoor incandescent bulbs or daylight fluorescent bulbs may contribute to UVA exposure, but it is less important to protect lenses from indoor sources than outdoor sources. Some authors have suggested that protection from indoor light sources may even be unnecessary. Calzavara-Pinton *et al.* (1994) found that patients who were given PUVA despite refusing to wear protective lenses developed conjunctival hyperemia and decreased lacrimation but no lens opacities. No increase in cataracts in patients who have been treated with PUVA and who have used proper eye protection has been documented, but because eye changes may take a long time to develop, ongoing vigilance is advised.

Adjunctive agents for oral PUVA

Numerous adjunctive therapies have been used with oral PUVA, including topical steroids, anthralin, emollients, methotrexate, etretinate, and UVB. The role of these adjunctive therapies is to hasten clearing of lesions while minimizing side-effects. Calcipotriene (Dovonex) absorbs in the ultraviolet B and C range, and its concentration in skin is reduced by UVA exposure. Tar products absorb in the UVA range, and anthralin absorbs in the UVB and UVC ranges. Dihydroxyacetone (DHA), the chemical in self-tanning lotions, binds to the stratum corneum and forms a UVA-protective pigment. DHA use during PUVA allowed higher UVA exposures with minimal burns in a pilot study.

Topical combination therapy

As soon as oral PUVA therapy became widely used, practitioners attempted to modify standard PUVA protocol to accelerate clearing of psoriasis. Topical corticosteroids produce a more rapid clearing, but recurrences of psoriasis may occur sooner. When clobetasol propionate is used in conjunction with PUVA therapy, greater improvement is noted, but the rate and time of relapse is uncertain. Topical coal tar treatment does not seem to reduce the time to clearing and should generally be avoided during PUVA phototherapy because a painful photosensitivity reaction known as "tar smarts" can occur. Anthralin is clinically useful, but patients are often noncompliant with this form of therapy in the outpatient setting because it is irritating and inelegant. Both calcipotriene and tazarotene are well accepted and lower the doses needed for clearing with PUVA, although patients must be warned to use tazarotene sparingly and be on guard for possible irritating effects. We typically prescribe a topical steroid to use in conjunction with tazarotene therapy. Topical flurandrenolide tape (Cordran tape) may be used during PUVA therapy as the transmission is good in the UVA range. (The tape absorbs in the UVB range and should be removed for UVB phototherapy.)

Systemic combination therapy

1 Methotrexate has been used to shorten the number of PUVA treatments necessary to clear extensive psoriasis. Methotrexate and PUVA doses can be kept considerably lower when both agents are used together as compared to either modality alone. Whether this effect is additive or synergistic is not known. An interesting side-effect noted by this combination therapy is enhanced phototoxicity

in some patients. This effect is reminiscent of a UVB-methotrexate type of "recall" reaction. Lack of repigmentation of areas cleared of psoriasis was one of the side-effects noted with this form of therapy. Both of these findings suggest that methotrexate may be having an effect on normal melanocyte function. The incidence of squamous cell carcinomas is increased when both of these agents are used.

2 The use of retinoids in conjunction with PUVA (called "re-PUVA" treatment) appears to give the most encouraging results. Both acitretin and etretinate have been studied in multicenter trials. In one protocol, patients were given 50 mg of acitretin or 50 mg of etretinate daily for 2 weeks prior to UVA exposure then started on PUVA therapy at a dosage of 25 mg of either retinoid, daily. UVA light was given three times weekly until remission was noted. Acitretin-PUVA treatment was superior to placebo-PUVA treatment, and etretinate-PUVA showed some benefit over placebo-PUVA in terms of lesion score. Etretinate reaches peak effects after 3 weeks of therapy with conventional dosage regimens and only slow increases in UVA dosage are then possible because of enhanced phototoxicity. If PUVA and etretinate therapy are given at a dosage of 1 mg/kg/day and are started at the same time, effective doses of UVA for maximal PUVA response can be achieved earlier in treatment. Eighty percent of patients are 100% cleared by the end of the sixth week of therapy by this method. RePUVA can reduce the number of treatments needed for clearing by up to one-third and decrease total PUVA cumulative dosage by up to one-fourth of what would be required by simple PUVA therapy alone.

5-MOP oral PUVA has been used with retinoids in an analogous fashion to 8-MOP PUVA. If etretinate is given at a dose of 0.5 mg/kg/day for 14 days prior to beginning PUVA, with 5-MOP at a dosage of 1 mg/kg/day, excellent clearing of psoriasis is seen, with a reduction in the total joules needed to achieve clinical remission. This innovation may be superior to 8-MOP RePUVA because of the lower radiance of UVA needed to achieve clearance. We have found the use of adjunctive retinoids, such as acitretin, to lower the cumulative doses of PUVA needed to control psoriasis and feel that retinoids increase efficacy and safety while lowering overall costs of phototherapy.

3 Ultraviolet B light has been used in combination with PUVA therapy. Ultraviolet B light is thought to control the rapid proliferation of keratinocytes in psoriasis by producing thymine dimers in DNA. The thymine dimers may inhibit DNA synthesis much like the

photo-adducts formed during PUVA therapy. A study of conventional PUVA therapy and ultraviolet B light revealed more rapid clearing of psoriasis on the PUVA-UVB treated side of the body. Combined UVB and PUVA treatment may reduce total cumulative UV radiation needed to clear psoriasis, although further studies to gauge the side-effects of such combination therapy are needed.

Topical PUVA

Topical PUVA has several theoretical advantages over oral PUVA. Small areas can be treated without subjecting uninvolved areas to unnecessary medicines, and systemic adverse effects are negligible. Topical PUVA is often impractical because severe phototoxic reactions can occur if patients use the psoralen in an unsupervised setting. Supervision of topical PUVA by office staff is labor intensive. The commercially available topical psoralens are also very expensive.

Topical PUVA has been used widely in the treatment of vitiligo. The modern use of topical psoralens has been pioneered by researchers in the Scandinavian countries. Vehicles for topical PUVA include cream, lotion, ointment or bath-water delivery systems. Lotions and creams often give uneven distribution of the psoralen and are, therefore, less widely used than bath-water delivery.

Pharmacokinetics of topical psoralens

The degree of photosensitization achieved by a particular psoralen can differ when comparing oral and topical routes. Curiously, 8-MOP causes more photosensitivity than TMP when given orally, but TMP bath delivery leads to greater photosensitivity than 8-MOP bath delivery. This may be due to greater lipid solubility of TMP.

After topical application of an alcohol-based 8-MOP solution, most 8-MOP is bound to the stratum corneum but topical 1% 8-MOP ointment can give rise to serum levels comparable to that of oral administration. Side-effects of nausea and cataract formation are generally absent with topical PUVA because of the low serum levels.

Mechanism of action of topical psoralens

The mechanism of action of topical PUVA therapy is analogous to oral PUVA. DNA cross-linking occurs and DNA synthesis is inhibited, thereby providing an antiproliferative effect to the skin. Patients seem to show only photosensitivity in the areas exposed to the psoralen and do not show distant effects, although some studies have indicated that serum levels similar to oral administration can be achieved. 8-MOP is the most widely used psoralen for topical delivery in the United States. 8-MOP treatment can be given to the total body by bath-tub immersion or to localized areas such as the hands or feet by soaks in basins.

Bath PUVA for extensive psoriasis

Bath-water delivery of 8-MOP or methoxsalen can be as effective as oral 8-MOP therapy, but requires up to fourfold less cumulative amounts of ultraviolet A dose to achieve clearing. Both bath-PUVA and broad-band UVB induced complete remission in about 70% of patients, but the duration of remission was significantly longer for bath-PUVA (8.4 vs. 5.1 months). Various protocols may be used. Base your selection on the one that works best for you, your patients, and staff.

1 One protocol uses 8-MOP lotion (Oxsoralen 1% Lotion). Thirty ml of the Oxsoralen 1% lotion is added to 80 liters of bath water at body temperature. The resultant 8-MOP concentration is 3.75 mg/l.

2 An alternative solution is made when 50 mg of Oxsoralen capsules are solubilized in hot water and added to the bath. The patient bathes for 15 minutes, is wiped dry, and is then given total body UVA irradiation at doses determined by skin type. Patients with type I skin are given 0.2 J/cm^2 and patients with type II are given 0.5 J/cm^2. Ultraviolet A irradiation is increased as tolerated with subsequent treatments. Dosage increases are given at the same increments as with oral PUVA to make dosing easier for nursing staff. The maximal dose of UVA needed is usually between 1 and 2 J/cm^2.

3 Another simple method of preparing a psoralen bath is to add 15 ml of the 1% Oxsoralen Solution to 80 liters of bath water to give a concentration of 1.875 mg/l. Because of this lower concentration, patients need to stay in the bath water for 30 minutes to maximize photosensitization.

4 A bath water concentration of 2.64 mg/l with a 5-minute immersion time has also been found to be effective.

It is not necessary for patients to wear protective UVA goggles on the day of the treatment. To ensure that the dosage of the clear

Oxsoralen Lotion added to the bath water is uniform, a food coloring dye can be added to the stock solution so that colorimetric indication of correct Oxsoralen Lotion dosing can be visually assessed grossly by nursing personnel.

Our patients have not experienced gastrointestinal side-effects from this form of therapy, although erythema and pruritus have been noted by about one-third of patients. An occasional patient will notice persistent photosensitivity up to 12 hours after bathing. In a study of 13 patients receiving 8-MOP bath delivery, 8-MOP levels were below the limit of detection of the HPLC assay (<10 ng/ml) at every time point from 0.5–6 h after treatment.

Trimethylpsoralen

Topical TMP or trioxsalen may be more effective than topical methoxsalen treatment. The systemic effect of trioxsalen bath preparations is negligible. Only 1/10 of the UVA dosage of systemic PUVA treatment is required with the bath-water delivery of TMP. This form of therapy shows great promise for selected patients with renal or hepatic failure or in those who cannot tolerate long treatment times. A half-body comparison of TMP bath PUVA and narrowband UVB showed that the latter was more effective at clearing chronic plaque psoriasis in patients with type I–III skin.

An unusual pattern of phototoxic burning may occur from prolonged contact of undissolved TMP crystals with skin and bath tub; a problem resolved by changing positions while soaking, and agitating the water.

5-Methoxypsoralen

Bath-water delivery of 5-MOP was shown to be comparable in efficacy to 8-MOP for palmar and plaque-type psoriasis at final concentrations of 0.0003% (wt/vol). 5-MOP was more phototoxic than 8-MOP in this system. Patients developed darker tans significantly earlier with 5-MOP.

6-Methyl-angelicans

Ultraviolet A light combined with topical 6-methyl-angelican treatment may prove superior to topical PUVA therapy according to one study. Pigmentation, but no phototoxicity, occurred with this regimen offering another advantage over topical PUVA.

Side-effects of topical PUVA

The acute cutaneous side-effects of topical PUVA therapy are much the same as oral therapy, although allergic contact or photocontact reactions may occur. The risk of excess squamous cell carcinoma is considered to be very low because of much lower cumulative UVA dosages. Gastrointestinal side-effects are not seen, and cataract formation from topical PUVA has not been reported to our knowledge. Even though systemic absorption may be small, we do not treat pregnant or lactating patients with this therapy.

Bath tubs need to be filled and cleaned, and this makes full body treatment with bath PUVA impractical for most private offices. Bath-water PUVA, however, can be efficiently used in the treatment of localized palmoplantar pustulosis or palmoplantar psoriasis. Serum levels after local soaks of palmoplantar psoriasis approximated 1/40 the level of oral administration in one study.

Bath PUVA protocols for localized palmar or plantar disease

A simple regimen is to add 0.4 ml of 8-MOP 1% solution (Oxsoralen 1% Lotion) to 1.5 liters of lukewarm bath water (about 37°C). The patient bathes the involved extremity in the resultant 3.7 mg/l 8-MOP solution for 20 minutes (Fig. 14.2). Alternatively, 1 ml of 1% Oxsoralen Lotion may be dissolved in 2 liters of water and the patient soaks for 30 minutes. The patient then receives UVA with a starting dose of 0.5 J/cm^2. The irradiance is then increased at 0.25 J/cm^2/treatment as tolerated until clearing occurs. Treatments are given 2–3 times weekly. Although a fluorescent light source (F40T12BL) may be used, good results have also been reported with high-pressure metal halide lamps (Dermalight 2001).

If one treatment is missed, the dose is held at the previous irradiance. If two treatments are missed, the dose is decreased to the second to last dose received, and so on.

An interesting effect of topical bath-water delivery is that photo-sensitivity can last for up to 72 hours. Topical PUVA may lead to the production of mono-adducts which are cleared slowly from the skin. UVA irradiation can still provoke sensitivity days after soaking. This observation suggests that several UVA exposures can be given after one bath-water treatment with psoralens, and this approach has been used in the treatment of a patient with palmoplantar eczema. This method frees up time for the nurses and patients because the long soak can be omitted. The expense of the psoralen solution is also

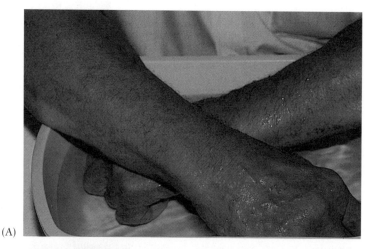

(A)

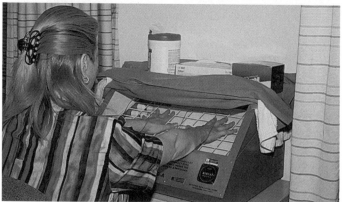

(B)

Figure 14.2 Soaking hands in 8-MOP solution (A) followed by exposure to UVA in a hand/foot unit (B) in the treatment of palmar psoriasis with bath PUVA.

saved. It is likely that similar adjustments in the interval of bath-water delivery will be useful in the management of palmoplantar psoriasis. TMP has been used for bath-water delivery of PUVA in cloudy seasons in order to exploit the greater photosensitization of TMP to hasten clearance. 8-MOP is used at other times when unwanted phototoxic reactions are more likely to occur. Not all researchers have found topical PUVA to be superior to placebo in the treatment of palmoplantar pustulosis, but this probably depends on the topical formulation used. Bath PUVA is associated with fewer acute problems than oral PUVA and is well accepted by patients.

It may be difficult to administer outside of a phototherapy center because of the need for more space and time than is available in the typical dermatology outpatient setting.

Combination therapies used with bath PUVA

Just as with oral PUVA, various adjunctive therapies have been used with bath PUVA to speed the clearing of psoriasis. Adjunctive agents include emollients, topical steroids, and retinoids. The addition of etretinate at a dosage of 1 mg/kg/day can enhance the effects of bath PUVA. The only side-effects noted were redness. The lower UVA dosage needed to attain clearing of psoriasis makes this an excellent treatment for psoriatic lesions. It does not seem to matter whether the retinoid administered is acitretin or etretinate because both give comparable results when used with bath PUVA.

Light sources

Artificial indoor light sources are most commonly used to produce UVA. The fluorescent sunlamp and black light units use low pressure mercury vapor which emits 254 nm radiation. Special substances, known as phosphors, are used to coat the glass tube containing the gas, and these phosphors absorb the emitted radiation and re-emit the radiation at a longer wavelength. The F40 T12 PUVA lamp is a commonly used light source capable of readily inducing a minimally perceptible phototoxic erythema. Most fluorescent UVA systems have a peak emission at 352 nm, but units with peak emission around 325 nm may prove more effective. One study showed clearing of psoriasis with PUVA at 335 nm to be twice as effective as irradiation at 365 nm.

A unit which can administer both UVA and UVB is most economical for smaller practices with limited space. Most practitioners feel that fluorescent systems for the delivery of ultraviolet A light are of greatest utility, because the fluorescent bulbs are relatively inexpensive, easily exchanged for ones with different phosphors (should a different emission wavelength be desired), and relatively cool. The advantages and disadvantages of fluorescent lamp UVA cabinets are the same as listed for UVB cabinets in Chapter 13, including inconsistent dosimetry for different anatomic sites.

High pressure mercury halide systems show a greater vertical uniformity of dose than fluorescent systems. Radiometry units are available to ensure adequate UVA irradiance. Uniformity of irradiance is important in PUVA therapy, and the lowest reading should not be less than 70% of the highest reading along the vertical axis of the chamber, and more than 80% of the highest reading along the horizontal plane. A patient viewing window, latches that can be opened from the inside by patients, thermoregulation with a fan or sufficient airflow, a nonskid floor, hand rails, as well as electrical grounding are all important safety features of a phototherapy cabinet.

Newer types of fluorescent lamps are being developed. The TL-01 monochromatic lamp (Philips) emits a wavelength at 311 nm, which avoids the other theoretically more carcinogenic wavelengths and is therapeutic when combined with psoralens.

Summary

PUVA therapy is an effective form of treatment for psoriasis. After conventional topical therapies or ultraviolet B light have failed, PUVA therapy should be considered as a possible next step for treatment of psoriasis. Relative contraindications to PUVA include concomitant photosensitivity diseases, cutaneous squamous cell carcinoma, a history of melanoma, and cataracts. Bath-water delivery shows much promise for localized disease. Bath treatment for extensive disease is as effective as oral PUVA but is more cumbersome and time consuming. Localized bath-water delivery of PUVA to the palms and soles is the treatment of choice for recalcitrant palmoplantar psoriasis and palmoplantar pustulosis.

Selected references

Anderson T. F., Voorhees J. J. (1980) Psoralen photochemotherapy of cutaneous disorders. *Ann Rev Pharmacol Toxicol* 20, 235–257.

Calzavara-Pinton P. G., Carlino A., Manfred E. *et al.* (1994) Ocular side effects of PUVA-treated patients refusing eye sun protection. *Acta Derm Venereol* 186 (Suppl), 164–165.

Calzavara-Pinton P. C., Zane C., Carlino A., De Panfilis G. (1997) Bath-5-methoxypsoralen-UVA therapy for psoriasis. *J Am Acad Dermatol* 36, 945–949.

Collins P., Wainwright N. J., Amorim I. *et al.* (1996) 8-MOP PUVA for psoriasis: a comparison of a minimal phototoxic dose-based regimen with a skin-type approach. *Br J Dermatol* 135, 248–254.

Coven T. R., Murphy F. P., Gilleaudeau P. *et al.* (1998) Trimethylpsoralen bath PUVA is a remittive treatment for psoriasis vulgaris. Evidence that epidermal immunocytes are direct therapeutic targets. *Arch Dermatol* **134**, 1263–1268.

Dawe R. S., Cameron H., Yule S. *et al.* (2003) A randomized controlled trial of narrowband ultraviolet B vs. bath psoralen plus ultraviolet A photochemotherapy for psoriasis. *Br J Dermatol* **148**, 1194–1204.

Gupta A. K., Stern R. S., Swanson N. A., Anderson T. F. (1988) Cutaneous melanomas in patients treated with psoralens plus ultraviolet A: a case report and the experience of the PUVA follow-up study. *J Am Acad Dermatol* **19**, 67–76.

Karrer S., Eholzer C., Akermann G. *et al.* (2001) Phototherapy of psoriasis: Comparative experience of different phototherapeutic approaches. *Dermatol* **202**, 108–115.

Kirby B., Buckley D. A., Rogers S. (1999) Large increments in psoralen-ultraviolet A (PUVA) therapy are unsuitable for fair-skinned individuals with psoriasis. *Br J Dermatol* **140**, 661–666.

Koo J. (1999) Systemic sequential therapy for psoriasis: a new paradigm for improved therapeutic results. *Am Acad Dermatol* **41**(Suppl. 3, part 2), 25–28.

Kornreich C., Zheng Z. S., Xue G. Z., Prystowsky J. H. (1996) A simple method to predict whether topical agents will interfere with phototherapy. *Cutis* **57**, 113–118.

Koulu L. M., Jansen C. T. (1988) Antipsoriatic, erythematogenic, and Langerhans cell marker depleting effect of bath-psoralens plus ultraviolet A treatment. *J Am Acad Dermatol* **18**, 1053–1059.

Lebwohl M., Ali S. (2001) Treatment of psoriasis: topical therapy and phototherapy. *J Am Acad Dermatol* **45**, 487–502.

Lebwohl M., Drake L., Menter A. (2001) Consensus conference: Acitretin in combination with UVB or PUVA in the treatment of psoriasis. *J Am Acad Dermatol* **45**, 544–553.

Lever L. R., Farr P. M. (1994) Skin cancers or premalignant lesions occur in half of high dose PUVA patients. *Br J Dermatol* **131**, 215–219.

Lindelof B., Sigurgeirsson B., Tegner E., Larko O. *et al.* (1991) PUVA and cancer: a large scale epidemiological study. *Lancet* **338**, 91–93.

Lindelof B., Sigugeirsson B., Tegner E. *et al.* (1999) PUVA and cancer risk: the Swedish follow-up study. *Br J Dermatol* **141**, 108–112.

Lowe N. J., Weingarten D., Bourget T., Moy L. S. (1986) PUVA therapy for psoriasis: comparison of oral and bath water delivery. *J Am Acad Dermatol* **14**, 754–760.

Lowe N. J., Urbach F., Bailin P., Weingarten D. P. (1987) Comparative efficacy of two dosage forms of oral methoxsalen in psoralens plus ultraviolet A therapy of psoriasis. *J Am Acad Dermatol* **16**, 994–998.

McNeely W., Goa K. L. (1998) 5-methoxypsoralen. A review of its effect in psoriasis and vitiligo. *Drugs* **56**, 667–690.

Nanda S., Grover C., Reddy B. S. (2003) PUVA-induced lichen planus. *J Dermatol* **30**, 151–153.

Ortel B., Liebman E. J., Honigsmann H., Taylor C. R. (1998) Oral psoralen photochemotherapy. In: Roenigk H. H. Jr, Maibach H. I. (eds) *Psoriasis*, 3rd edn. Marcel Dekker, New York, 543–557.

Parrish J. A., Fitzpatrick T. B., Tanenbaum L., Pathak M. A. (1974) Photochemotherapy of psoriasis with oral methoxsalen and longwave ultraviolet light. *N Engl J Med* **291**, 1207–1211.

Peritz A. E., Gasparro F. P. (1999) Psoriasis, PUVA, and skin cancer—molecular epidemiology: The curious question of T → A transversions. *J Invest Dermatol Symposium Proc* 1999, **4**, 11–16.

Setaluri V., Clark A. R., Feldman S. R. (2000) Transmittance properties of flurand renolide tape for psoriasis: helpful adjunct to phototherapy. *J Cutan Med Surg* **4**, 196–198.

Stern R. S. (2001) The PUVA Follow up Study. The risk of melanoma in association with long-term exposure to PUVA. *J Am Acad Dermatol* **44**, 755–761.

Stern R. S., Laird N. (1994) The carcinogenic risk of treatment for severe psoriasis. *Cancer* **73**, 2759–2764.

Stern R. S., Nichols K. T., Vakeva L. H. (1997) Malignant melanoma in patients treated for psoriasis with methoxsalen (psoralen) and ultraviolet A radiation (PUVA). *N Engl J Med* **336**, 1041–1045.

Taylor C. R., Kwangsukstith C., Wimberly J. *et al.* (1999) Turbo-PUVA: dihydroxyacetone-enhanced photochemotherapy: a pilot study. *Arch Dermatol* **135**, 540–544.

Tzaneva S., Honigsmann H., Tanew A. (2002) A comparison of psoralen plus ultraviolet A (PUVA) monotherapy, tacalcitol plus PUVA and tazarotene plus PUVA in patients with chronic plaque-type psoriasis. *Br J Dermatol* **147**, 748–753.

Virvidakis K. E., Brokalakis J. D., Singhellakis P. N., Mountokalakis T.D. (1988) Effect of PUVA on intestinal calcium absorption. *Br J Dermatol* **118**, 219–221.

Weinstock M. A., Coulter S., Bates J. *et al.* (1995) Human papillomavirus and widespread cutaneous carcinoma after UVA photochemotherapy. *Arch Dermatol* **131**, 701–704.

Wolff K., Fitzpatrick T. B., Parrish J. A., Gschnait F., Gilchrest B., Honigsmann H., Pathak M. A., Tannenbaum L. (1976) Photochemotherapy for psoriasis with orally administered methoxsalen. *Arch Dermatol* **112**, 943–950.

Zanolli M. D., Feldman S. R., Clark A. R., Fleischer A. B. Jr. (2000) *Phototherapy Treatment Protocols for Psoriasis and other Phototherapy Responsive Dermatoses*. Parthenon, New York.

15 Retinoids

Charles Camisa

Introduction

Retinoids are chemicals that are naturally or synthetically derived from vitamin A (retinol). They all have anti-inflammatory, antikeratinizing, and antiproliferative effects on skin. Indeed, the systemic toxicity of retinoids, with the exception of idiosyncratic reactions, is that of hypervitaminosis A. The advent of synthetic retinoids for dermatologic therapy was welcomed by all clinicians with anticipation and excitement. Because the possible modifications of the vitamin A molecule's three main building units (the cyclic end group, the polyene side-chain, and the polar end group) (Fig. 15.1) seemed unlimited, the potential for synthesizing retinoids suitable for many diseases existed. More than 2500 retinoids have been screened with the goal of dissociating therapeutic action from the toxic effects of hypervitaminosis A using a chemically induced mouse skin papilloma model.

The "first-generation" of retinoids are the compounds resulting from manipulation of the polar end group of the polyene side-chain such as all-*trans*-retinoic acid (tretinoin) and 13-*cis*-retinoic acid (isotretinoin). Systemic isotretinoin is most effective for severe forms of acne, but it also temporarily improves inherited disorders of keratinization such as Darier's disease (keratosis follicularis) and lamellar ichthyosis. It has a rather limited role in the treatment of psoriasis (vide infra).

The "second generation" of retinoids results from replacing the cyclic end group with a series of ring systems. The best known example is the *p*-methoxytrimethylphenyl ethyl ester analogue of retinoic acid (etretinate), which was approved by the FDA for treatment of psoriasis in 1986. Its first-order metabolite, acitretin, has also been studied intensively as psoriasis treatment. It is apparently

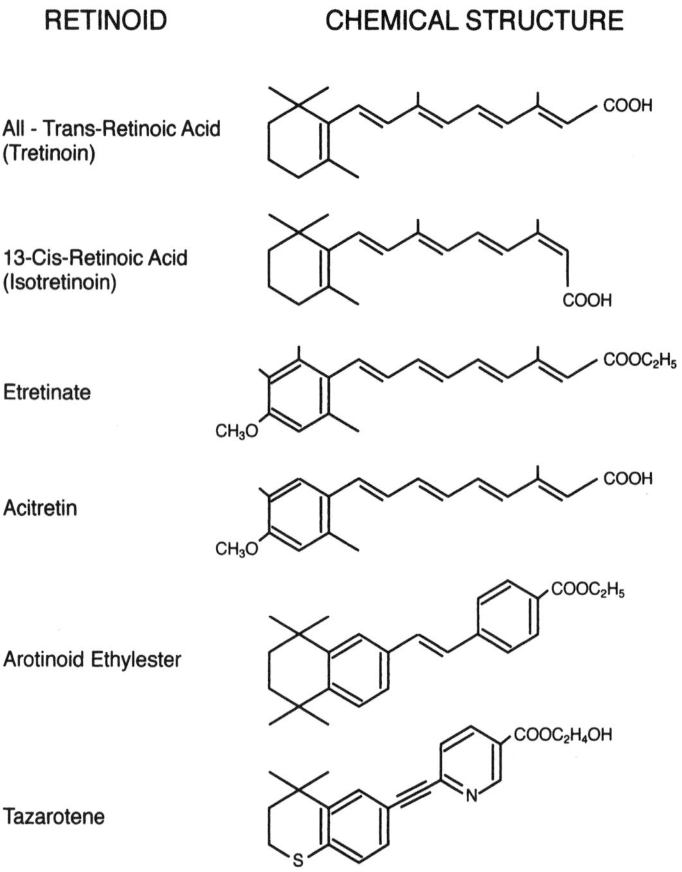

RETINOID   CHEMICAL STRUCTURE

All - Trans-Retinoic Acid
(Tretinoin)

13-Cis-Retinoic Acid
(Isotretinoin)

Etretinate

Acitretin

Arotinoid Ethylester

Tazarotene

Figure 15.1 Chemical structures of selected retinoids.

therapeutically equivalent to etretinate and received FDA approval
in 1996.

The "third generation" of retinoids consists of analogues with
various forms of cyclization of the polyene side-chain including the
arotinoids or benzoic acid derivatives of retinoic acid. Arotinoid ethyl
ester is 8000 times more potent than tretinoin in the papilloma
regression assay but is also 800 times more active in causing hypervitaminosis A. It has been used successfully to treat recalcitrant
psoriasis in limited trials but has not become commercially available.

The initial optimism with which the retinoids were received—
comparisons to the "corticosteroid era" of medicine were made—
has been dampened by problems with teratogenicity and the long
terminal half-life of etretinate. The therapeutic results with etretin-

ate and acitretin in the treatment of psoriasis have been good to excellent, especially in combination with other conventional treatments. With the exception of teratogenicity, the side-effects, while numerous, are generally not serious. The disappointments have been with response to monotherapy, lack of a durable remission, and the fact that, after more than 30 years of retinoid research, only four systemic drugs have been approved in the U.S. A new in vitro assay of retinoid effects on human keratinocyte cultures has been developed that may be more relevant for predicting activity in the treatment of psoriasis. Keratin profiles and the extent of envelope formation are assessed.

Absorption and metabolism

Bioavailability of the 40 mg isotretinoin (Accutane) capsule is 25%. Peak blood concentrations occur at 2–3 hours after ingestion. The blood concentration profile after oral administration can be described with a linear two compartment pharmacokinetic model. The terminal elimination half-life ranges from 10 to 20 hours. The major metabolite found in the blood and urine of patients on chronic therapy is 4-oxo-isotretinoin. After 6 hours, blood concentrations of the metabolite exceed those of the parent drug. The apparent half-life of 4-oxo-isotretinoin ranges from 11 to 50 hours. Enterohepatic circulation may be a component of isotretinoin pharmacokinetics. Isotretinoin is 99.9% bound to plasma albumin.

Etretinate has an absolute bioavailability of 40% following oral administration of the capsule; the bioavailability is significantly increased when taken with whole milk or a high-lipid diet. Peak plasma concentrations occur at about 4 hours. The carboxylic acid, metabolite acitretin, is formed by enzymatic hydrolysis of the ester in the gut, liver, and blood. Etretinate undergoes significant first-pass metabolism to acitretin prior to reaching the systemic circulation such that the metabolite appears in the blood before and exceeds the concentration of the parent drug.

After single-dose oral administration the apparent half-life for elimination of etretinate and acitretin is 6–13 hours; however, during chronic therapy, because etretinate is stored in adipose tissue, the terminal half-life is approximately 120 days. The data are consistent with a linear pharmacokinetic model with a deep peripheral compartment.

In a study of 47 patients receiving long-term etretinate therapy, seven had detectable serum drug levels (0.5–12 ng/ml) 2.1–2.9

years after discontinuing therapy. For comparison, during a 6-month course of treatment with doses ranging from 25 mg to 100 mg daily, the maximum serum concentrations ranged from 102 to 389 ng/ml. Patients with a greater amount of body fat tended to have higher serum concentrations and slower elimination of etretinate. Etretinate is more than 99% bound to plasma proteins, mainly lipoproteins, and acitretin is predominantly bound to albumin. Animal studies indicated biliary excretion, enterohepatic circulation, and substantial uptake of etretinate by the liver. Liver concentrations of etretinate in patients receiving the drug for 6 months were generally higher than concomitant plasma concentrations, and tended to be higher in livers with moderate or severe fatty infiltration.

Acitretin (Soriatane), the main active metabolite of etretinate, was developed to avoid the accumulation in adipose tissue and the slow elimination after discontinuation of the parent drug. The bioavailability of acitretin is 60% and is markedly increased with food intake. The peak plasma concentration is reached 2–6 hours after ingestion. During repeated dosing, the steady-state plasma concentration of 13-*cis*-acitretin is higher than all-*trans*-acitretin. The relatively short half-lives of acitretin (about 50 hours) and its 13-*cis*-isomer (75 hours) are such that, within 3 weeks of cessation of therapy, neither can be detected in plasma (<5 ng/ml). A new high-performance liquid chromatography assay detected etretinate in plasma and subcutaneous fat of a woman 4.3 years after stopping acitretin. Therefore, acitretin may be esterified to etretinate, a reaction that is enhanced by alcohol consumption and possibly excess body fat. The prevalence of detectable etretinate is higher in fat than in plasma among both current acitretin users and patients who have discontinued acitretin.

Mechanism of action

How synthetic retinoids improve psoriasis has not been elucidated. In order for retinoids to have biologic effects, there must be uptake from the plasma by cells, transport and metabolism in the cytoplasm, and interaction with receptors in the nucleus.

Recent major advances in our understanding of the biology of retinoids include the identification of compounds that are specific to receptor subtypes and preferentially bind to nuclear retinoic acid receptors (RAR-α, -β, -γ) or retinoid X receptor (RXR). The RARs bind to DNA and control the transcription of many target genes.

Different retinoids have different affinities for the various RARs. Therefore, it might be possible to segregate the therapeutic from the toxic effects. A new acetylenic retinoid tazarotene, is selective for gene transcription through RAR-γ (the major subtype in skin) and RAR-β and is inactive through RXR. It improves psoriasis by normalizing keratinocyte differentiation, by antiproliferative effects, and by decreasing expression of inflammatory markers.

Another important advance is the recognition of two cellular retinoic acid-binding proteins (CRABPs), CRABP I and II, that differ in their affinity for retinoid ligands and tissue distribution. CRABPs in turn control the amount of retinoid made available for binding to RARs in the nucleus. The response of a disease to synthetic retinoids might depend on the relative amounts of CRABP I and II expressed by the involved cells. For example, psoriatic epidermis synthesizes much more CRABP II than does normal epidermis, and CRABP II apparently does not bind isotretinoin. Isotretinoin, very effective for acne yet weakly active in psoriasis vulgaris, reduces sebaceous gland size and inhibits sebocyte proliferation. Isotretinoin also inhibits the conversion of retinol to dehydroretinol in epithelia. The aromatic retinoids do not exert any of these effects. Neither isotretinoin nor the aromatic retinoids alter plasma retinol levels.

Anti-inflammatory effects of retinoids have been demonstrated. For example, they inhibit neutrophil functions in vitro such as lysosomal enzyme release, superoxide anion production, antibody-dependent cytotoxicity, as well as chemotaxis in the presence of serum. Topical and systemic administration of retinoids reduces the intraepidermal accumulation of polymorphonuclear leukocytes after epicutaneous application of leukotriene TB_4. Kaplan *et al.* showed that etretinate therapy of psoriasis significantly reduced epidermal polyamine levels after 4 weeks before any significant decrease in epidermal DNA synthesis was detected, suggesting that this action might be responsible in part for the subsequent clinical improvement.

Clinical studies

Topical

Topical tretinoin cream is modestly effective for psoriasis but its use is limited by skin irritation. Isotretinoin cream 0.1% did not improve psoriasis in one placebo-controlled trial. Tazarotene (Tazorac), the first compound in a new generation of receptor-selective acetylenic retinoids, was formulated into a gel and applied once daily. In one study, 0.1% and 0.05% tazarotene gel applied once daily for 12 weeks produced 65% and 50% improvement, respectively, compared to 30% with vehicle gel; the differences were statistically significant. The patients were followed for an additional 12 weeks without therapy; success was sustained among 43% of the patients who received 0.05% tazarotene gel and 24% of the patients who received 0.1% tazarotene gel. Skin irritation (burning, itching, redness) was the main dose-related side-effect and was reported by about 20% of patients. Adverse effects led to a 10% dropout rate. Perceived advantages of tazarotene include:

1 Gel formulation may be applied to scalp.
2 No facial dermatitis reported (the drug is also approved for acne vulgaris).
3 There is minimal systemic absorption (about 5%).
4 It is applied once daily.
5 There is a possible sustained response.
6 A cream formulation is now available.
7 Combination with mid- and high-potency topical corticosteroids improves efficacy and reduces local irritation.

In a 2-week paired comparison study, the combination of tazarotene gel and calcipotriene ointment was equivalent to clobetasol ointment. Tazarotene gel 0.1% applied once daily for 2 weeks, followed by thrice weekly along with UVB phototherapy, improves and accelerates the efficacy of either UVB plus vehicle or UVB alone. Clinical studies with oral tazarotene are in progress.

Systemic

Double-blind studies showed both etretinate and acitretin to be significantly superior in efficacy to placebo in the treatment of psoriasis. In most studies of plaque-type psoriasis, 70–80% of patients had good to excellent (>50% clearing) results after 4–6 months of continuous treatment. Clinical improvement became significant in a dose-dependent fashion after 8 weeks of therapy. The optimal dose was 0.6–0.7 mg/kg/day, equivalent to 50–75 mg/day. All patients showed mucocutaneous side-effects with dose-dependent severity. A maintenance dose is necessary because psoriasis generally relapses 2–3 months after the discontinuation of therapy.

The aromatic retinoids are also effective for generalized pustular, palmoplantar pustular, and erythrodermic psoriasis. In one study, etretinate at 0.75 mg/kg/day was much more efficacious in achieving moderate to complete control of chronic plaque psoriasis than was isotretinoin at 1.5 mg/kg/day. However, in patients with generalized pustular psoriasis, isotretinoin (1.5–2.0 mg/kg/day) was effective at rapidly abating the pustulation and systemic symptoms. Additional therapy was required to induce complete clearing. In some patients, etretinate improved symptomatic psoriatic arthropathy, decreasing the pain and stiffness such that less anti-inflammatory medication was required.

Combinations with UVL

To achieve a greater therapeutic effect with lower toxicity, the retinoids have been combined with ultraviolet B (UVB) or psoralen with ultraviolet light A (PUVA). The rationale is that the desquamation and thinning of psoriatic plaques produced by retinoids would bring about a more rapid response to ultraviolet radiation. The combination of acitretin 50 mg daily for 12 weeks, and suberythemogenic UVB, three times a week, was superior to acitretin alone, which was superior to UVB plus placebo. The group treated with UVB and acitretin received a lower cumulative ultraviolet dose than did the group treated with UVB and placebo. In another trial, more aggressive UVB was combined with a lower dose of acitretin (25–35 mg/day) or placebo. At the end of 8 weeks, 60% of patients in the combination-treatment group and 24% in the control group attained 75% clinical improvement. For the same degree of improvement the cumulative UVB energy received was 40% less in the combination-treatment group.

Photochemotherapy (PUVA) has been combined with etretinate, acitretin, or isotretinoin as concurrent treatment or with prior retinoid treatment, also known as *re-PUVA*. Dubertret *et al.* "cleared" the psoriasis in 36 of 37 patients in less than 10 weeks with the combination of etretinate, 1 mg/kg/day, and PUVA three times a week. After skin clearing, PUVA was given once weekly for 2 months to two groups who were randomized to receive either etretinate, 0.5 mg/kg/day, or placebo as maintenance treatment for one year. The patients receiving placebo were twice as likely to have a relapse as the etretinate group. The investigators further showed that etretinate maintenance seemed most beneficial for those patients whose psoriasis cleared rapidly with PUVA; that is, requiring less than 18 treatments. Acitretin 0.5 mg/kg/day for 4 weeks combined with bath PUVA is also effective for severe psoriasis including pustular and erythrodermic psoriasis.

In 2001, a consensus conference recommended giving low-dose acitretin (25 mg/day or 0.3–0.5 mg/kg/day) for 2 weeks before initiating UVB or PUVA therapy. After clearing, institute maintenance therapy for 4 weeks at 75–90% of the final UV light dose. It is important to remember to reduce the dose of UVB or PUVA by 50% when adding a retinoid to ongoing suboptimal UV light therapy. Conversely, reduce the dose of failing retinoid monotherapy by 50% before introducing UVB or PUVA in order to avoid causing erythema of the thinned epidermis.

Palmoplantar psoriasis

The combination of PUVA-etretinate (0.6 mg/kg/day) was more effective than either PUVA or etretinate alone in recalcitrant palmoplantar pustulosis, clearing 78% of the sites compared to 25% or 17%, respectively. No untreated site cleared. Relapses generally occurred within 1–3 months after treatment was stopped. When acitretin 1 mg/kg/day or placebo was given for 5 days alone before the initiation of PUVA therapy, which was given four times weekly, and the combination was continued, complete clearing or marked improvement occurred in 22 (96%) of 23 and 20 (80%) of 25 patients, respectively. The acitretin-PUVA group required 29% fewer exposures and a 42% lower cumulative UVA dose than did the placebo-PUVA group. Similarly, when lower dosages of acitretin (50 mg, then 25 mg daily) or placebo were given prior to and during PUVA, significantly more patients in the acitretin-PUVA group (70% vs. 40%) achieved 75% improvement yet required a lower total UVA dose. The acitretin-PUVA combination was superior to placebo-PUVA in the treatment of severe palmoplantar psoriasis. Acitretin 25 mg/day was given for 3 weeks before PUVA was started, and continued. Whether re-PUVA utilizing isotretinoin, 0.5–1 mg/kg/day given for one week prior to the initiation of PUVA, is as effective for this indication as etretinate plus PUVA is controversial.

Arotinoids

Several successful therapeutic trials using the arotinoid ethyl ester and its metabolite arotinoid acid for the treatment of psoriasis have been reported. These drugs may have pronounced anti-inflammatory effects on psoriatic arthropathy and do not seem to produce significant elevations of serum lipids. The efficacy of etretinate and arotinoid ethyl ester in the treatment of psoriasis are comparable.

Conventional emollients and topical therapy may enhance the efficacy of systemic retinoids, allowing a reduction in dosage and dose-related mucocutaneous toxicity. The effect of etretinate and anthralin was additive in patients who were previously resistant to anthralin. The combination of etretinate, 0.5–0.66 mg/kg/day, with triamcinolone 0.1% and salicylic acid 5% cream, was superior to either agent alone. Retinoids may facilitate the penetration of anthralin and corticosteroids. The combination of calcipotriene with either etretinate or acitretin gave significantly better clearing than retinoid monotherapy.

Adverse effects

The toxicity of retinoids is essentially that of hypervitaminosis A. Side-effects are common, and some should be expected in all patients who receive therapeutic doses. Patients should be warned not to take supplementary vitamin A beyond the 5000 units ordinarily supplied in multiple-vitamin tablets. Fortunately, most of the unwanted effects such as cheilitis are nuisances made tolerable by emollients or by reducing the dosage, and are completely reversible with cessation of therapy. Theoretical concerns, such as long-term cardiovascular risks, may be mitigated by screening for other risk factors, frequent monitoring of blood lipid levels, and early dietary, medical, or dose-reduction intervention. The severity of idiosyncratic hepatotoxic reactions may be limited by close monitoring of liver enzyme levels and early discontinuation of therapy. Finally, the most serious adverse effect of all, teratogenicity, may be completely avoided by simply not prescribing retinoids for women of child-bearing potential. In practice, such a conservative stance can be modified with the precautions discussed below.

Mucocutaneous toxicity

The most common and frequently troublesome side-effects of oral retinoids relate to the skin and mucous membranes because of changes in the stratum corneum, decreased sebum production, and increased insensible water loss. Any or all of the mucocutaneous

Mucous membranes	
Dry lips, cheilitis	
Dry mouth, thirst	
Dry nasal mucosa, epistaxis	
Dry eyes, irritation, conjunctivitis	

Skin
Dry skin, xerosis
Pruritus
Palm, sole peeling
Fingertip peeling
Skin fragility
Sticky skin
Dermatitis
Flare of psoriasis

Hair and nails
Hair loss
Change in hair texture
Paronychia
Nail dystrophies
Periungual pyogenic granulomas

Table 15.1 Mucocutaneous side-effects of retinoids.

side-effects listed in Table 15.1 could occur in an individual patient with any degree of severity. Cheilitis is the hallmark of retinoid therapy. Without it, one may assume that the patient is noncompliant or that the dosage prescribed is subtherapeutic. Another problem associated with dry lips not frequently mentioned, especially in older patients with dentures, is angular cheilitis, fissures at the angles of the mouth colonized by *Candida* species. It is for this reason that I recommend frequent emolliation of the lips with petrolatum or Aquaphor healing ointment *without* hydrocortisone and treatment of the fissures with nystatin ointment or clotrimazole cream. Concomitant oral candidiasis, if present, must also be treated with nystatin suspension oral rinses, clotrimazole troches, or systemic fluconazole.

Several cutaneous findings may be explained by ultrastructural or kinetic studies of retinoid-treated skin. About 15–30% of patients complain of a "sticky" or "clammy" feel to their skin. The skin may appear more shiny, pink, and smooth than before treatment. A mucous-like material that stains positively with periodic acid–Schiff (PAS) has been detected in an intracellular and intercellular loca-

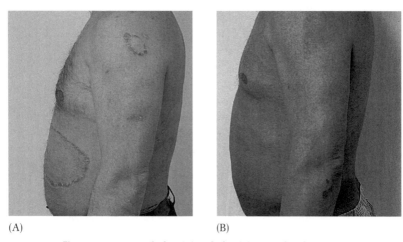

(A)   (B)

Figure 15.2 Patient before (A) and after (B) 9 months of treatment with acitretin 75 mg/day.

tions in the epidermis of etretinate- and arotinoid-treated psoriatics. Increased skin fragility, noted in 20–60% of patients in various studies, may be related to dehiscence of desmosomes between adjacent keratinocytes seen by electron microscopy. It is uncertain whether the development of granulation tissue in the nail folds or rare cases of blistering and ulceration represent clinical manifestations of skin fragility.

During the first month of therapy with retinoids, there may be a flare-up of psoriasis, seen as an expansion of established psoriatic plaques, or the appearance of new papulosquamous lesions. There are several possible explanations for this. I believe it is seen more frequently in patients with severe disease who are withdrawn from other therapies that had previously maintained stability of their disease. Thus, extension of disease and new lesions could be explained by the natural progression of disease. This phenomenon is observed less frequently in practice because patients whose disease is severe enough to warrant systemic therapy are usually not given a "washout" period and may receive adjunctive therapy along with retinoids. As chronic plaque psoriasis resolves during etretinate or acitretin therapy, however, it is common to observe central thinning followed by clearing with centrifugal spread of the scaling border, which closely resembles tinea corporis ("ringworm") (Fig. 15.2). The apparent worsening of psoriasis prior to clearing with etretinate may be due to a simultaneous decrease in the mitosis in involved skin and an increase in the uninvolved skin, both of which have been demonstrated in cell cultures. Another explanation for the worsening of psoriasis during retinoid therapy, especially if it occurs later in the course, is the development of an eczematoid eruption that may be confused with psoriasis. It can occur anywhere but has a predilection for the backs of hands and arms. It may be improved by applying topical steroids or by reducing the retinoid dosage. The development of this so-called *retinoid dermatitis* is highly suggestive of an atopic diathesis. Miscellaneous rare cutaneous complications of etretinate have been reported and include erythroderma, toxic epidermal necrolysis, and generalized edema.

Hair loss is definitely more common and more marked, in the range of 50–70%, at higher dosages in patients receiving the aromatic retinoids compared to those receiving isotretinoin. It takes several months to evolve and is believed to be a telogen effluvium. The hair loss is not limited to the scalp, but that is where it is most noticeable and distressing, particularly to women. Alopecia is reversible and may be improved by reducing the dose. A smaller percentage of patients notice a change in hair texture. Occasionally straight hair becomes more curly or kinked or demonstrates pili torti. These latter changes may not be reversible. Chronic paronychia, granulation tissue in the lateral nail folds, and nail dystrophies occur in 10–40% of patients. The latter may include softening of the nailplate, Beau's lines, onychomadesis, proximal onychoschizia, and distal onycholysis if there is also desquamation of fingertip skin. Fingernail growth rates of psoriatic patients, already higher than in normal control subjects, are further increased during etretinate therapy.

Ophthalmologic toxicity

Twenty to 50% have ocular side-effects in the form of dry eyes, conjunctivitis, or eye irritation, probably as a result of changes in meibomian gland function, an altered lipid layer, and instability of the tear film. Frequent use of artificial tears may decrease the irritation, but contact lens users may have to decrease wearing time. The dry eye tends to be colonized with *Staphylococcus aureus*, and purulent conjunctivitis may develop. Scrubbing the eyelids with baby shampoo and applying ophthalmic antibiotic ointments may be indicated. While corneal opacities usually do not affect vision, it may be prudent to reduce the dose or discontinue treatment if they develop. Synthetic retinoids can cause symptomatic decreased night vision, probably as a result of interfering with the visual cycle (rhodopsin dissociated by light to opsin and all-*trans*-retinal).

Problems with decreased night vision or excessive glare while driving have been encountered during therapy with isotretinoin and aromatic retinoids. Patients with symptoms of color or night vision dysfunction should be referred to an ophthalmologist. Dark adaptometry may be the preferred test for monitoring night blindness. In affected patients, vision gradually returns to normal after treatment is stopped.

Visual disturbances associated with persistent global headaches should alert the physician to the rare occurrence of papilledema or pseudotumor cerebri. The retinoid should be discontinued and treatment undertaken in consultation with the ophthalmologist or neurologist. Patients should not receive tetracycline or minocycline in conjunction with retinoids because they may increase the risk of pseudotumor cerebri.

Musculoskeletal toxicity

Muscle cramps and arthralgias are quite common during retinoid therapy. In a 5-year prospective follow-up of 956 patients taking etretinate, 236 noted a joint problem and 79 patients self-reported joint improvement. The latter group were significantly more likely to be high-dose etretinate users. Painless muscle stiffness has occurred in patients taking etretinate. A patient with exfoliative dermatitis developed nonspecific myopathy during etretinate treatment. Examination of a muscle biopsy specimen indicated segmental muscle necrosis. Muscle pain and weakness developed in three patients during etretinate therapy, and the authors (Hodak *et al.*) concluded that etretinate can induce reversible skeletal muscle damage. Muscle weakness with elevated aldolase and creatine phosphokinase levels developed in a patient taking acitretin. Electromyography showed severe myopathic changes, but a biopsy specimen showed no inflammation. Considerable improvement occurred within a month of stopping the drug.

Bony changes including demineralization, thinning of the long bones, cortical hyperostosis, periosteitis, and premature closure of epiphyses have been identified in individuals with chronic hypervitaminosis A.

Since the initial report of a diffuse idiopathic skeletal hyperostosis (DISH)-like syndrome in four patients receiving long-term high dose isotretinoin, it has become clear that small pointed excrescences may develop on the anterior margins of one or more vertebral bodies after only 4 months of therapy. There was generally no correlation between the radiographic finding of small spurs and musculoskeletal signs or symptoms.

Similar DISH-like spine involvement was observed in 11 (29%) of 38 patients receiving etretinate (mean dose, 0.8 mg/kg/day) for 5 years. However, extraspinal tendon and ligament calcifications of feet (76%), pelvis (53%), and knees (42%) were much more common. About half the patients had no symptoms referable to the site of radiographic abnormality.

Acitretin may produce similar bony changes and ligamentous calcification. Kilcoyne found that 14% of patients showed progression of spinal spurs at two sites after 3 years of therapy. He further enumerated problems with the design of prospective radiographic studies of psoriatic patients. Because DISH of the spine is ordinarily associated with aging and psoriatic patients tend to be older, with preexisting arthritic changes, there should be control groups consisting of age- and sex-matched normal subjects and psoriatics who are followed for progressive changes over time without retinoid therapy.

Well-established guidelines for monitoring skeletal toxicity in adults are lacking. Some investigators recommend annual lateral radiographs of the spine and a single lateral view of the ankle. Others recommend pretreatment radiographs with follow-up attention only to areas of skeletal pain or restricted mobility.

Long-term etretinate but not isotretinoin therapy has been associated with osteoporosis of peripheral sites (cortical bone) but not the spine (predominantly trabecular bone). One study used the standard techniques to measure bone mineral density (BMD), single- and dual-photon absorptiometry. However, the study is controversial for a number of reasons:

1 Most of the patients did not have psoriasis.
2 No assessment of pretreatment BMD was made.
3 Skeletal hyperostosis and extraspinal tendon and ligament calcifications may have caused technical difficulties.

Several other studies have yielded conflicting conclusions. A group of 13 psoriatic patients who received etretinate for 3.7 years had significantly decreased BMD of the lumbar spine compared to a

Table 15.2 Strategies to minimize retinoid-induced skeletal toxicity.

1 Select alternative therapy for children less than 16 years of age
2 Use the lowest possible dose of retinoid to achieve the desired result
3 Avoid long-term treatment whenever possible
4 If long-term maintenance with retinoids is required, give a drug-free holiday for three or more months after every 9 months of therapy
5 Order radiographs of symptomatic regions
6 For perimenopausal women, consider estrogen replacement therapy, calcium and vitamin D supplementation, a bisphosphonate such as aledronate (Fosamax), and pretreatment bone densitometry

control group of psoriatics using topical corticosteroids. Eighteen female patients with palmoplantar pustulosis had significantly lower BMD of the forearm and spine compared to control subjects. The severity correlated with the duration of disease, suggesting that the osteoporosis is related to the primary pathologic process or that treatment with topical corticosteroids under occlusion may be contributory. Another three patients were treated with etretinate and acitretin for about 15 years. They all developed typical hyperostoses of the spine, calcanei, acetabulum and extraspinal calcifications that were monitored for 9 years. There were no clinical symptoms or signs of progression, regression, or functional impairment. Moreover, bone densitometry revealed no signs of osteoporosis. Monitoring for osteoporosis should be done in patients with the standard risk factors: female, post-menopausal, Caucasian, low-weight, and chronic use of systemic corticosteroids.

In summary, many patients will develop vertebral osteophytes and bony bridging of vertebral bodies during chronic retinoid therapy. DISH-like spinal changes are less frequent with etretinate and acitretin than with isotretinoin, but extraspinal calcifications may be more common. Fortunately, in most cases these changes are not clinically significant and are not contraindications to further treatment (Table 15.2). The relationship between osteoporosis and chronic retinoid treatment of psoriasis has not yet been fully elucidated.

Liver toxicity

Elevated levels of liver enzymes, aspartate aminotransferase (AST), alanine aminotransferase (ALT), and lactic dehydrogenase (LDH), occur in about 20% of patients treated with synthetic retinoids. Most of the changes are slight to moderate, are asymptomatic, and normalize during therapy or after it is discontinued. In clinical studies of etretinate in the U.S., however, 10 (1.5%) of 652 patients developed evidence of clinical or histologic hepatitis possibly or probably related to the drug. This finding was confirmed in a post-marketing long-term prospective study of 956 patients. While most cases of acute clinical hepatitis resolved with cessation of therapy, sequelae, such as chronic active hepatitis and hepatitis-related deaths, have occurred. These may represent idiosyncratic reactions to etretinate. Chronic etretinate therapy did not cause significant histologic alterations of the liver in a group of patients preselected for potential hepatotoxicity and followed prospectively for 3 years. A 2-year prospective study of acitretin-treated patients did not demonstrate biopsy-proven hepatotoxicity. Therefore, it is not necessary to perform liver biopsies on a routine basis in patients treated with long-term etretinate or acitretin therapy.

Alteration of lipid metabolism

The retinoids cause hyperlipidemia. In the short term, as in isotretinoin treatment of acne or the induction phase of re-PUVA with etretinate or acitretin, reversible laboratory parameters probably have no adverse effect on the risk of cardiovascular disease. However, lipid abnormalities may be clinically significant during long-term therapy of psoriasis, especially if patients have other risk factors such as a personal or family history of a lipid abnormality, obesity, diabetes, smoking, and alcoholism. Moreover, two independent surveys of a total of 57 patients with psoriasis suggested an increased risk of atherosclerosis based on significantly decreased high-density lipoprotein cholesterol (HDL-C) and significantly elevated total cholesterol and low-density lipoprotein cholesterol (LDL-C), respectively, compared to healthy control subjects. In the 5-year follow-up of 956 psoriasis patients treated with etretinate, the incidence of myocardial infarction or diabetes was not greater than expected in the population. Etretinate does not alter the insulin requirements of diabetics. Serum triglycerides and cholesterol were elevated in 45–65% and 0–16%, respectively, of patients treated with etretinate or acitretin. Decreases in HDL-C occurred in 30–37% of patients.

Experimental evidence in humans seems to support the hypothesis that retinoids induce increased hepatic production of

Table 15.3 Strategies to reduce hyperlipidemia.

1 Reduce weight
2 Limit alcohol intake
3 Cease smoking
4 Reduce simple sugar intake
5 Increase aerobic exercise
6 Take fish oil supplements
7 If triglycerides attain 600 mg/dl, reduce the dose or discontinue therapy
8 Take lipid-lowering drugs, e.g. gemfibrozil, atorvastatin calcium

apolipoprotein C-III (apo C-III), which acts by delaying catabolism of triglyceride-rich particles and interferes with apo E-mediated clearance of these particles from the plasma. Retinoids modulate HDL levels (by inducing apo A-I and apo A-II production) and by effects on genes that control HDL catabolism. Plasma HDL levels are inversely correlated with triglyceride levels. Strategies to reduce retinoid-induced hyperlipidemia should be implemented if the triglyceride level attains 400 mg/dl. (Table 15.3). One should not allow triglyceride levels to reach 800 mg/dl because of the risk of acute pancreatitis and eruptive xanthomas. It may be necessary to consult a dietitian or an endocrinologist if the use of lipid-lowering drugs is contemplated. Gemfibrozil (Lopid) is useful in patients with hyperlipidemia due to acitretin who were recalcitrant to dietary manipulation and dose reductions. Triglyceride and cholesterol levels were significantly reduced, but the LDL/HDL ratio remained unchanged.

Fish oil supplements (3 g of omega-3 fatty acids daily) given to patients receiving etretinate or acitretin significantly decreased triglyceride levels in every patient (mean, 27%). There was a mean increase in HDL-C levels of 11%. Fish oil had no effect on total cholesterol, apo B, or LDL-C levels. Fish oil supplementation may be a valuable adjunctive measure to ameliorate the lipid changes in patients receiving long-term retinoid therapy. The combination of low-dose etretinate (0.3–0.5 mg/kg/day) with eicosapentaenoic acid 1800 mg/day produced significantly better clearing of psoriasis than etretinate alone. A regimen of a low-fat isocaloric diet supplemented with fish oil concentrate (15 ml daily) combined with an aerobic exercise program could conceivably reverse most of the deleterious retinoid-induced lipid perturbations. If fish oil supplements are used as a source of omega-3 fatty acids, one should select the cholesterol-free brands of Max-EPA (R.P. Scherer, Clearwater, FL) or Cardi-Omega 3 (Thomson Medical Co., New York, NY).

Teratogenicity

Retinoids are potent teratogens. Isotretinoin and etretinate can cause spontaneous abortions and birth defects when given to women who are pregnant or, in the case of etretinate, even when conception occurs up to 24 months after the drug is discontinued. The anomalies described in the literature include small or absent ears, cleft palate, microphthalmos, micrognathia, central nervous system malformations such as hydrocephalus, conotruncal heart defects and aortic arch abnormalities, retinal or optic nerve abnormalities, and thymic defects. It is possible that a major mechanism of retinoid teratogenesis is a deleterious effect on cephalic neural-crest cell activity at the critical period of embryogenesis. It is estimated that, of all fetuses exposed during the first trimester who reach delivery, about 25% will have a major congenital anomaly. Acitretin must be considered a possible teratogen in humans because it is embryotoxic or teratogenic in animal species.

All three synthetic systemic retinoids are contraindicated during pregnancy and breast-feeding. In the case of isotretinoin, more fetal exposures and malformations have occurred than for etretinate. While the only *labeled* indication for isotretinoin in the U.S. is severe cystic acne, it may be prescribed for fully informed women of child-bearing potential with severe psoriasis when it is appropriate in the best judgment of the dermatologic consultant. Conception is safe one or more cycles after discontinuation of isotretinoin because of its relatively brief elimination half-life. The guidelines for prescribing isotretinoin have been published by the manufacturer in the promotional and package insert material. Briefly, the guidelines are:

1 Begin using two effective contraceptive methods simultaneously 1 month before and continue until 1 month after therapy.

2 Obtain a negative sensitive pregnancy test at the qualification visit and a negative pregnancy test on the second day of the next normal menstrual period.

3 Repeat the serum pregnancy test monthly during therapy and obtain negative result before refilling the prescription.

As discussed earlier, etretinate is stored in the adipose tissue and released slowly for months or years after discontinuation of therapy.

Table 15.4 Retinoid use in women with childbearing potential.

1 Do *not* use etretinate

2 If a retinoid is the next logical alternative, acitretin may be used but all precautions against pregnancy must be taken for 3 years after therapy is stopped

3 Alcohol must not be consumed during treatment with acitretin and 2 months after therapy is stopped

4 Isotretinoin may be effective for pustular psoriasis at 1.5–2.0 mg/kg/day, but maintenance with isotretinoin, PUVA, or MTX is necessary

5 Isotretinoin is not very effective for plaque psoriasis as monotherapy or combined with UVB. Therefore, consider using isotretinoin or acitretin in a re-PUVA regimen

Low levels of etretinate were detected in the blood of five out of 47 patients up to 2.9 years after therapy. Three of 37 pregnancies occurring within 24 months of concluding etretinate therapy resulted in congenital anomalies. There is probably an etretinate blood and fat level below which the risk of fetal malformations is equivalent to the background rate. Until that level is known and the measurements can be obtained in patients, it is risky to prescribe etretinate to a fertile woman.

Much of the work done that proved acitretin to be superior to placebo and as efficacious as etretinate, either alone or in combination with ultraviolet light, was based on the pharmacokinetic premise that acitretin was not stored in the fat and had a short terminal half-life. If proven to be true, it would have allowed acitretin to be prescribed for fertile woman with severe psoriasis while following the established contraception guidelines for isotretinoin. It is now known that the ethylesterification of acitretin takes place and is correlated with the amount of alcohol intake. In one 35-year-old woman who admitted to sporadic moderate alcohol intake, etretinate could be measured in plasma and fat 52 months after the last acitretin dose. Two acitretin-treated women in the study by Maier and Honigsmann, in whom no etretinate was detected, gave birth to healthy children 25 and 40 months after stopping the drug. Neither drank any alcohol. No positive correlation between excess body weight and the amount of etretinate biotransformation was found. The prescribing guidelines for acitretin are the same as for isotretinoin with the notable exceptions of strict alcohol abstinence during treatment and for 2 months after stopping therapy and a post-therapy contraceptive period of *3 years* (Table 15.4).

How to use synthetic retinoids

Retinoids are complex and potent drugs. They should only be prescribed by physicians who are experienced in the treatment of moderate to severe plaque-type psoriasis, localized or generalized pustular psoriasis, and erythrodermic psoriasis. The prescriber must also be thoroughly familiar with the acute and chronic toxicity of retinoids and understand the risk of teratogenicity. Consultation with a dermatologist is usually in order. The package insert states that acitretin "should be reserved for patients who are unresponsive to other therapies or whose clinical condition contraindicates the use of other treatments." Whereas MTX and cyclosporine are more effective than acitretin as monotherapy, I would select the retinoid first in the appropriate clinical setting, to avoid the long-term risk to the liver and kidney, respectively. If UVB or PUVA is available and practical, however, I would consider using it before choosing a retinoid or possibly combining the retinoid with ultraviolet light.

The patient information brochures published and distributed by Roche Laboratories should be read by patients before they are prescribed the drug. A good strategy is to order baseline laboratory studies while the patient reviews the brochure at home, and discuss results and answer any remaining questions about the drug and treatment plan on the next visit (Table 15.5).

There has been discussion in the literature regarding the dosage of etretinate and acitretin, that is, whether to start high and taper or start low and work the dose upward. The latter method is predicated on combining the retinoid with efficacious UV therapy, while the former allows retinoid monotherapy to be effective. After working with both methods for both drugs, I favor a starting dose of about 0.3 mg/kg/day taken once daily with the largest meal of the day. The dosage is gradually increased monthly to a maximum of 0.75–1.0 mg/kg/day, based on clinical response, adverse effects, and laboratory results. I usually prescribe concomitant anthralin (highest concentration tolerated), calcipotriene, or group II topical corticosteroids for recalcitrant lesions. The psoriasis recrudesces within 3 months of stopping acitretin.

The optimal combination is retinoid therapy for 1–2 weeks followed by PUVA or UVB phototherapy. This technique allows clearing to occur earlier and at a lower total energy exposure than the respective light therapy alone. The retinoid can be stopped and the light continued at a decreased frequency for maintenance of

Table 15.5 Recommended monitoring guidelines for etretinate and acitretin.

1 Baseline complete blood cell count, liver function tests, 12-hour fasting lipid profile, electrolytes, blood urea nitrogen, creatinine, and urinalysis (liver biopsy is *not* ordered)

2 Repeat liver function tests and fasting lipid measurements every 2 weeks until levels have stabilized

3 Repeat full battery every 3 months during therapy

4 Monitor clinical efficacy monthly until disease has stabilized, then every 2–3 months

5 Ophthalmologic consultation is *not* routinely ordered. Reserve for purulent conjunctivitis, corneal opacities, decreased night-vision or increased glare, papilledema, or suspected pseudotumor cerebri. Only the latter is a contraindication to further retinoid therapy

6 X-rays are *not* routinely ordered. Reserve for persistently symptomatic bones or joints. The findings of vertebral osteophyte formation, spinal ligament calcification, or extraspinal tendon or ligament calcification do not preclude further use of retinoids

7 Measurements of bone mineral density are *not* routinely ordered

8 Strategies to reduce long-term bony toxicity and the cardiovascular risk of sustained unfavorable LDL-C to HDL-C ratio include intermittent courses of retinoids (6–9 months, separated by 1–3 months off drug), reduced maintenance dosage, low-fat diet and fish oil supplementation, and concomitant administration of lipid-lowering agents

remission. Re-PUVA (systemic or bath) should be used for recalcitrant palmoplantar pustulosis.

Patients with pustular psoriasis usually respond more rapidly than plaque or erythrodermic psoriasis. For erythrodermic psoriasis, the recommendation is to start with a lower dose of etretinate or acitretin (0.25–0.33 mg/kg/day) and gradually increase upwards by similar increments. This method is intended to avoid the early development of "retinoid dermatitis," which, if superimposed upon erythroderma could worsen both the appearance and symptoms of the disease. The dose needed for maximal improvement, however, is usually the same as that for plaque psoriasis.

Selected references

Anstey A., Hawk J. L. M. (1997) Isotretinoin-PUVA in women with psoriasis. (Letter to editor). *Br J Dermatol* **136**, 798–799.

Brazzell R. K., Coburn W. A. (1982) Pharmacokinetics of the retinoids isotretinoin and etretinate. *J Am Acad Dermatol* **6**, 643–651.

Chandraratna R. A. (1997) Tazarotene: The first receptor-selective topical retinoid for the treatment of psoriasis. *J Am Acad Dermatol* **37** (2 Pt 3), S12–S17.

Chandraratna R. A. S. (1996) Tazarotene—first of a new generation of receptor-selective retinoids. *Br J Dermatol* **135**, 18–25.

Danno K., Sugie N. (1998) Combination therapy with low-dose etretinate and eicosapentaenoic acid for psoriasis vulgaris. *J Dermatol* **25**, 703–705.

DiGiovanna J. J., Sollitto R. B., Abangan N. *et al.* (1995) Osteoporosis is a toxic effect of long-term etretinate therapy. *Arch Dermatol* **131**, 1263–1267.

Dubertret L., Chastang C., Beylot C. *et al.* (1985) Maintenance treatment of psoriasis by Tigason: a double-blind randomized clinical trial. *Br J Dermatol* **113**, 323–330.

Duvic M. (1998) Pharmacologic profile of tazarotene. *Cutis* **61** (Suppl. 2), 22–26.

Giannetti A., Coppini M., Bertazzoni M. G. *et al.* (1999) Clinical trial of the efficacy and safety of oral etretinate with calcipotriol cream compared with etretinate alone in moderate-severe psoriasis. *J Eur Acad Dermatol Venereol* **13**, 91–95.

Herrmann G., Jungblut R. M., Goerz G. (1997) Skeletal changes after long-term therapy with systemic retinoids. (Letter to editor) *Br J Dermatol* **136**, 469–470.

Hodak E., David M., Gadoth N., Sandbank M. (1987) Etretinate-induced skeletal muscle damage. *Br J Dermatol* **116**, 623–626.

Kaplan R. P., Russell D. H., Lowe N. J. (1983) Etretinate therapy for psoriasis: clinical responses, remission times, epidermal DNA and polyamine responses. *J Am Acad Dermatol* **8**, 95–102.

Kilcoyne R. F. (1991) The skeletal effects of retinoids and their relationship to DISH. *Fifth International Psoriasis Symposium Proceedings. San Francisco, CA July 1991*, 117.

Koo J. Y., Lowe N. J., Lew-Kaya D. A. *et al.* (2000) Tazarotene plus UVB phototherapy in the treatment of psoriasis. *J Am Acad Dermatol* **43**, 821–828.

Krueger G. G., Drake L. A., Elias P. M. *et al.* (1998) The safety and efficacy of tazarotene gel, a topical acetylenic retinoid in the treatment of psoriasis. *Arch Dermatol* **134**, 57–60.

Larsen F. G., Steinkjer B., Jakibsen P. *et al.* (2000) Acitretin is converted to etretinate only during concomitant alcohol intake. *Br J Dermatol* **143**, 1164–1169.

Lebwohl M., Ali S. (2001) Treatment of psoriasis. Part 2. Systemic therapies. *J Am Acad Dermatol* **45**, 649–661.

Lebwohl M., Drake L., Menter A. *et al.* (2001) Consensus conference: Acitretin in combination with UVB or PUVA in the treatment of psoriasis. *J Am Acad Dermatol* **45**, 544–553.

Lebwohl M. (2000) Strategies to optimize efficacy, duration of remission, and safety in the treatment of plaque psoriasis by using tazarotene in combination with a corticosteroid. *J Am Acad Dermatol* **43**, 543–546.

Lowe N. J., Prystowsky J. H., Bourget T. *et al.* (1991) Acitretin plus UVB therapy for psoriasis. Comparisons with placebo plus UVB and acitretin alone. *J Am Acad Dermatol* 24, 591–594.

Magis N. L., Blummel J. J., Kerkhof P. C., Gerritsen R. M. (2000) The treatment of psoriasis with etretinate and acitretin: a follow up of actual use. *Eur J Dermatol* 10, 517–521.

Maier H., Honigsmann H. (2001) Assessment of acitretin-treated female patients of childbearing age and subsequent risk of teratogenicity. (Letter to editor). *Br J Dermatol* 145, 1028–1029.

Muchenberger S., Schopf E., Simon J. C. (1997) The combination of oral acitretin and bath PUVA for the treatment of severe psoriasis. *Br J Dermatol* 137, 587–589.

Nymann P., Kollerup G., Jemec G. B., Grossman E. (1996) Decreased bone mineral density in patients with pustulosis palmaris et plantaris. *Dermatol* 192, 307–311.

Okada N., Nomura M., Morimato S. *et al.* (1994) Bone mineral density of the lumbar spine in psoriatic patients with long term etretinate therapy. *J Dermatol* 21, 308–311.

Reynoso-von Prateln C., Martinez-Abundis E., Balcazar-Munoz B. R. *et al.* (2003) Lipid profile, insulin secretion, and insulin sensitivity in psoriasis. *J Am Acad Dermatol* 48, 882–885.

Roenigk H. H. Jr, Callen J. P., Guzzo C. A. *et al.* (1999) Effects of acitretin therapy on the liver. *J Am Acad Dermatol* 41, 584–588.

Rosen K., Mobacken H., Swanbeck G. (1987) PUVA, etretinate, and PUVA-etretinate therapy for pustulosis palmplantaris. *Arch Dermatol* 123, 885–889.

Ruzicka T., Sommerburg C., Braun-Falco O. *et al.* (1990) Efficiency of acitretin in combination with UVB in the treatment if severe psoriasis. *Arch Dermatol* 126, 482–486.

Soriatane Package Insert, Roche Laboratories, January 2001.

Staels B. (2001) Regulation of lipid and lipoprotein metabolism by retinoids. *J Am Acad Dermatol* 45, 5158–5167.

Stern R. S., Fitzgerald E., Ellis C. N. *et al.* (1995) The safety of etretinate as long-term therapy for psoriasis: Results of the etretinate follow-up study. *J Am Acad Dermatol* 33, 44–52.

Tanew A., Guggenbichler A., Honigsmann H. *et al.* (1991) Photochemotherapy for severe psoriasis without or in combination with acitretin: a randomized double-blind comparison study. *J Am Acad Dermatol* 25, 682–684.

Van de Kerkhof P. C., Cambazard F., Hutchinson P. E. *et al.* (1998) The effect of addition of calcipotriol ointment (50 micrograms/g) to acitretin therapy in psoriasis. *Br J Dermatol* 138, 84–89.

Vanizor Kural B., Orem A., Cimsit G. *et al.* (2003) Evaluation of the atherogenic tendency of lipids and lipoprotein content and their relationships with oxidant-antioxidant system in patients with psoriasis. *Clin Chim Acta* 328, 71–82.

16   Methotrexate

Charles Camisa

Methotrexate (MTX) was first used for psoriasis in 1958. Since then, it has become the most common antimetabolite prescribed by dermatologists for psoriasis.

MTX is a folic acid antagonist. It competes with folic acid for binding sites on the intracellular enzyme dihydrofolate reductase (DHFR), which converts dihydrofolate to tetrahydrofolate. Tetrahydrofolate is the active form of folic acid that is necessary for thymidine synthesis and for the donation of methyl groups in purine synthesis. The affinity of MTX for binding sites on DHFR is 100,000 times greater than that of folic acid. The inhibition of folic acid reduction effectively inhibits the DNA synthesis (S) phase of the cell cycle. Psoriatic epidermis is more susceptible to the action of MTX because it has a larger fraction of cells in the S phase and a shorter cell cycle than normal epidermis. Therefore, if MTX were present in keratinocytes for approximately 36 hours, it might be expected to inhibit most of the proliferating psoriatic cells while affecting only about 10% of the normal keratinocytes.

Proliferating lymphoid cell lines were 1000 times more sensitive to the growth inhibitory effects of MTX than were normal human keratinocytes in cultures. Moreover, at concentrations of MTX attained in vivo during treatment, more than 95% of proliferating lymphoid cells were killed compared to less than 10% of epidermal cells. These findings suggest that in patients with psoriasis, lymphoid cells are more likely to be the major cellular target of MTX than keratinocytes.

Metabolism

MTX is readily absorbed from the gastrointestinal tract at the doses routinely employed in psoriasis treatment. Intramuscular injections of MTX are rapidly and completely absorbed. The terminal half-life is about 10 hours. In general, doses between 7.5 mg and 25 mg weekly can be administered either orally or parenterally to the same patient with the expectation of equivalent efficacy and toxicity. There may be considerable interpatient variability in MTX blood levels based on the rate of absorption, rate of excretion, and exchange between plasma proteins and tissues. MTX is retained in tissues, particularly the kidneys and liver, for weeks or months presumably bound as polyglutamates to intracellular DHFR.

Metabolism of MTX does not seem to occur to a significant degree, and most of the drug is excreted by the kidneys. About 90% of MTX is excreted in the urine unchanged within 24 hours by glomerular filtration and active tubular secretion. Therefore, renal insufficiency magnifies the toxicity of low doses of MTX. A small amount of oral MTX is excreted in the feces, proportional to the dosage, probably through the biliary tract.

Drug interactions

MTX toxicity may be increased in cases of folic acid deficiency due to malabsorption or malnutrition. Drugs which impair folic acid absorption, such as barbiturates and nitrofurantoin, should be avoided. Moreover, drugs that inhibit DHFR should not be given concomitantly with MTX: trimethoprim-sulfamethoxazole, triamterene, and pyrimethamine.

Fifty to 70% of MTX is bound to albumin and may be competitively displaced from binding sites by certain drugs, including salicylates, sulfonamides, probenecid and phenytoin which may increase free MTX. These interactions are usually not clinically relevant in the treatment of psoriasis.

Drugs that also undergo tubular secretion, such as aspirin, probenecid, phenylbutazone, penicillin, ascorbic acid, and sulfonamides, may prolong excretion and expose patients to toxic levels of MTX. Toxicity can also occur with concomitant use of nonsteroidal anti-inflammatory drugs (NSAIDs) with higher doses of MTX. Ketoprofen, piroxicam, and flurbiprofen do not appear to affect MTX disposition and may be used in combination with low doses of MTX. Any drug that has the potential to reduce glomerular filtration rate (e.g. cyclosporine, aminoglycoside antibiotics) should be used with caution in combination with MTX.

Efficacy

Double-blind studies confirmed the superiority of MTX over placebo in improving the skin manifestations, joint symptoms, and function in psoriatics. Good to excellent responses (50–100% clearing of psoriasis) have been found in 70% of patients with severe disease using a single weekly oral dose of MTX (Fig. 16.1). When Roenigk *et al.* treated 204 patients with 25 mg of oral MTX weekly, the estimated mean body surface area of involvement decreased from 67% to 5% in 3–6 weeks. Rees *et al.* (in 1967) obtained good to excellent results in 50% of patients with weekly injections of 15–35 mg. Nausea is the dose-limiting symptom for parenteral MTX use.

In 1971, Weinstein and Frost first reported the dosing of MTX, 2.5–7.5 mg orally at 12-hour intervals for a total of three doses at weekly intervals. This schedule was based on experimental knowledge of the kinetics of keratinocyte proliferation and the rationale of using cell cycle-specific drugs for cancer. The same therapeutic effect was achieved with a smaller total weekly dose compared to a single oral or IM weekly dose, with less nausea. Recent long-term follow-up results have shown that about 80% of patients achieve sustained clearance or near clearance with low weekly oral dosages of 5–15 mg. After 16 weeks of treatment with MTX 15–22.5 mg/week, 43 patients with moderately severe psoriasis vulgaris achieved a 63% reduction in PASI score. The results were not statistically different from a parallel group of patients treated with cyclosporine 3–5 mg/kg/day.

Toxicity

The most commonly encountered adverse effects of MTX are nausea, anorexia, fatigue, headaches, and alopecia. At the doses normally used for psoriasis treatment, oral erosions (ulcerative stomatitis) and ulcerations of psoriatic lesions generally do not occur and are indicative of toxic serum levels due to drug interactions, dehydration, or deterioration of renal function. Bone marrow depression is more likely to occur under these circumstances.

Skin and mucous membrane toxicity

Stomatitis, oral ulcerations or ulceration of psoriatic lesions is indicative of toxic levels of MTX. MTX-induced necrolysis presents clinically as toxic epidermal necrolysis or erythema multiforme major revealing necrotic epithelium and blister formation. Two separate patterns of skin ulcerations may be associated with MTX toxicity. In type 1, painful erosions and ulcerations of psoriatic plaques develop shortly after MTX therapy is initiated. Histologically, epidermal necrosis and a dermal lymphocytic infiltrate are present. The ulcerations heal rapidly after reduction of the MTX dose or cessation of treatment. There is a danger of misinterpreting the erosions as a flare of preexisting psoriasis and increasing the dose of MTX. Type 2 ulcerations more closely mimic stasis ulcerations and take many weeks to heal.

Myelosuppression

Leukopenia and thrombocytopenia are the most serious acute side-effects of MTX. In the U.K. between 1969 and 1993, myelosuppression from MTX was listed as the cause of death in 19 patients compared to three deaths attributed to hepatotoxicity. If the white blood cell count or platelet count drops below 3500 or 100,000 per microliter, respectively, MTX should be discontinued until the cause is found. The nadir for leukocytes and platelets is 8–11 days after the dose is given. It generally takes about 3 weeks for the bone marrow to recover. Granulocyte colony-stimulating factor (G-CSF) infusion is indicated as soon as bone marrow toxicity becomes evident. While this has not been confirmed, elevated mean corpuscular volume (MCV) is indicative of folic acid deficiency and may be predictive of cytopenia. Low–normal pretreatment plasma and red blood cell (RBC) folate levels are predictive of future overall toxicity during MTX therapy.

Folic acid levels and supplementation

Folic acid levels, plasma and RBC, are significantly lower in patients receiving MTX for rheumatoid or psoriatic arthritis. The degree of folic acid depletion depends on the weekly administered dose of MTX (not the cumulative total). Folic acid depletion also leads to significant decreases in RBC vitamin B_{12} levels. Folic acid supplementation is recommended during MTX therapy because it prevents megaloblastic anemia and significantly lowers overall toxicity scores. The recommended dose of folic acid has not been standardized, but the following doses apparently do not compromise the therapeutic efficacy of MTX: 1–5 mg daily or 5.5 mg/day for 5 days of the week.

Carcinogenicity

There is no well-documented report of a carcinogenic potential for the skin or viscera, but there have been case reports of non-Hodgkin's B-cell lymphomas, developing during MTX treatment of rheumatoid arthritis (RA) or dermatomyositis. Some of these lymphomas resolved completely after the drug was stopped. Therefore, the cytotoxic effect of MTX combined with infection by oncogenic viruses such as Epstein–Barr virus may pose an additional risk in patients with autoimmune diseases including psoriasis.

Teratogenicity

Anecdotal reports implicated MTX treatment as either teratogenic or abortifacient in pregnant women. It may cause transient infertility in men. MTX should not be used by pregnant women, and pregnancy should be prevented in female patients during MTX therapy and for 3 months after the drug is stopped.

Photosensitivity

Photosensitivity does not occur with MTX, but there are rare examples of "sunburn recall." If a patient sustains a sunburn or a UVB burn, MTX therapy should be withheld for at least a week.

Pulmonary toxicity

The pulmonary complications of MTX are rarely encountered in psoriasis patients. No evidence of pulmonary fibrosis was detected in 27 patients with psoriatic arthritis who received a median cumulative dose of 2240 mg over 52 months. Acute interstitial pneumonitis due to hypersensitivity or as a direct toxic reaction to MTX is apparently more common than liver disease in patients with rheumatoid arthritis. It was diagnosed in 3% of patients during 2 years of MTX treatment and could not be detected earlier by periodic pulmonary function tests. The most common clinical presentation is a nonproductive cough and dyspnea with or without fever. It is nonresponsive to leucovorin rescue, but withdrawal of MTX and administration of corticosteroids may be therapeutically useful.

Hepatotoxicity

Hepatotoxicity is the primary clinical concern when long-term treatment of psoriasis is planned. Mild elevations (less than twice the upper limit of normal) of transaminases are expected during therapy, but enzyme levels do not correlate with hepatic fibrosis. In a study of long-term, oral, weekly MTX therapy in patients with rheumatoid arthritis, chronic low-grade elevations of serum aspartate aminotransferase (AST) at 3–4 years of therapy correlated with an increase in the hepatic histologic grade. These results taken together with the less common occurrence of liver disease in RA patients compared to psoriasis patients receiving MTX led to a discrepancy between safety monitoring recommendations promulgated by the American College of Rheumatology (ACR) and the American Academy of Dermatology (AAD). For example, the ACR does not recommend liver biopsy during treatment unless 5/9 or 6/12 AST levels in a 12-month period are elevated or serum albumin concentration decreases below normal. Many rheumatologists have adopted the same guidelines for monitoring patients with psoriatic arthritis. In 1998, a consensus conference of dermatologists modified its guidelines to mitigate conflict between specialists of the two disciplines who are most likely to consult on a case of severe psoriasis with arthropathy. The main change from 1988 is that the baseline liver biopsy is no longer recommended unless there are important risk factors. The initial liver biopsy is done after 1–1.5 g and repeated after 3.0 and 4.0 g cumulative doses. Liver biopsy is not indicated at all in the following situations:

1 In elderly patients (not specifically defined).
2 During acute illness.
3 If there are medical contraindications.
4 In patients with limited life expectancy.

The guidelines notwithstanding, a single abnormal liver biopsy specimen obtained during therapy does not necessarily imply that progressive disease will occur if MTX administration is continued. The incidence of cirrhosis as first reported was probably inflated because pretreatment liver biopsies that might have revealed pre-existing liver disease were not performed. The now-abandoned regimen of low daily doses of MTX increased the duration of exposure of hepatocytes to MTX, thereby increasing toxicity. Other major risk factors for hepatotoxicity that may not have been excluded or minimized include alcoholism, obesity, diabetes, renal insufficiency, and concomitant usage of drugs that increase the serum levels or decrease the clearance of MTX.

The incidence of cirrhosis occurring in psoriasis patients reportedly range from 0 to 20%, but the risk of cirrhosis developing before a total cumulative dose of 1.5 g is reached is minimal. MTX was continued in some patients with cirrhosis, without progression and sometimes even with regression of fibrosis. It is uncertain whether this finding represents a regeneration of liver or simply sampling errors. On the other hand, several patients required liver transplantation after developing MTX-induced cirrhosis.

Long-term, low-dose, once-weekly MTX may be less hepatotoxic than previously thought. Of 49 patients undergoing two sequential liver biopsies after the cumulative MTX dose reached 2.5 g and 5.0 g, there was no change in 28, deterioration in nine, and improvement in 12. Of the 11 patients found to have fibrosis at the first liver biopsy, none deteriorated and five showed significant improvement; none had cirrhosis. Of 55 patients who had at least one liver biopsy, fibrosis was seen in seven (13%) and cirrhosis in two (4%). There was no correlation between histologic grade and cumulative dose, duration of MTX therapy, or abnormal liver function tests. No deaths or life-threatening side-effects were attributable to MTX during 22 years of follow-up.

The preferred method for assessing pretreatment liver status and monitoring for MTX hepatotoxicity remains the percutaneous liver biopsy via the aspiration or suction needle technique, or a disposable spring-triggered cutting needle. The latter, called the Trucut needle, has the advantage of a shorter time interval within the liver. Although generally considered safe, a liver biopsy is not without some risk. In a series of over 68,000 procedures, the overall complication rate was 2.2%. The most serious complications that might require hospitalization or result in death include shock, pneumothorax, hemoperitoneum, and biliary peritonitis. The mortality varies from 0 to 0.12% with an average of 0.03%. Zachariae reported five cases of perforation of the gall bladder in over 2000 liver biopsies, but there were no deaths. Serious hemorrhagic complications were more frequent after biopsy with the Trucut needle than with the Menghini-type needles. The cost of an uncomplicated liver biopsy in the U.S. is about $1800 and is much higher if followed by a complication.

Noninvasive alternative methods have been studied. Radionuclide liver scans have been shown to be unreliable. Hepatic ultrasound may be a better screening test for severe toxicity. While the rate of false positive (with normal histology) and false negative (with Grade IIIA or less severity) results was high, ultrasound reliably detected Grade IIIB or cirrhosis that would interdict further MTX under the current guidelines. Moreover, a normal liver ultrasound screening subsequent to a normal histology may allow for safely lengthening the interval between liver biopsies. Ultrasound also enhances the safety of the liver biopsy procedure by allowing the operator to select the site that is the shortest distance between the skin and liver and thus easily avoid the lung, bowel loops, and large vessels in the liver. Dynamic hepatic scintigraphy, which measures the portal venous contribution to total hepatic blood flow, is very accurate (>95%) in predicting normal biopsy findings but poor for predicting moderate to severe portal fibrosis (25%).

Zachariae *et al.* demonstrated that serum elevations of the aminoterminal propeptide of type III procollagen (PIIINP) are correlated with liver fibrosis or cirrhosis in patients without arthropathy. They proposed that PIIINP levels measured by a commercial radioimmunoassay (Orion Diagnostica) be used for screening patients for liver fibrogenesis after the first biopsy when the total cumulative dose has reached 1.5 g, in order to reduce the number of additional biopsies performed. A single measurement does not detect all patients with fibrosis, but the yield is increased if PIIINP levels are serially measured every 3–4 months. Continuously normal levels can result in a reduction of liver biopsies. On the other hand, liver biopsy would be indicated in patients with persistently elevated levels.

How to treat a patient with MTX

MTX is a very effective treatment for psoriasis with potentially life-threatening effects. Before therapy with MTX is initiated, one must consult with a physician who is well-versed in the pharmacokinetics, drug interactions, treatment guidelines, and toxicity monitoring. The known risks and benefits of MTX are discussed and compared to the reasonable alternatives. It is helpful to provide written material concerning MTX to the patient to read at home and share with family members. Examples of such materials include the National Psoriasis Foundation brochure on systemic medications, the package insert, and MTX Patient Instructions from the AAD Guidelines.

Patient selection

MTX is indicated for severe or disabling psoriasis that is not responsive to other forms of therapy. Usually the patient has not responded
to topical and UVB phototherapy and is a candidate for systemic
treatment. Unless already tried, systemic treatment would include
PUVA, acitretin, and MTX. MTX has the advantage because the
tablets are taken orally once weekly and it does not require frequent
visits to the office for ultraviolet light treatments. A patient may
choose not to take MTX for fear of the liver biopsy and cirrhosis.
MTX may be considered for women of childbearing potential.

While each patient is evaluated individually with regard to disease severity, and symptoms, level of physical and social disability,
patients with minor plaque disease or predominantly nail psoriasis
without arthritis or functional impairment should not be treated
with MTX. In preselecting a patient for MTX, one should consider the indications (Table 16.1) and relative contraindications
(Table 16.2) to reduce the potential toxicity of MTX.

If the patient is a candidate for MTX, a complete history and
physical examination (Table 16.3) and laboratory evaluations
(Table 16.4) are performed.

I request that patients enter into a verbal contract that includes
a commitment to abstain from alcohol, to take the medicine exactly
as prescribed, to inform me of any new medication, preferably before
it is taken, to keep all follow-up appointments, and to undergo
laboratory tests as ordered. Finally, patients are advised that, after a
cumulative dose of 1–1.5 g MTX therapy, they may have to undergo
a liver biopsy in order for therapy to continue. During this time, I
can determine whether the patient can tolerate the drug, whether it
is efficacious, and whether the patient is reasonably compliant. I
generally do not order liver biopsies in patients older than 60 years.

Table 16.1 Indications for methotrexate: moderate to severe psoriasis.

1 Extensive plaque-type psoriasis involving 10% or more of body surface area
2 Disabling plaque-type psoriasis involving face, hands, feet
3 Psoriatic erythroderma
4 Generalized pustular psoriasis
5 Localized pustular psoriasis (e.g. palmoplantar pustulosis, acrodermatitis continua)
6 Complicated psoriasis, i.e. flaring after withdrawal of a previously effective
medication
7 Psoriatic arthritis with skin disease

Table 16.2 Relative contraindications for MTX.

1 Pregnancy or current desire to become pregnant
2 Alcoholism
3 Active hepatitis
4 Cirrhosis
5 Active infections
6 Chronic renal failure
7 Primary or secondary immunodeficiency
8 Active peptic ulcer disease
9 Blood dyscrasias
10 Unreliable for compliance or follow-up visits

Table 16.3 Risk factors for preexisting liver disease.

1 History of excessive alcohol intake
2 History of substance abuse including exposure to hepatotoxic chemicals
3 Persistently elevated transaminases
4 History of hepatitis A, B or C
5 Family history of heritable liver disease
6 Diabetes mellitus
7 Obesity (also increases risk of complications from liver biopsy procedure)

Table 16.4 Pre-methotrexate laboratory evaluations.

1 Complete blood count including red cell indices and leukocyte differential
2 Platelet count
3 Kidney function tests
4 Urinalysis
5 Liver function tests
6 HIV antibody screen (if risk factors can be ascertained)
7 Chest x-ray (optional)
8 Folic acid and vitamin B_{12} levels (optional)

Routine safety monitoring

The following are performed to monitor the safety of the treatment:
1 Complete blood cell count is determined after 1 week and then monthly. If significant leukopenia or thrombocytopenia develops, MTX is discontinued for 2–3 weeks.
2 Kidney and liver function tests are performed after 1 month and then every 3 months (plan blood test on the day before the next dose of MTX, to reduce transaminase levels).

3 More frequent monitoring may be advisable during acute illnesses, when increasing doses, and during concomitant drug therapy.

Planning the liver biopsy

Schedule the biopsy for 1–2 weeks after the last dose of MTX to reduce any acute morphologic alterations. Immediately prior to liver biopsy, a complete blood cell count, platelet count, prothrombin time, and activated partial thromboplastin time are measured. The pathologist should be informed of the clinical situation and be familiar with drug-induced liver abnormalities. The trichrome stain is utilized to detect fibrosis. The grading system in Table 16.5 should be used. If the first liver biopsy specimen is Grade I or II, the next liver biopsy is planned after an additional cumulative dose of 1.5 g MTX. Table 16.6 helps to predict the next biopsy. If the biopsy shows Grade III A, then the liver biopsy is repeated after 6 months of continuous MTX therapy regardless of the cumulative dose. I prefer not to give MTX to patients who have Grade III B or IV findings, but it may be unavoidable, in extraordinary cases.

Table 16.5 Grading system for liver biopsy and whether to continue MTX.

Grade I	Normal or mild fatty infiltration, nuclear variability, or portal inflammation; continue MTX
Grade II	Moderate to severe fatty infiltration, nuclear variability, portal tract expansion or inflammation; continue MTX
Grade III A	Fibrosis, mild; continue MTX and repeat liver biopsy in 6 months
Grade III B	Fibrosis, moderate to severe; discontinue MTX
Grade IV	Cirrhosis; discontinue MTX

Table 16.6 When to perform a liver biopsy.

Regular weekly dose (mg)	Months to 1.5 g cumulative dose and next liver biopsy
7.5	50
10.0	38
15.0	25
20.0	19
25.0	15

Table 16.7 Special warnings for methotrexate.

---

1 Low daily doses of MTX must never be used for psoriasis

2 Slow intravenous drips of MTX should never be used for psoriasis

3 It is rarely necessary to give MTX more than once per week for psoriasis, even for hospitalized patients

---

How to dose MTX

MTX is administered as a single weekly oral or parenteral dose. Special warnings for MTX dosing are listed in Table 16.7. The oral dosage may be divided over a 24-hour period once weekly. MTX is available as oral 2.5 mg tablets and parenteral isotonic liquid at 25 mg/ml with or without preservative. Most patients take the tablets. There is a trend away from parenteral therapy. Intramuscular or intravenous bolus injections are reserved for the occasional patient who cannot follow the oral dosing schedule or who is unreliable in keeping follow-up appointments for laboratory testing. Some patients with erratic absorption of oral MTX demonstrate a better therapeutic response with parenteral MTX. Others have less gastrointestinal symptoms with the injection.

The method of intermittent dosing over a 24-hour period is utilized by the majority of dermatologists, but it seems to confer no therapeutic advantage and is theoretically more hepatotoxic than a single weekly oral or parenteral bolus. For consistency, I prescribe MTX to be taken on Mondays at 8 am and 8 pm, and on Tuesday at 8 am, on an empty stomach if possible. The doses may be different at the different times; for example, a patient taking 10 mg weekly takes 2.5, 5.0, and 2.5 mg. Some patients are able to overcome the nausea induced by a single 15 mg dose, for example, by taking 5 mg 12 hours apart or by taking MTX with food, although the latter probably reduces bioavailability of the drug. I routinely prescribe folic acid supplementation, 1 mg daily, because it mitigates gastrointestinal (nausea, diarrhea, liver enzymes) toxicity of MTX without altering the efficacy and prevents megaloblastic anemia due to folic acid deficiency.

Dosage recommendations

After the pre-MTX consultation, education, and physical and laboratory examinations are completed (but not necessarily the liver biopsy), MTX is started with a single oral dose of 5 mg or 7.5 mg.

The complete blood cell count is checked for an idiosyncratic reaction before the next dose is given. This dose is continued weekly for one month. The dose is increased by 2.5 mg per week each month after complete blood cell (CBC) counts and other tests are performed as indicated. The physician should dispense only enough MTX for 1 or 2 weeks beyond the next scheduled visit without refills. Monthly intervals between increments in dose allow enough time for a therapeutic response and dose-related adverse reactions to develop. It is usually not necessary to induce complete clearing of psoriasis because it risks overmedicating the patient. I encourage the concomitant use of topical emollients, keratolytics, corticosteroids, anthralin, and tar shampoos for resistant localized plaques. If nausea should become a dose-limiting symptom, one can begin dividing the weekly dosage into three doses, 12 hours apart. Some food can be taken with the pills if nausea persists. The goal is to achieve adequate control of psoriasis, to overcome the physical and psychosocial disability of psoriasis with the lowest dose possible. The total dose needed usually does not exceed 30 mg weekly: 25 mg or less is sufficient for most, but doses up to 37.5 mg may be needed by a few patients. Elderly patients usually require lower mean doses as there is progressive deterioration in creatinine clearance associated with aging.

After stability of residual psoriasis (or clearing) is attained, an attempt to taper the dose in monthly 2.5 mg decrements should be made. Increasing the interval between doses of MTX from 7 to 10 or 14 days serves the same purpose but makes for inconsistencies in office practice patterns and changes an established schedule for the patient. The psoriasis may be expected to replapse within weeks to months, depending on the type and severity of the disease. There is no "rebound flare-up" of psoriasis as some believe, and there is no "resistance" to MTX when it is reinstated. The therapeutic to toxicity ratio of MTX renders interruption of long-term therapy (i.e. rotational therapy) a philosophically sound idea, but it is risky for some patients. Of 10 well-controlled patients receiving MTX for 12 years, three relapsed in 4 weeks, while seven did not need MTX for 11 weeks. Short-term (1–3 months) intermittent MTX therapy has been advocated as a strategy to reduce the cumulative dose and thereby delay or avoid the need for a liver biopsy.

Overdosage of MTX

Because of the inherently low doses of MTX used for psoriasis, it is rare to encounter in practice a true overdosage that requires inter-

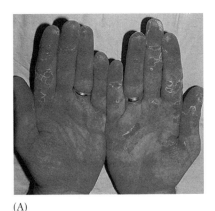
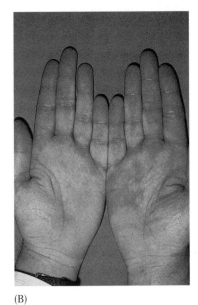

(A) (B)

Figure 16.1 Psoriasis of the palms before (A) and after (B) 10 weeks of treatment with methotrexate 15 mg per week.

vention other than decreasing or withholding the next dose and routine laboratory monitoring. The most likely clinical scenarios that may result in overdosage requiring intervention are as follows:

1 A noncompliant patient increases his or her own dose deliberately to improve efficacy or rate of response. The patient may complain of burning or ulceration of psoriasis lesions.

2 A patient develops acute renal failure or an unrelated acute illness with dehydration without reducing the dose of MTX. This is usually revealed by routine laboratory monitoring or by a call to the physician from the local emergency room because of leukopenia.

3 The patient is given another drug that increases the serum level of MTX or prolongs the excretion of MTX, thereby increasing the toxicity of MTX. Trimethoprim-sulfamethoxazole is frequently the "other drug." Patients may complain of a sore mouth.

Leucovorin calcium (citrovorum factor, folinic acid) can bypass the metabolic block produced by MTX and supply the active form of folic acid that cells require. Leucovorin should be readily available in the office or clinic as it must be given as promptly as possible, preferably within 4 hours of the last dose of MTX. As the time interval between MTX and leucovorin administration increases, the effectiveness of leucovorin as an antidote diminishes so that, by 24 hours, it is doubtful that leucovorin will have any effect except in patients with severely depressed creatinine clearance.

In general, if an overdose with MTX is suspected, the clinician should give an intramuscular injection of leucovorin equal to the last dose of MTX or 25 mg, whichever is greater. Then blood is sampled to assess hematologic and kidney function parameters and MTX level. In patients with renal impairment, the leucovorin dosing is repeated every 6 hours until the MTX level is 0.1 micromolar or less. Neither hemodialysis nor peritoneal dialysis improve MTX elimination. The patient with dehydration should be rehydrated with normal saline and observed. In patients with massive over-dosage, admission to a hospital is justified for leucovorin rescue. Alkalinization of the urine prevents precipitation of MTX in the renal tubules. G-CSF infusion should be considered if severe neu-tropenia develops.

Combination therapy

Patients pretreated with MTX followed by combined MTX and ultraviolet light generally experienced more rapid clearing with lower doses of UVB or UVA, probably by decreasing scaling and induration of plaques and altering the photo-optical properties of the skin, making it favorable for UVL penetration.

In one study, MTX, 15 mg weekly, was given for 3 weeks, and then UVB three times weekly was started. MTX was discontinued when the psoriasis cleared, and UVB therapy was continued at twice-weekly maintenance. The psoriasis in all 26 patients cleared with a combination of a mean cumulative MTX dose of 112 mg and 12 UVB exposures over 7 weeks. The UVB dose at clearing was less than half that noted in 20 patients treated with UVB alone. The total number of phototoxic episodes was not increased by the combina-tion of MTX with UVB, and MTX recall of UV light-induced eryth-ema (photoreaction) was not observed in any patient.

Similarly, MTX combined with PUVA resulted in clearing in 93% of patients with 9.3 PUVA treatments and a final dose of 6.2 J/cm^2, about one-third of that required without MTX. The mean cumulat-ive dose of MTX was only 93 mg. PUVA is more likely to maintain clearance alone than is UVB, but the two potent therapies should be used together only in patients who did not respond to UVL alone or who required high final maintenance doses. A significant adverse effect of MTX combined with PUVA was prolonged phototoxicity.

The combination of MTX and acitretin should be used, if at all, with caution in patients with severe forms of psoriasis, erythrodermic or pustular, who cannot be controlled with either drug alone or in the conversion from one treatment to the other. Additive hepatotoxicity is the main concern, but the toxic hepatitis uncommonly observed with retinoids and the fibrosis induced by chronic administration of MTX seem to be due to different mechanisms. In a study of six psoriasis patients treated chronically with the combination of intramuscular MTX and etretinate, the maximal plasma concentration of MTX was significantly increased compared to that in a matched control group receiving only MTX. The levels of etretinate and metabolites were not affected by MTX administration. Higher maximal MTX plasma concentrations might predispose patients to more mucous membrane, cutaneous, hematologic, and hepatic toxicity.

MTX was combined with cyclosporine to treat 19 patients with psoriasis (15 with arthropathy) who were recalcitrant to either one of the drugs alone. In each case, the combination resulted in good control of both the skin and joint manifestations at lower doses of each agent than would have been used for monotherapy.

Topical methotrexate

Topical formulations of methotrexate 0.1–10% in aqueous cream, petrolatum, and dimethyl sulfoxide were ineffective when applied to psoriasis for 7–14 days, as were intradermal injections of 0.1–1.0% solutions. A more recent study of 1% MTX gel formulation containing Azone (laurocapram), a skin penetration enhancer, applied once daily for 8 weeks, demonstrated significant antipsoriatic effect (scaling, thickness) compared to vehicle. Only 2/296 plasma samples showed detectable levels of MTX. Another topical MTX gel 0.25% formulation in hydroxy cellulose 1% was significantly more effective at clearing psoriasis than placebo gel when applied twice daily 5 days per week for 4 weeks. Although the two studies are not directly comparable, they suggest that, with the optimal concentration of MTX and vehicle, it is feasible to enjoy at least some of the therapeutic benefit of MTX on psoriasis without the risk of systemic toxicity or costly laboratory monitoring.

Selected references

Ameen M., Taylor D. A., Williams I. P. *et al.* (2001) Pneumonitis complicating methotrexate therapy for pustular psoriasis. *J Eur Acad Dermatol Venereol* **15**, 247–249.

Belzunegui J., Intaxausti J. J., De Dios J. R. *et al.* (2001) Absence of pulmonary fibrosis in patients with psoriatic arthritis treated with weekly low-dose methotrexate. *Clin Exp Rheumatol* **19**, 727–730.

Boffa M. J., Chalmers R. J. G., Haboubi N. Y. *et al.* (1995) Sequential liver biopsies during long-term methotrexate treatment for psoriasis: a reappraisal. *Br J Dermatol* **133**, 774–778.

Clark C. M., Kirby B., Morris A. D. *et al.* (1999) Combination treatment with methotrexate and cyclosporin for severe recalcitrant psoriasis. *Br J Dermatol* **141**, 279–282.

Cueller M. L., Espinoza L. R. (1997) Methotrexate use in psoriasis and psoriatic arthritis. *Rheum Dis Clin North Am* **23**, 797–809.

Ellman M. H., Telfer M. C., Turner A. F. (1992) Benefit of G-CSF for methotrexate-induced neutropenia in rheumatoid arthritis. *Am J Med* **92**, 337–338.

Guzzo C., Kaidby K. (1995) Recruitment recall of sunburn by methotrexate. *Photodermatol Photoimmunol Photomed* **11**, 55–56.

Hassan W. (1996) Methotrexate and liver toxicity: role of surveillance liver biopsy: conflict between guidelines for rheumatologists and dermatologists. *Ann Rheum Dis* **55**, 273–275.

Haustein U. F., Rytter M. (2000) Methotrexate in psoriasis: 26 years' experience with low-dose long-term treatment. *J Eur Acad Dermatol Venereol* **14**, 382–388.

Heydendael V. M., Spuls P. I., Opmeer B. C. *et al.* (2003) Methotrexate versus cyclosporine in moderate-to-severe chronic plaque psoriasis. *N Engl J Med* **349**, 658–665.

Jeffes E. W. B., McCullough J. L., Pittelkow M. R. *et al.* (1995) Methotrexate therapy of psoriasis: Differential sensitivity of proliferating lymphoid and epithelial cells to the cytotoxic and growth-inhibitory effects of methotrexate. *J Invest Dermatol* **104**, 183–188.

Kazlow D. W., Federgrun D., Kurtin S., Lebwohl M. G. (2003) Cutaneous ulceration caused by methotrexate. *J Am Acad Dermatol* **49** (Suppl. 2), S197–S198.

Kumar B., Saraswat A., Kaur I. (2002) Short-term methotrexate therapy in psoriasis: a study of 197 patients. *Int H Dermatol* **41**, 444–448.

Larson F. G., Nielsen-Kudsk F., Jakobsen P. *et al.* (1990) Interaction of etretinate with methotrexate pharmaco-kinetics in psoriatic patients. *J Clin Pharmacol* **30**, 802–807.

Lawrence C. M., Dahl G. C. (1984) Two patterns of skin ulceration induced by methotrexate in patients with psoriasis. *J Am Acad Dermatol* **11**, 1059–1065.

Leeb B. F., Witzmann E. O., Studnicka-Benke A. *et al.* (1995) Folic acid and cyanocobalamin levels in serum and erythrocytes during low-dose methotrexate therapy of rheumatoid arthritis and psoriatic arthritis patients. *Clin Exp Rheumatol* **13**, 459–463.

Morgan S. L., Baggott J. E., Vaughn W. H. *et al.* (1994) Supplementation with folic acid during methotrexate therapy for rheumatoid arthritis. A double-blind, placebo-controlled trial. *Ann Intern Med* **121**, 833–841.

Morison W. L., Momtaz T. K., Parrish J. A., Fitzpatrick T. B. (1982) Combined methotrexate-PUVA therapy in the treatment of psoriasis. *J Am Acad Dermatol* **6**, 46–51.

Paul C., LeTourneau A., Cayuela J. M. *et al.* (1997) Epstein-Barr virus-associated lymphoproliferative disease during methotrexate therapy for psoriasis. *Arch Dermatol* **133**, 867–871.

Paul B. S., Momtaz T. K., Stern R. S. *et al.* (1982) Combined methotrexate ultraviolet B therapy in the treatment of psoriasis. *J Am Acad Dermatol* **7**, 758–762.

Primka E. J. III, Camisa C. (1997) Methotrexate-induced toxic epidermal necrolysis in a patient with psoriasis. *J Am Acad Dermatol* **36**, 815–818.

Rees R. B., Bennett J. H., Maibach H. I., Arnold H. L. (1967) Methotrexate for psoriasis. *Arch Dermatol* **95**, 2–11.

Roenigk H. H. Jr, Auerbach R., Maibach H. *et al.* (1998) Methotrexate in psoriasis: consensus conference. *J Am Acad Dermatol* **38**, 478–485.

Roenigk H. H., Bergfeld W. F., Curtis G. H. (1969) Methotrexate for psoriasis in weekly oral doses. *Arch Dermatol* **99**, 86–93.

Roenigk H. H., Auerbach R., Maibach H. I., Weinstein G. D. (1988) Methotrexate in psoriasis: revised guidelines. *J Am Acad Dermatol* **19**, 145–156.

Schiff E. R., Schiff L. (1993) Needle biopsy of the liver. In: Schiff L., Schiff E. R. (eds) *Diseases of the Liver*, 7th edn. JB Lippincott, Philadelphia, 216–225.

Sutton L., Swinehart J. M., Cato A., Kaplan A. S. (2001) A clinical study to determine the efficacy and safety of 1% methotrexate/Axone (MAZ) gel applied topically once daily in patients with psoriasis vulgaris. *Int J Dermatol* **40**, 464–467.

Syed T. A., Hadi S. M., Qureshi Z. A. *et al.* (2001) Management of psoriasis vulgaris with methotrexate 0.25% in a hydrophilic gel: a placebo-controlled, double-blind study. *J Cut Med Surg* **5**, 299–302.

Tracy T. S., Worster T., Bradley J. D. *et al.* (1994) Methotrexate disposition following concomitant administration of ketoprofen, piroxicam, and flurbiprofen in patients with rheumatoid arthritis. *Br J Clin Pharmacol* **37**, 453–456.

Van Dooren-Greebe R. J., Kuijpers A. L. A., Mulder J. *et al.* (1994) Methotrexate revisited: effects of long-term treatment in psoriasis. *Br J Dermatol* **130**, 204–210.

Viraben R., Brousse P., Lamant L. (1996) Reversible cutaneous lymphoma occurring during methotrexate therapy. *Br J Dermatol* **135**, 116–118.

Weinstein G. D., Frost P. (1971) Methotrexate for psoriasis. A new therapeutic schedule. *Arch Dermatol* **103**, 33–38.

Zachariae H. (2000) Liver biopsies and methotrexate: a time for reconsideration? *J Am Acad Dermatol* **42**, 531–534.

17 Cyclosporine, tacrolimus, and pimecrolimus

Charles Camisa

Introduction

Cyclosporine is a cyclic polypeptide consisting of 11 amino acids isolated from a soil fungus in 1972. Cyclosporine and tacrolimus inhibit the calcineurin/nuclear factor of activated T-cells' (NFAT) signaling pathway. This action directly interferes with T-cell activation and communication with antigen-presenting cells by inhibiting the synthesis or expression of interleukin (IL)-1 and IL-2 and IL-2 receptor (IL-2R) without suppressing the bone marrow. In psoriatic lesions, cyclosporine also inhibits the epidermal cytokine network, which leads to decreased expression of IL-I β, IL-8, IL-2R, and E-selectin, reduction in infiltrating activated T-cells expressing CD3+CD25+ and CD3+HLA-DR+ and clinical improvement. Cyclosporine is superior to azathioprine, cyclophosphamide, and corticosteroids in the prevention of graft rejection in patients receiving allogeneic organ transplants. Besides psoriasis, cyclosporine has efficacy in treating the mucocutaneous manifestations of putative autoimmune diseases such as atopic dermatitis, lichen planus, pyoderma gangrenosum, and Behçet's disease.

Metabolism

Oral cyclosporine is absorbed rapidly from the small intestine, but the absorption is incomplete (about 30%) and highly variable (4–89%). The bioavailability of the soft gelatin capsules is equivalent to that of the oral solution. Peak plasma concentrations are achieved in 2–4 hours.

A microemulsion formulation of cyclosporine (Neoral) increases the bioavailability of the drug by increasing the absorption. In several pharmacokinetic studies, the time to maximal concentration decreased (from 2.3 to 1.4 hours), maximal drug concentration increased about 60%, and the area under the steady-state blood concentration time curve (AUC) increased about 50%. There was less interpatient variability for the microemulsion formulation than for soft gelatin capsules as a result of the more consistent and predictable absorption of cyclosporine from the microemulsion formulation.

The drug is metabolized extensively in the liver by the microsomal P-450 3A4 oxidase system. The metabolites are primarily excreted into the bile and enter the enterohepatic circulation. About 6% of the dose is excreted in the urine, and only 0.1% of the dose is excreted as unchanged cyclosporine. There is great variability in the metabolism of cyclosporine, with an average terminal half-life of 19 hours (range, 10–27 hours).

Cyclosporine is widely distributed in all body tissues. Due to its lipophilic nature, it remains in the tissues long after dosing has been discontinued. In blood the distribution is concentration-dependent; that is, at high concentrations leukocytes and erythrocytes become saturated. In the plasma, approximately 90% of cyclosporine is bound to lipoproteins. The individual variation in plasma concentration can be accounted for in part by differences in concentrations of high- and low-density lipoproteins. Bioavailability of the drug appears to increase during the first two weeks of oral administration apparently after the "first-pass effect," as tissues become saturated and as the enterohepatic recirculation reaches equilibrium.

Cyclosporine in psoriasis

The first reports of cyclosporine's remarkable efficacy in psoriasis were the serendipitous results of treating patients for psoriatic arthritis and allogeneic kidney transplantation. Over the next 15 years, numerous reports of open and controlled studies of cyclosporine in the treatment of thousands of patients with psoriasis helped to define the selection, dosing, toxicity, and monitoring of patients taking this drug.

In 1986, Ellis *et al.* established the efficacy of high-dose cyclosporine in a double-blind study, showing that 14 mg/kg/day was significantly better than placebo at improving psoriasis ($p < 0.0001$) after 4 weeks of treatment. The onset of subjective and objective improvement occurred rapidly, as early as after 1 and 7 days, respectively. The authors recognized that high-dose cyclosporine was not the optimal regimen for psoriasis, but the study was important because it confirmed efficacy as well as the significant toxicities to be monitored in future protocols employing lower doses for longer periods of time. They demonstrated statistically significant elevations in diastolic blood pressure, serum creatinine, blood urea nitrogen, bilirubin, cholesterol, triglycerides, potassium, and uric acid. Magnesium levels were reduced. Liver enzymes were not affected.

Subsequent dose-finding studies performed in multiple centers in Europe and the U.S. have given consistent results. "Success" was defined as a reduction in the psoriasis area and severity index (PASI) score of 75% or more or a score of 8 or less after 3 or more months of cyclosporine treatment for severe plaque-type psoriasis. Success rates were about 21%, 54%, and 88% for 1.25, 2.5 or 3, and 5 mg/kg/day. When the cyclosporine dose was escalated from a starting dose of 1.25 or 2.5 mg/kg/day, it reached a dose of 5 mg/kg/day for 28% of patients because of their insufficient therapeutic response at the lower doses. After 8 weeks of fixed-dose therapy, psoriasis was clear or almost clear in 0%, 36%, 65%, and 80% of patients receiving placebo or 3, 5, or 7.5 mg/kg/day cyclosporine, respectively.

A meta-analysis of three major German studies was performed to evaluate the efficacy of cyclosporine (1.25, 2.5, and 5.0 mg/kg/day), etretinate (0.53 mg/kg/day), and placebo. Cyclosporine was significantly superior to placebo (at all doses) and superior to etretinate at 2.5 and 5.0 mg/kg/day. Quality of life was improved by cyclosporine treatment according to the Dermatology Life Quality Index (DLQI) at the beginning and end of each treatment course. The overall DLQI scores improved ($p < 0.001$) along with significant decreases in PASI and itch scores ($p < 0.001$).

Cyclosporine does not cure psoriasis and does not induce remissions that are more durable than PUVA or the Ingram regime, for example. Therefore, continuous cyclosporine administration or conversion to alternative systemic therapy is necessary in order to maintain prolonged remission. After clearing psoriasis with cyclosporine 5 mg/kg/day for 16 weeks, 58% of patients were adequately and safely maintained at 3 mg/kg/day for 6 months. An alternative to long-term continuous therapy is intermittent short courses until clearance or for a maximum of 12 weeks. The cyclosporine dose is then abruptly stopped or tapered over a 4 week period (1 mg/kg/day per week). Over a 2 year period, there was no significant difference in the total time in remission between the two groups. The median time to relapse was 115 days after the first treatment course. The median time to relapse for both placebo and cyclosporine 1.5 mg/kg/day is 6 weeks. Although rare cases of a generalized pustular flare of psoriasis have occurred, discontinuation of cyclosporine or continuation of a suboptimal maintenance dose allows skin lesions to recur at a rate and severity consistent with the natural history of an individual's disease.

Toxicity

The mild common adverse effects of cyclosporine are generally well tolerated and accepted by patients (Table 17.1). These symptoms are dose-dependent and usually disappear upon cessation of therapy.

As with all immunosuppressive medications, there is a theoretical increased risk of infections and malignancy, particularly lymphoma, squamous cell carcinoma, and Kaposi's sarcoma. The incidence of lymphoma in transplant patients is about 0.1–0.4%, but is lower in patients with autoimmune diseases (<0.1%). In a 5-year prospective follow-up study of 1252 patients from 11 countries with psoriasis treated with cyclosporine for an average of 1.9 years, malignancies were diagnosed in 47 (3.8%) patients. The overall two-fold higher incidence of any malignancy was caused by a six-fold higher incidence of nonmelanoma skin cancers, primarily squamous cell carcinoma.

Many patients with severe psoriasis are already at risk for squamous cell carcinoma because of previous exposure to arsenic, x-rays, solar radiation, therapeutic UVB, and PUVA. In the same cohort of 1252 patients there were 13 skin cancers and two melanomas (relative risk = 12.4). The rate of incidence of skin tumors in psoriasis treated with cyclosporine has been calculated to be 0.5–0.8/1000 patients per month. Previous exposure to PUVA, retinoids, and methotrexate increased the relative risk of

Table 17.1 Minor dose-related cyclosporine side-effects.

1 Gingival hyperplasia
2 Hypertrichosis affecting face, scalp, and extremities
3 Tremor
4 Paresthesia
5 Headache
6 Nausea

developing nonmelanoma skin cancer. No cases of Kaposi's sarcoma were observed. The risk of malignancy was significantly increased in patients receiving more than 2 years' treatment with cyclosporine compared with those receiving less than 2 years. There was a significantly higher risk of developing leukemia (7.3), but only three patients in the cohort were affected in this way.

The frequency and severity of bacterial, viral, and opportunistic infections in psoriatics appears not to be increased by cyclosporine alone. Infections in psoriatics occur at the same rate with placebo, cyclosporine, or etretinate and are uncomplicated.

The two most important side-effects of cyclosporine, requiring baseline evaluation, constant monitoring, and intervention (medical treatment, dose reduction, or discontinuation of cyclosporine) are nephrotoxicity and hypertension.

Nephrotoxicity

Cyclosporine produces widespread vasoconstriction leading to systemic hypertension and decreased renal blood flow. In a group of psoriatics treated with cyclosporine 5 mg/kg/day who showed significant reductions in glomerular filtration rate (GFR) and renal blood flow, circulating angiotensin II levels were significantly elevated, but plasma renin activity, aldosterone, and atrial natriuretic peptide were not altered. Hypoperfusion of the kidney leads to early nephrotoxicity, decline in the GFR, and the development or exacerbation of hypertension.

The increase in serum creatinine and urea concentrations is a direct reflection of decreased glomerular filtration rate. The percent increase in serum creatinine and blood urea nitrogen (BUN) is dose dependent. Lewis *et al.* and Ellis *et al.* independently reported the median decline in GFR, measured as the percentage of clearance of I-125 iothalamate sodium, to be 16% in patients receiving an average dose of either 3.3 or 5.2 mg/kg/day. The GFR increased toward its baseline level, concomitant with a reduction in average dose over a period of 1–3 months.

1 Interstitial fibrosis
2 Tubular atrophy
3 Arteriolar hyalinosis
4 Glomerular sclerosis

Table 17.2 Cyclosporine-induced nephropathy.

It is apparent that after 2 or more years of continuous cyclosporine therapy at the doses required to control severe psoriasis, nearly all patients will develop some features of cyclosporine-induced nephropathy (Table 17.2).

In the study of Zachariae *et al.*, after 2 years of cyclosporine treatment (2.5–6.0 mg/kg/day), all 25 kidney biopsies demonstrated features of cyclosporine nephropathy compared to pretreatment biopsies. The severity of the morphologic findings progressed with the length of therapy such that, after 4 years, 24/25 had arteriolar hyalinosis and 11 had moderate to severe interstitial fibrosis. The severity of the structural injury correlated with a reduction in GFR. In a separate study of 20 patients receiving an average dose of 2.8 mg/kg/day for 6 years, nine (45%) of 20 patients showed persistent *increases* of serum creatinine of >30%; and seven (35%) of 20 patients showed persistent *decreases* of GFR of >30%. Powles *et al.* emphasized that there is individual patient variability as to when nephrotoxicity begins, its speed of progression, and the extent of improvement after stopping cyclosporine.

If the severity and recalcitrance of psoriasis, taken together with the impact on the patient's quality of life, indicates that cyclosporine treatment continue beyond 2 years, then the kidney function must be monitored by sequential renal biopsies and GFR determinations in addition to serum creatinine. There is consensus among investigators that, while changes in renal function do not always reflect morphologic changes, if serum creatinine rises to more than 30% above an individual patient's baseline value, then the dose of cyclosporine should be reduced. The likelihood of developing nephropathy can be minimized by limiting the dose of cyclosporine to a maximum of 5 mg/kg/day and adhering to the lowest possible maintenance dose for the shortest possible duration.

Hypertension

Cyclosporine induces a dose-related rise in diastolic blood pressure equal to about 1 mmHg for every 1 mg/kg/day of drug. Hypertension (systolic BP >160 mmHg or diastolic >95 mmHg) develops in 10–15% of patients within weeks of initiating treatment at 2–5 mg/kg/day and in one-third of patients after 1 year of treatment. Sixteen (57%) of 28 patients treated for longer than 4 years developed hypertension. This suggests that the risk of developing hypertension increases with either duration of cyclosporine

Table 17.3 Some commonly prescribed drugs that affect the plasma level of cyclosporine.

Inhibit metabolism and increase cyclosporine levels	Induce cytochrome P-450 enzymes and diminish cyclosporine levels
Bromocriptine	Phenytoin
Danazol	Phenobarbital
Ketoconazole	Carbamazepine
Fluconazole	Rifampin
Itraconazole	Intravenous trimethoprim
Erythromycin	Sulfamethoxazole
Verapamil	
Nicardipine	
Diltiazem	
Methyltestosterone	
Oral contraceptives	

treatment or with cumulative cyclosporine dose. It is usually controlled medically and is reversible after cyclosporine is stopped.

Drug interactions

Several commonly prescribed drugs can alter the concentration of cyclosporine in blood or enhance certain cyclosporine toxicities by different mechanisms. The plasma level of cyclosporine is influenced by drugs that compete for or induce hepatic microsomal P450 3A4 activity (Table 17.3). Concomitant administration of potentially nephrotoxic drugs may accentuate cyclosporine's effects by compromising renal blood flow or by a direct tubulo-interstitial effect: aminoglycoside antibiotics, amphotericin B, trimethoprim, vancomycin, melphalan, ranitidine, and nonsteroidal anti-inflammatory drugs. The addition of immunosuppressive drugs, such as corticosteroids, azathioprine, mycophenolate mofetil, and cyclophosphamide, to cyclosporine increases the risk of severe infections and malignancies.

Topical cyclosporine

The high tissue levels required for successful local cyclosporine psoriasis therapy cannot be achieved with topical preparations because cyclosporine penetrates poorly through skin. Topical formulations of 5% in oil and ointment base applied to psoriasis with and without plastic film occlusion for 6 hours per day had no effect. Intralesional injections of cyclosporine 17 mg/ml improved psoriatic plaques without affecting distant plaques. Pain on injection was the most common side-effect. Topical therapy with cyclosporine is ineffective, and intralesional injections, while potentially efficacious, are impractical.

Combination therapy

PUVA

PUVA was added to cyclosporine therapy after relapse occurred upon reduction of dose or if cyclosporine, 5 mg/kg/day, was considered ineffective as monotherapy. Combination therapy was effective in only 1/4 of patients. The well-documented increased risk of cutaneous squamous cell carcinoma with PUVA is potentiated by cyclosporine. Therefore, combination treatment with cyclosporine and PUVA is not recommended.

Retinoids

With a protocol similar to that described above, etretinate was added to the therapy in five patients. No additive therapeutic effect of etretinate to cyclosporine therapy was observed. All five patients demonstrated reversible increases in serum creatinine levels (19–56%).

Isotretinoin has been used to treat severe acne in kidney and heart transplant patients taking cyclosporine. The acne improved without evidence of graft rejection or cyclosporine toxicity. Cyclosporine trough levels remained within the recommended therapeutic range, with the usual dosage adjustments required during monitoring. Therefore, while isotretinoin has limited usefulness in plaque-type psoriasis, there may be instances in women of childbearing potential, with pustular psoriasis, or with cyclosporine-induced nephrotoxicity where combination therapy might be desirable. The chief concern here is hyperlipidemia, a potential side-effect of both cyclosporine and retinoids.

Methotrexate

The combination of MTX and cyclosporine therapy has been considered dangerous because the target organ of toxicity for one drug is the predominant organ of excretion of the other (liver/kidney). However, the combination has proved significantly more effective than either agent alone in reducing the incidence of acute graft-versus-host disease in patients receiving allogeneic bone marrow transplantation. The combination of cyclosporine and methotrexate was effective in the treatment of psoriatic arthritis that was resisitant to prior second-line agents. Clark *et al.* successfully treated 19 patients with severe, recalcitrant psoriasis and psoriatic arthritis with the combination who had not responded to the maximum tolerated dose of either methotrexate or cyclosporine monotherapy. Impairment of renal function developed in six (32%) out of 19 patients and did not normalize in three patients following a reduction in the dose of cyclosporine. This combination should probably be reserved for exceptional cases of psoriasis or psoriatic arthritis or when converting or rotating from one to the other drug.

Topical corticosteroids

Griffiths *et al.* employed cyclosporine with and without the super-potent topical corticosteroid clobetasol propionate. The combination cleared psoriasis faster (3.5 weeks vs. 6 weeks) than cyclosporine alone, and there was no significant difference in relapse rates or side-effects. Such an approach would be more valuable if it allowed for a lower starting dose of cyclosporine.

Anthralin

Short-contact (20 min) anthralin was applied to one side of the body of patients receiving cyclosporine, 5 mg/kg/day. The patients who responded more slowly to cyclosporine showed a significantly better response on the anthralin-treated side as early as 4 weeks; the response persisted through 16 weeks. Anthralin alone does not prevent relapse of psoriasis after stopping cyclosporine, but it may induce a quicker response in some patients, especially when lower starting dosages of cyclosporine are used.

Calcipotriene

The combination of calcipotriene with cyclosporine improves the risk to benefit ratio of the cyclosporine because it improves the efficacy of lower starting doses. Grossman *et al.* demonstrated that ≥90% improvement in PASI score occurred in 50% of patients with the combination of calcipotriene ointment applied twice daily plus cyclosporine, 2 mg/kg/day, compared to 12% of patients who received placebo plus cyclosporine.

How to use cyclosporine

Consultation

Cyclosporine is a potent and toxic drug for patients with severe psoriasis. Before initiating therapy, physicians should consult a dermatologist with experience in the management of patients taking cyclosporine. In patients with normal baseline renal function, monitoring is straightforward, and it is usually not necessary to consult a nephrologist.

Selection of patients

Patients with extensive or disabling plaque-type, erythrodermic, or pustular psoriasis, or psoriatic arthritis who have not responded to, cannot tolerate, or cannot obtain approved systemic therapies including PUVA, methotrexate, acitretin, and biologic agents, can be considered for cyclosporine treatment. Contraindications and relative contraindications are displayed in Tables 17.4 and 17.5.

Table 17.4 Contraindications for cyclosporine.

1 Abnormal renal function
2 Uncontrolled hypertension
3 Primary or secondary immunodeficiency
4 Severe hepatic dysfunction
5 Pregnancy or lactation
6 Serious infection
7 Drug or alcohol abuse
8 Noncompliant to safety monitoring schedule

Table 17.5 Relative contraindications for cyclosporine.

---

1 Immunosuppressive or carcinogenic treatments, including PUVA and UVB, should not be given during cyclosporine therapy because of the increased risk of skin cancer

2 Whenever possible, drugs known to interfere with the metabolism of cyclosporine and drugs known to be nephrotoxic including NSAIDs should be avoided

3 Patients with a previous or concomitant noncutaneous malignancy should obtain clearance from their general practitioner or oncologist before receiving cyclosporine

---

Evaluation of patient prior to initiation of cyclosporine

The patient should receive (preferably written) educational material about cyclosporine, and the physician or consultant should discuss the risk to benefit ratio for the individual. If the decision is made to proceed with cyclosporine treatment, the patient should undergo a complete history and physical examination including routine screening tests for cancer where appropriate (rectal examination, stool guaiac test, cervical cytologic smear, chest x-ray film, mammogram) and a thorough examination of the integument to include the oral cavity and genitalia for tumors, as well as an estimation of body surface area involved, type of psoriasis, and degree of itch and disability. Blood pressure should be measured on two or more occasions prior to therapy. Routine laboratory tests include 12-hour fasting serum electrolyte, liver enzyme, and lipid levels, complete blood cell count, and urinalysis. A baseline serum creatinine level should be measured on two or more occasions. It is not necessary to measure GFR or calculate creatinine clearance because these are difficult to perform on outpatients and are not generally used to monitor nephrotoxicity during therapy except in controlled experimental protocols.

Initiation of cyclosporine therapy

Several studies showed that administration of 3 mg/kd/day for 3 months significantly improves psoriasis in the majority of patients. Using this conservative approach, 30–40% of patients will not have to receive a higher dose of cyclosporine thereby reducing the risk of

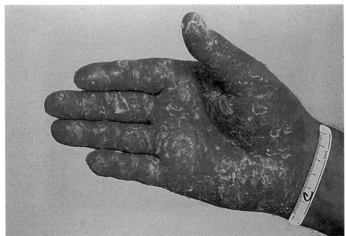

(A)

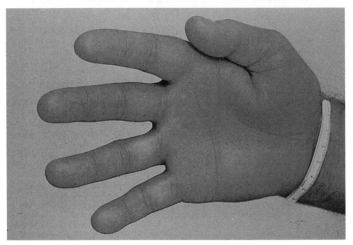

(B)

Figure 17.1 Severe disabling pustular psoriasis of the palms before (A) and after (B) 6 months of treatment with cyclosporine 5 mg/kg/day.

nephrotoxicity. In patients in whom it is desirable to obtain a more rapid response to therapy, such as those with acute inflammatory forms of psoriasis, hospitalized patients, and patients with disabling arthropathy, it is appropriate to use a higher starting dose not to exceed 5 mg/kg/day (Fig. 17.1). Because the plasma half-life is less than 24 hours, cyclosporine is administered in divided doses 12 hours apart.

In selected patients, the concominant use of potent topical corticosteroids, short-contact anthralin therapy, or calcipotriene ointment may accelerate the response to cyclosporine.

The microemulsion formulation of cyclosporine (Neoral) is more rapidly absorbed, has greater bioavailability, and less pharmacokinetic variability than the soft gelatin capsule (Sandimmune). The mean dose required to control psoriasis is about 10% lower with Neoral. A more predictable response and perhaps fewer dosage adjustments may facilitate high-dose, short courses of intermittent therapy.

Maintenance dose of cyclosporine

If the patient started at 3 mg/kg/day and continued this dose for 3 months, taper or increase the dose by 0.5–1 mg/kg/day monthly depending upon the response. If 5 mg/kg/day produces an insufficient therapeutic response, the combination therapy discussed above should be considered, or alternative therapy should be sought. If the patient initially responds well to 2.5–5.0 mg/kg/day, consider reducing the dose to 1.25 mg/kg/day for maintenance. If the patient's psoriasis is well maintained at ≤1.5 mg/kg/day, stoppage of cyclosporine should be considered as less than half the patients will relapse in 6 months. If the psoriasis flares during the taper, the clinician should revert to the previous higher dose and consider chronic maintenance. Provided that the monitoring recommendations are followed, cyclosporine may be used safely continuously for at least 2 years. An alternative approach that may reduce the nephrotoxicity risk is to treat patients intermittently for 3 months, stopping therapy and only retreating upon relapse.

Renal monitoring

During the first 3 months of cyclosporine therapy, blood pressure and serum creatinine levels should be assessed every 2 weeks. After that, if these parameters are acceptable and stable, a monthly determination will suffice.

The maximal serum creatinine level is most closely associated with decreased GFR and serious structural changes in the kidney. Cyclosporine-induced nephropathy developed in only 7% of patients with a maximal increase in serum creatinine of less than 30%

above baseline values and in 59% of patients with an increase of 100% or more.

1 If serum creatinine rises above 30% of the baseline value (*not* the upper limit of the normal range), the dose of cyclosporine must be reduced.

2 If the reduced cyclosporine dose decreases the creatinine value to a "safe" level but the psoriasis fails to improve, then cyclosporine monotherapy should be considered a therapeutic failure.

3 If the reduced cyclosporine dose is *not* able to decrease the creatinine value to a "safe" level (<30% above baseline value) after 1 month, cyclosporine should be discontinued; it may be restarted later at an even lower dose.

4 If the serum creatinine level rises into the abnormal range, but is still *less* than 30% above baseline levels, a nephrology consultation should be obtained.

5 Rotate to an alternative treatment after 2 years of cumulative cyclosporine therapy. (Intermittent short courses of cyclosporine lengthen the total duration of the therapy.)

6 If cyclosporine is required for maintenance beyond 2 years, then nephrology consultation should be obtained and kidney biopsy contemplated.

It is believed that cyclosporine increases the synthesis of thromboxane A2, a potent vasoconstrictor. In the hope of decreasing thromboxane A2 production, fish oil concentrate 12 g (containing eicosapentaenoic acid and docosahexaenoic acid in a ratio of 3 : 2) added to the diet may attenuate cyclosporine-induced nephropathy.

What is the role of cyclosporine blood levels in psoriasis?

There is no role for cyclosporine blood levels in the routine monitoring of uncomplicated cases. Exceptions are patients taking medications that affect cyclosporine metabolism or patients having an insufficient clinical response. In the treatment of psoriasis, there is no significant correlation between cyclosporine level and efficacy or renal dysfunction, but there is a trend for patients with hypertension and nephrotoxicity to have higher trough levels. As a general rule, cyclosporine trough levels of 50–100 ng/ml are efficacious for psoriasis and levels over 200 ng/ml are more likely to be associated with hypertension and nephrotoxicity. Monitoring of dosing, efficacy, and toxicity of cyclosporine are summarized in Table 17.6.

Table 17.6 Monitoring of cyclosporine dosing, efficacy, and toxicity.

---

1 Monitor the dose of cyclosporine taken by writing detailed limited prescriptions
2 Monitor efficacy by examining the skin, recording estimated extent of body involvement and asking patients about subjective symptoms such as pruritus at periodic follow-up visits
3 Monitor minor toxicity by examining for gingival hyperplasia and hypertrichosis and asking about headache, tremor, and nausea
4 Monitor serious toxicity by measuring blood pressure and serum creatinine level every 2 weeks until dosage stabilized, and then monthly
5 Whole-blood cyclosporine trough levels by monoclonal radioimmunoassay are optional

---

How to treat hypertension

Hypertension commonly develops during cyclosporine therapy. The documentation of systolic pressure of 160 mmHg or diastolic pressure of 95 mmHg on two or more occasions requires intervention. If the clinical situation permits reducing the dose or stopping cyclosporine, that should be done first. If medical treatment of hypertension is contemplated, consultation with a nephrologist may be obtained, but the physician experienced with cyclosporine can usually treat hypertension.

The calcium channel-blocking agents are the drugs of choice for treating cyclosporine-induced hypertension. They are "renal protective" because they cause preferential vasodilation of renal afferent arterioles with increases in GFR and renal blood flow. Some calcium channel-blocking agents such as nicardipine and verapamil increase cyclosporine levels by interfering with its disposition, and this effect must be considered before selecting a drug.

Sustained-release nifedipine tablets decreased and maintained blood pressure in all 13 cyclosporine-treated patients. Nine of 13 demonstrated an increase in blood urea nitrogen levels. Amlodipine 5 mg daily reversed cyclosporine-induced hypertension and nephrotoxicity by increasing GFR and urinary kallikrein levels. Patients should be informed that both cyclosporine and the calcium channel-blocking agents can cause gingival hyperplasia.

It is best to avoid the diuretics. Potassium-sparing agents like triamterene may aggravate cyclosporine-induced hyperkalemia. Diuretics like thiazides and furosemide increase the risk of hyperuricemia (and gout) and worsening azotemia. Angiotensin-converting enzyme inhibitors have limited efficacy when used alone and may aggravate hyperkalemia and acidosis.

Tacrolimus

The macrolide lactone tacrolimus previously known as FK506 is an immunosuppressive drug that is chemically unrelated to cyclosporine but also inhibits T-lymphocyte activation and the synthesis and expression of cytokines by a similar mechanism. Tacrolimus is approved for the prevention of organ rejection in patients receiving allogeneic liver transplants. Because the IL-8/IL-8 receptor pathway may be important in the pathogenesis of psoriasis, it is of great interest that tacrolimus decreases IL-8 mRNA in primary keratinocyte cultures in a dose-dependent manner. In tacrolimus-treated psoriatic plaques, expression of IL-8 mRNA was lost, but IL-8R message persisted. Circulating IL-8 levels seemed to correlate with disease activity.

Seven patients with psoriasis, four receiving organ transplants, were reported to have cleared completely by 4 weeks with full anti-rejection doses of tacrolimus. The remissions were sustained for 5.5–14 months. Improvement of psoriatic arthritis occurred simultaneously. Efforts to reduce the dose of tacrolimus resulted in relapse of psoriasis. Examination of serial biopsies from active psoriatic plaques revealed rapid disappearance of dermal inflammatory cells and neutrophils in the stratum corneum. Hyperkeratosis and acanthosis were slower to return to normal. Immunophenotypic analysis during remission showed reductions in epidermal and dermal CD4+, CD8+, CD25+ (IL-2R+) activated T-cells; striking rise in CD1+ epidermal Langerhans' cells; and reduction but persistence of CD54 (ICAM-1) and E-selectin expression on vascular endothelium. These results are similar to those reported for cyclosporine.

Tacrolimus is 10–100 times more potent than cyclosporine; the chief concern is that the serious adverse effects of this agent will be the same as those of cyclosporine: hypertension and nephrotoxicity. The three psoriasis patients who did not receive transplants experienced serum creatinine increases of 27–111% (mean 68%) above baseline. Mild neurotoxicity was noted; infections, hypertrichosis, and gingival hyperplasia were not observed.

In 1996, a double-blind placebo-controlled trial showed that tacrolimus was effective at improving severe plaque-type psoriasis (reducing PASI 83%) after 9 weeks at doses of 0.05–0.15 mg/kg/day.

Diarrhea and paresthesia were more common in the tacrolimus-treated patients than in the placebo group. Mild hypertension (4%) and mild–moderate renal dysfunction (7%) developed infrequently. Additional studies with larger numbers of patients treated long-term are necessary to elucidate optimal dosing schedules and the toxicity profile of systemic tacrolimus in the treatment of psoriasis.

Topical tacrolimus ointment, 0.03 and 0.1%, is safe and effective for atopic dermatitis and oral lichen planus. A psoriasis microplaque assay system, which employs a discrete 17 mm descaled lesion under occlusion, demonstrated that tacrolimus 0.3% ointment was superior to vehicle and equivalent to a mid-potency corticosteroid and calcipotriene. However, after 6 weeks' application of tacrolimus 0.3% ointment or placebo ointment once daily to psoriatic plaques, without occlusion, there was no significant difference in efficacy. Methods to enhance the skin penetration of tacrolimus such as liposomal delivery may enhance its topical anti-psoriatic effect.

Pimecrolimus

The novel ascomycin macrolactam derivative pimecrolimus, formerly known as SDZ ASM 981, is a selective inflammatory cytokine release inhibitor with low potential for systemic immunosuppression. It is safe and effective for atopic dermatitis and is FDA-approved for that indication in a 1% cream formulation. Pimecrolimus 1% is nearly as effective as clobetasol 0.05% ointment in the psoriasis microplaque assay described above. In a phase I/II double-blind placebo-controlled study, pimecrolimus 20 mg twice daily and 30 mg twice daily reduced the PASI score by 60 and 75%, respectively, after 4 weeks. There was no significant effect on serum creatinine, GFR, or renal blood flow during this brief period. The only consistent side-effect noted was a transient feeling of warmth occurring about 40 minutes after ingestion of the drug; it was well tolerated by the patients.

Selected references

Al-Daraji W. I., Grant K. R., Ryan K. *et al.* (2002) Localization of calcineurin/NFAT in human skin and psoriasis and inhibition of calcineurin?NFAT activation in human keratinocytes by cyclosporin A. *J Invest Dermatol* **118**, 779–788.

Burns M. K., Ellis C. N., Eisen D. *et al.* (1992) Intralesional cyclosporine for psoriasis. *Arch Dermatol* **128**, 786–790.

Clark C. M., Kirby B., Morris A. D. *et al.* (1999) Combination treatment with methotrexate and cyclosporin for severe recalcitrant psoriasis. *Br J Dermatol* **141**, 279–282.

DeSilva B. D., Benton E. C., Tidman M. J. (1999) Generalized pustular psoriasis following withdrawl of oral cyclosporin treatment for palmoplantar pustulosis. *Clin Exp Dermatol* **24**, 10–13.

Economidou J., Barkis J., Demetriou Z. *et al.* (1999) Effects of cyclosporin A on immune activation markers in patients with active psoriasis. *Dermatol* **199**, 144–148.

Edwards B. D., Chalmers R. J., O'Driscoll J. B. *et al.* (1994) Angiotensin II is a risk factor for cyclosporin nephrotoxicity in patients with psoriasis. *Clin Nephrol* **41**, 350–356.

Ellis C. N., Fradin M. S., Hamilton T. A., Coorhees J. J. (1995) Duration of remission during maintenance cyclosporine therapy for psoriasis. *Arch Dermatol* **131**, 791–795.

Ellis C. N., Fradin M. S., Messana J. M. *et al.* (1991) Cyclosporine for plaque-type psoriasis. Results of a multidose, double-blind trial. *N Engl J Med* **324**, 277–284.

Ellis C. N., Gorsulowksy D. C., Hamilton T. A. *et al.* (1986) Cyclosporine improves psoriasis in a double-blind study. *JAMA* **256**, 3110–3116.

Erkko P., Granlund H., Nuutinen M., Reitamo S. (1997) Comparison of cyclosporin A pharmacokinetics of a new microemulsion formulation and standard oral preparation in patients with psoriasis. *Br J Dermatol* **136**, 82–88.

European FK506 Multicentre Psoriasis Study Group (1996) Systemic tacrolimus (FK506) is effective for the treatment of psoriasis in a double-blind, placebo-controlled study. *Arch Dermatol* **132**, 419–423.

Faerber L., Braeutigam M., Weidinger G. *et al.* (2001) Cyclosporine in severe psoriasis. Results of a meta-analysis in 579 patients. *Am J Clin Dermatol* **2**, 41–47.

Gottlieb S. L., Heftler N. S., Gilleaudeau P. *et al.* (1995) Short-contact anthralin treatment augments therapeutic efficacy of cyclosporine in psoriasis: A clinical and pathologic study. *J Am Acad Dermatol* **33**, 637–645.

Griffiths C. E. M., Powles A. V., Baker B. S. *et al.* (1988) Combination cyclosporin A and topical corticosteroid in the treatment of psoriasis. *Transplant Proc* **30** (Suppl. 4), 50–52.

Grossman R. M., Chevret S., Abi-Rached J. *et al.* (1996) Long-term safety of cyclosporine in the treatment of psoriasis. *Arch Dermatol* **132**, 623–269.

Grossmann R. M., Thivolet J., Claudy A. *et al.* (1994) A novel therapeutic approach to psoriasis with combination calcipotrial ointment and a very low-dose cyclosporine: results of a multicenter placebo-controlled study. *J Am Acad Dermatol* **31**, 68–74.

Heydendael V. M. R., Spuls P. I., Ten Berge I. J. M. *et al.* (2002) Cyclosporin trough levels: is monitoring necessary during short-term treatment in psoriasis? A systemic review and clinical data in trough levels. *Br J Dermatol* **147**, 122–129.

Ho V. C., Griffiths C. E., Berth-Jones J. *et al.* (2001) Intermittent short courses of cyclosporine microemulsion for the long-term management of psoriasis: a 2-year cohort study. *J Am Acad Dermatol* **44**, 643–651.

Koo J. (1998) A randomized, double-blind study comparing the efficacy, safety and optimal dose of two formulations of cyclosporin, Neoral and Sandimmun, in patients with severe psoriasis OLP302 Study Group. *Br J Dermatol* **139**, 88–95.

Lemster B. H., Carrol P. B., Rilo H. R. *et al.* (1995) IL-8/IL-8 receptor expression in psoriasis and the response to systemic tacrolimus (FK506) therapy. *Clin Exp Immunol* **99**, 148–154.

Lewis H.M., Powles A.V., Garioch J.J. *et al.* (1992) Six years experience of cyclosporin A in the treatment of chronic plaque psoriasis. *Br J Dermatol* **127** (Suppl. 40), 18.

Mahrle G., Schulze H.-J., Farber L. *et al.* (1995) Low-dose short-term cyclosporine versus etretinate in psoriasis: improvement of skin, nails, and joint involvement. *J Am Acad Dermatol* **32**, 78–88.

Markham T., Watson A., Rogers S. (2002) Adverse effects with long-term cyclosporin for severe psoriasis. *Clin Exp Dermatol* **27**, 111–114.

Meisgassner J. G., Stutz A. (1992) Immunosuppressive macrolides of the type FK506: a novel class of topical agents for treatment of skin diseases? *J Invest Dermatol* **98**, 851–855.

Nakayama J., Koga T., Furue M. (1998) Long-term efficacy and adverse event of nifedipine sustained-release tablets for cyclosporinA-induced hypertension in patients with psoriasis. *Eur J Dermatol* **8**, 563–568.

Nasr I. S. (2000) Topical tacrolimus in dermatology. *Clin Exp Dermatol* **25**, 250–254.

Olivieri I., Salvarani C., Cantini F. *et al.* (1997) Therapy with cyclosporine in psoriatic arthritis. *Semin Arthritis Rheum* **27**, 36–43.

Paul C. F., Ho V. C., McGeown C. *et al.* (2003) Risk of malignancies in psoriasis patients treated with cyclosporine: a 5 year cohort study. *J Invest Dermatol* **120**, 211–216.

Powles A. V., Hardman C. M., Porter W. M. *et al.* (1998) Renal function after 10 years' treatment with cyclosporin for psoriasis. *Br J Dermatol* **138**, 443–449.

Raman G. V., Campbell S. K., Farrer A. *et al.* (1998) Modifying effects of amlodipine on cyclosporinA-induced changes in renal function in patients with psoriasis. *J Hypertension* **16** (Suppl.), 539–541.

Rappersberger K., Komar M., Ebelin M.-E. *et al.* (2002) Pimecrolimus identifies a common genomic anti-inflammatory profile, is clinically highly effective in psoriasis and is well tolerated. *J Invest Dermatol* **119**, 876–887.

Remitz A., Reitamo S., Erkko P. *et al.* (1999) Tacrolimus ointment improves psoriasis in a microplaque assay. *Br J Dermatol* **141**, 103–107.

Ruzicka T., Bieber T., Schopf E. *et al.* (1997) A short-term trial of tacrolimus ointment for atopic dermatitis. *N Engl J Med* **337**, 816–821.

Shupack J., Abel E., Bauer E. *et al.* (1997) Cyclosporine as maintenance therapy in patients with severe psoriasis. *J Am Acad Dermatol* **36** (3 Part 1), 423–432.

Stoot T. J., Korstanje M. J., Bilo H. J. G. *et al.* (1989) Does fish oil protect renal function cyclosporin-treated psoriasis patients? *J Int Med* **226**, 437–441.

Thomson A. W., Nalesnik M. A., Rilo H. R. *et al.* (1993) ICAM-1 and E-selectin expression in lesional biopsies of psoriasis patients responding to systemic FK506 therapy. *Autoimmunity* **15**, 215–223.

Touw C. R., Hakkaart-Van Roijen L., Verboom P. *et al.* (2001) Quality of life and clinical outcomes in psoriasis patients using intermittent cyclosporine. *Br J Dermatol* **144**, 967–972.

Zachariae H., Kragballe K., Hansen H. E. *et al.* (1997) Renal biopsy findings in long-term cyclosporin treatment of psoriasis. *Br J Dermatol* **136**, 531–535.

Zonneveld I. M., Rubins A., Jablonska S. *et al.* (1998) Topical tacrolimus is not effective in chronic plaque psoriasis. A pilot study. *Arch Dermatol* **134**, 1101–1102.

18   Vitamin D_3 and analogues

Charles Camisa

Introduction

Vitamin D_3 is synthesized in the epidermis from 7-dehydro-cholesterol, when exposed to the ultraviolet B (UVB) spectrum (290–320 nm) of natural sunlight. It must then be bound to plasma vitamin D-binding protein and transported via the circulation to the liver and kidney for successive hydroxylations before it becomes active 1,25-dihydroxyvitamin D_3 (calcitriol). Calcitriol exerts its effects by inducing protein synthesis after binding to a specific chromosomal vitamin D receptor (VDR) and forming a dimer with the retinoid X receptor (RXR). Calcitriol affects systemic calcium homeostasis by its actions on several organs (Table 18.1). VDRs for calcitriol have also been demonstrated in normal human epidermis and cultured keratinocytes (KC) indicating that the skin is a target organ. Receptors have also been found in melanocytes, Langerhans' cells, fibroblasts, endothelial cells, activated T-lymphocytes, macrophages, and granulocytes.

Mechanism of action

In normal and nonlesional skin, VDR antigens are expressed in KC of all viable layers of the epidermis. In psoriasis, there is a significant

Table 18.1 Actions of vitamin D_3 in calcium homeostasis.

Parathyroid gland: inhibits parathyroid hormone production
Kidney: inhibits 1-alpha-hydroxylase, suppressing activation of vitamin D_3
Small intestine: stimulates absorption of calcium and phosphate
Bone: promotes both mineralization and osteolysis

increase in VDR expression in the basal and suprabasal layers as well as a marked increase in the density of VDR-positive intra-epidermal and perivascular T-cells and macrophages. Increased VDR expression of psoriatic KC may be a reflection of high proliferative activity and the altered differentiation pattern in psoriasis. The expression of VDR in basal KC is increased in lesional skin during calcitriol treatment. VDR messenger RNA is increased 2.4-fold in calcitriol-treated plaques. The response to vitamin D analogues may be determined by their ability to upregulate transcription or stability of the VDR gene.

The mechanisms of action of vitamin D_3 and analogues has been studied in cell cultures, organ cultures, animal models, and in living human skin. In normal human KC cultures, calcitriol inhibits cell proliferation and induces terminal differentiation. Growth inhibition caused by nontoxic concentrations of calcitriol was accompanied by marked inhibition of DNA synthesis and a decrease in the number of high-affinity receptors for epidermal growth factor/transforming growth factor (TGF)-alpha. The inhibition of growth of cultured KC from involved and uninvolved psoriasis skin was virtually complete at 10^{-6} M. Similarly, DNA synthesis was inhibited in KC cultures in a dose-response fashion from 10^{-8} to 10^{-6} M.

Normal differentiation of KC is induced by increasing free intracellular calcium. Very low concentrations of calcitriol (10^{-11} to 10^{-9} M) in normal human KC cultures caused rapid transient increases in intracellular free calcium independent of protein synthesis.

In skin organ cultures, both calcitriol and a new analogue 22-oxa-calcitriol suppressed the proliferation of normal and psoriatic KC in a concentration- and time-dependent manner. In the study, degeneration of the epidermis was characterized as "top-down necrosis" rather than apoptosis. Xenografts of psoriasis skin on SCID mice demonstrated improvement of clinical and histologic parameters after injections of calcitriol and cyclosporine. Both drugs also reduced the ability of activated autologous lymphocytes to change symptomless skin grafts toward psoriasis morphology.

When calcitriol was added to activated T-lymphocyte clones derived from psoriatic skin, there was dose-dependent inhibition of proliferation and production of interferon-gamma, IL-2, IL-4, and IL-5. TNF-alpha and granulocyte-macrophage colony stimulating factor (GM-CSF) were not inhibited. Inoue *et al.* assessed the effect of calcitriol on the production of cytokines by mitogen-stimulated peripheral blood mononuclear cells of psoriatic patients. Calcitriol

significantly inhibited interferon-alpha, interleukin-6, and inter-
leukin-8, but not tumor necrosis factor-alpha, in a dose-dependent
manner. However, a flow cytometric analysis of calcipotriene-
treated psoriasis indicated an inhibitory effect on the hyperproliferative basal KC rather than an effect on infiltrating leukocytes and
antigen-presenting cells. Calcitriol significantly decreased phagocytosis and the generation of reactive oxygen species by both normal
and psoriatic polymorphonuclear leukocytes (PML); chemotaxis of
only the psoriatic PML was significantly inhibited. The metabolic-
ally inactive vitamin D_2 had no effect in these assays. In summary,
calcitriol may exert its beneficial effects in psoriasis by inhibiting
proliferation of basal KC and lymphocytes and by down-regulating
the production of pro-inflammatory cytokines.

In an immunohistologic study of lesional biopsies during calcipotriene treatment, the earliest change noted was a decrease in
PMLs after 1 week. The number of actively cycling epidermal cells
(Ki-67-positive nuclei) showed a statistically significant decrease
after 2 weeks. There was a trend toward diminished cytokeratin
K16, a marker for aberrant differentiation, in the suprabasal layers
between weeks 4 and 12. The number of T-cells was decreased by
4 weeks. In this study, the antineutrophil and antiproliferative
effects of calcipotriene occurred first and persisted. Calcipotriene
upregulated expression of the VDR in the basal keratinocytes of
psoriatic lesions.

In an independent study of immunohistologic markers in
calcipotriene-treated psoriasis, there was no clinical change at day
3 but significant improvement at day 7. Kang *et al.* demonstrated
no significant change in the markers for CDla, C4, CD8, ICAM-1,
VCAM-1, E-selectin, and HLR-DR. However, IL-10 levels were
increased by 57% and IL-8 levels were decreased by 70% at day 3
compared to baseline. That these changes were documented before
clinical improvement occurred suggests a significant role for the
mechanism of action of calcipotriene. The anti-inflammatory type 2
cytokine interleukin-10 downregulates the expression of IL-8 and
its receptor, but IL-10 is not by itself effective in the treatment of
psoriasis.

In summary, the results of these two seminal studies indicate
that the earliest detected effects of calcipotriene are on markers of
proliferation and differentiation and downregulation of proinflammatory cytokines.

Clinical use of vitamin D₃

The development of vitamin D_3 analogues for the treatment of psoriasis illustrates the typical orderly progression of therapeutic research: serendipity, in vitro work, open pilot studies to assess toxicity and efficacy, double-blind placebo-controlled trials, development of topical formulations, and novel analogues with better safety and efficacy profiles, and the use of analogues in combination with other anti-psoriatic treatments.

Oral vitamin D₃

A patient receiving 1-alpha-hydroxy vitamin D for osteoporosis demonstrated dramatic clearing of her psoriasis. This was followed by several open studies using oral calcitriol, which showed promise, some dramatic results, and significant toxicity. Perez *et al.* treated 85 patients with oral calcitriol for 0.5–3 years. The usual therapeutic dose was 1.5–2.5 µg, administered as a single dose at bedtime because there is less calcium remaining in the gut for absorption. Eighty-eight percent of patients responded: 26.5% complete, 36.2% moderate, 25.3% slight. Nail involvement, pruritus and symptoms of arthritis improved. Plaque-type psoriasis and erythroderma seemed to respond better than pustular or thick guttate lesions.

The serum calcium and 24-hour urine calcium excretion rose 4% and 148%, respectively. The creatinine clearance decreased 13.4% at 6 months and then stabilized, but inulin clearance, a more accurate measure of glomerular filtration rate, was not significantly altered. Two (2.4%) patients developed radiopaque kidney stones. Bone mineral density was not affected after 2 years of therapy.

A placebo-controlled study of oral calcitriol alone has not been performed. However, calcitriol had no additive effect compared to placebo when combined with 21 erythemogenic ultraviolet B (UVB) treatments. Levels of 25-hydroxyvitamin D_3 were increased similarly in both groups, but the patients receiving calcitriol had higher 1,25-hydroxyvitamin D_3 levels as expected. One explanation for the lack of benefit of added calcitriol in this study is that UVB maximally induces cutaneous vitamin D metabolism, rendering exogenous administration superfluous.

Oral calcitriol is an expensive drug whose therapeutic and toxic levels are very close and may overlap in some patients. For this

Table 18.2 Contraindications to the use of oral calcitriol.

1 Personal history of kidney stones

2 Hypercalciuria

3 Mild renal failure

4 Patient taking supplementary calcium, vitamin D, or antacids containing calcium

Table 18.3 How to use oral calcitriol.

1 Measure baseline serum creatinine, blood urea nitrogen (BUN), calcium, phosphorus, and albumin levels, and 24-hour urinary calcium excretion; the maximum allowed throughout the treatment period is 250 mg for women and 300 mg for men

2 Initiate treatment as 0.5 μg at bedtime

3 Increase dose by 0.25 μg every 2 weeks based on calcium levels and skin condition to a maximum of 2.5 μg/day

4 Limit dietary calcium intake to less than 800 mg daily

5 Monitor 24-hour urinary calcium, and serum creatinine, BUN, albumin, calcium and phosphorus every 2 weeks while increasing the dose of calcitriol, and monthly after dose and calcium levels have stabilized

6 Order yearly renal ultrasound to monitor for nephrocalcinosis and kidney stones

reason, it is relegated to fourth-line adjuvant status for severe or recalcitrant cases of psoriasis. Contraindications and how to use calcitriol are shown in Tables 18.2 and 18.3.

Topical calcitriol

Double-blind left–right comparison studies were performed with calcitriol compounded in petrolatum 15 μg/g in 84 patients for 2.4 months. The improvement in the calcitriol-treated side was statistically better, 61% vs. 5%. There were 44% excellent and 36% moderate responses in the calcitriol-treated side. When extensive areas were treated with up to 10 g of ointment daily, no significant changes in serum or 24-hour urine calcium were detected. There was no increase in blood calcitriol or parathyroid hormone (PTH) levels.

When calcitriol 3 μg/g (Silkis ointment, Galderma Laboratories) was applied for 6 weeks at 50 g/week, there was no affect on parameters of systemic calcium homeostasis. An additional 253 patients were treated with 3 μg/g twice daily for up to 78 weeks. The PASI declined 53%, and there were no clinically relevant changes in mean serum levels of calcium, phosphorus, creatinine, calcitriol, PTH, or 24-hour urine calcium and creatinine clearance. No serious adverse events occurred during the study. About 15% experienced mild transient skin irritation. In subsequent safety studies of calcitriol ointment 3 µg/g, no sensitization, phototoxicity, or photoallergenicity was observed. Comparison with other topical psoriasis therapies demonstrated that: (1) calcitriol 3 µg/g applied twice daily is comparable in efficacy to short-contact anthralin therapy; (2) calcitriol applied *once* daily and betamethasone valerate 0.1% applied once daily was equivalent to betamethasone valerate applied *twice* daily; (3) when 90 g per week of either calcitriol 3 µg/g or calcipotriene was used to treat psoriasis, the PASI score was significantly more reduced by calcipotriene; and (4) in open studies, calcitriol ointment produced "definite improvement" or complete clearance in the majority of patients treated for psoriasis of the face, hairline, or retroauricular areas. Treatment of psoriasis with the combination of broadband UVB phototherapy plus calcitriol ointment compared to UVB plus vehicle ointment reduced the PASI scores by 65% vs. 43%, respectively. The cumulative UVB dose needed for clearing was reduced by one-third in the calcitriol-treated group. In summary, results indicate that calcitriol ointment 3 µg/g is moderately effective for chronic plaque psoriasis, safe, well tolerated and does not adversely affect systemic calcium and phosphorus homeostasis.

Vitamin D₃ analogues

Calcipotriene

An analogue of calcitriol, called calcipotriene (calcipotriol outside of the U.S.) acts via the same receptor but is 100 times less calciotropic than calcitriol. It is equally as effective in the induction of differentiation and the inhibition of proliferation of human KC in vitro. Double-blind placebo-controlled trials confirmed its efficacy and tolerability. Limited data show that it is more effective than vehicle in children 2–14 years of age. The optimal concentration was found to be 50 µg/g of ointment, and this product is now commercially available worldwide as Dovonex or Daivonex.

A double-blind right to left comparison of calcipotriene ointment 50 µg/g and betamethasone valerate 0.1% ointment (a group III corticosteroid) showed that calcipotriene was slightly superior for mild to moderate psoriasis vulgaris. At 6 weeks, the mean PASI reduction was 68.8% with calcipotriene and 61.4% with betamethasone ($p < 0.001$). Both preparations were well tolerated; the most common adverse event, lesional or perilesional irritation, was slightly but not significantly more common with calcipotriene. Calcipotriene is also more effective than coal tar or short-contact anthralin therapy. Calcipotriene ointment twice daily showed similar efficacy to fluocinonide 0.05% or betamethasone dipropionate plus salicylic acid ointment applied twice daily.

Once daily application of calcipotriene ointment is also more active than placebo, producing marked improvement in 59% vs. 12%. Calcipotriene in a cream formulation is available; it is comparable to a group V corticosteroid, decreasing the PASI score by about 48%. Facial irritation was reported in 10% of the calcipotriene users. The application of calcipotriene cream in the morning and the ointment in the evening may increase the patient's compliance with twice daily dosing.

Calcipotriene scalp solution applied twice daily was superior to placebo but not as effective as betamethasone valerate 0.1% solution, clearing or markedly improving 58% vs. 75% of patients, respectively. Scalp irritation was seen much more often with calcipotriene (26%) than with the corticosteroid solution (8%).

In short-term studies of the effects of topical calcipotriene 50 µg/g (3 g applied daily) on calcium metabolism, no increase in serum calcium, 24-hour urinary calcium, or change in other special markers of calcium or bone metabolism was detected. Despite an estimated 2.6–12% percutaneous absorption of calcipotriene, significant effects on systemic calcium homeostasis were not observed. Rare examples of hypercalcemia have been reported when more than 100 g calcipotriene ointment was applied in 1 week. In a study of efficacy and toxicity in patients with extensive psoriasis, a total of up to 500 g applied in 2 weeks reduced serum calcitriol and PTH levels in all patients. The mean serum and 24-hour urine calcium values rose during treatment and fell after withdrawal, but no patient developed hypercalcemia and some developed transient hypercalciuria. The PASI score was reduced by 65% in 28 patients so treated, and the relapse rate was comparable to that of the Ingram regime.

Calcipotriene ointment may be applied under occlusion. In a study of palmoplantar psoriasis, twice daily application gave the same improvement as twice weekly application under plastic occlusion after 6 weeks. In a different study, target psoriasis plaques were treated with calcipotriene ointment under hydrocolloid dressing occlusion once weekly. The average time to clearance was 3.6 weeks and the average remission time was greater than 8 weeks.

Combination therapy

Ultraviolet light and systemic therapy

In practice, it is popular to combine topical calcipotriene with ultraviolet light (UVL) therapy or systemic therapy. Although the combinations may allow for lower cumulative doses of UVB, UVA, acitretin, or cyclosporine over the short-term (generally 6–12 week studies), they do not significantly increase the number of patients who achieve marked improvement or clearance. For this reason, longer trials must be performed to determine whether the addition of calcipotriene to phototherapy or systemic drugs improves the risk–benefit ratio by decreasing the long-term toxicity.

Some caveats apply when calcipotriene is combined with UVL. Calcipotriene absorbs light in the UVB range and has the effect of increasing the minimal erythema dose. If patients are undergoing erythemogenic UVB, calcipotriene should be added cautiously because a "sunburn reaction" has been reported. The calcipotriene concentration on the skin is reduced after UVA exposure. If used in combination, calcipotriene must be applied after the UV exposure.

Topical corticosteroids

The combination of calcipotriene and potent topical corticosteroids is synergistic therapeutically and reduces the adverse effects of the corticosteroid (cutaneous atrophy and rebound) and calcipotriene (local cutaneous irritation). Many studies employing different regimens and different topical steroids have borne this out. For example, calcipotriene cream in the morning and betamethasone valerate cream in the evening was more effective and less irritating than calcipotriene cream twice daily. In another study, 2 weeks of twice daily calcipotriene was followed by 4 weeks of calcipotriene and betamethasone valerate or calcipotriene monotherapy. The combination was more effective. Clobetasol twice daily for 2 weeks followed by calcipotriene for 4 weeks was superior to calcipotriene for 6 weeks. A different short-term strategy utilizes betamethasone dipropionate in ointment vehicle (OV) once daily and calcipotriene twice daily on alternate weeks. The combination was more effective than the daily topical steroid for 4 weeks. After significantly improving mild to moderate psoriasis with calcipotriene ointment in the morning and halobetasol ointment in the evening, the duration of remission was extended by combining weekday calcipotriene with a weekend pulse therapy regimen of the superpotent topical steroid.

A new ointment vehicle has been developed in order to contain both calcipotriene (50 µg/g) and betamethasone dipropionate (0.5 mg/g). The combination ointment was more effective than either active constituent alone, whether it was applied once or twice daily, and had a more rapid onset of action. The combined formulation produced less local adverse reactions than either calcipotriene or the vehicle, but not betamethasone dipropionate alone.

Tacalcitol

Tacalcitol (1-alpha, 24-dihydroxyvitamin D_3) is another synthetic analogue of calcitriol. A double-blind right-to-left comparison of once-daily application of tacalcitol 4 µg/g ointment demonstrated significantly better ratings of erythema, thickness and scaling compared to application of the vehicle, starting at the week 2 evaluation. Local skin irritation was reported by 12% of patients. Patients were permitted to treat facial and flexural lesions. Of 30 patients treating lesions on the face, only two reported local irritation there. After 8 weeks, none of the laboratory parameters of calcium homeostasis were affected, including PTH. Tacalcitol (Curatoderm, Hermal) is registered for once daily application in Japan (2 µg/g) and some European countries (4 µg/g). A double-blind randomized trial compared tacalcitol once daily to calcipotriene twice daily during 8 weeks. Both ointments reduced the severity of psoriasis, but calcipotriene was significantly more effective. Both were well-tolerated.

The safety and efficacy of tacalcitol has been followed in a group of 304 patients with chronic plaque psoriasis involving 7–20% of the body surface area over a period of 18 months. The median PASI score decreased from 9.5 to 3.3. There were no significant changes in tests of calcium homeostasis. Discontinuation of treatment as a result of skin irritation occurred in 5.9% of patients.

In summary, tacalcitol ointment is a safe, well-tolerated, effective, long-term treatment of plaque-type psoriasis. Although it is less effective than calcipotriene, once daily application may improve compliance especially for patients with extensive and facial psoriasis. A higher concentration of tacalcitol (20 µg/g) is under study.

Maxacalcitol

Maxacalcitol (1-alpha, 25-dihydroxy-22-oxa-calcitriol) exhibits ten times greater efficacy at suppressing KC proliferation in vitro than calcipotriene and tacalcitol. It was applied to chronic plaque psoriasis once daily in varying concentrations (6–50 µg/g). All concentrations fared better than placebo, and at 8 weeks, maxacalcitol 25 µg/g once daily produced marked improvement or clearing of psoriasis in 55% of patients compared to calcipotriene applied once daily (46%). Longer-term studies and comparisons to calcipotriene twice daily and tacalcitol once daily are indicated.

Fluorinated calcitriol

Hexafluoro-calcitriol (hexafluoro-1,25-dihydroxyvitamin D_3) is a novel fluorinated derivative of calcitriol. It demonstrates increased potency and longer lasting effect in inhibiting proliferation of normal and psoriatic cultured KC, possibly owing to decreased metabolic inactivation and a much longer half-life in these cells. In a pilot double-blind left–right comparison, all 15 subjects improved significantly; two reported mild irritation. When larger areas were treated in an open fashion, 90% of patients showed moderate to marked improvement. There were no significant changes in the parameters of calcium homeostasis, including PTH levels.

Summary

The topical vitamin D_3 analogues, calcipotriene, tacalcitol, calcitriol, and others, are first-line therapy along with topical corticosteroids for mild to moderate cases of psoriasis vulgaris covering up to 20% of the body surface area. Most of the improvement occurs during the first 4–6 weeks of treatment and is maintained with continuous application. While mild irritant dermatitis of the face and anogenital area have been reported frequently, these unwanted effects generally do not lead to withdrawal of treatment, thus giving the clinician a safe and effective alternative for the hairline and body folds where potent topical corticosteroids are relatively contraindicated. Neither dermal atrophy nor tachyphylaxis occurred after 6–18 months' use of calcipotriene and tacalcitol. Allergic contact dermatitis to calcipotriene occurred in a few patients with possible cross-sensitivity to other vitamin D_3 analogues.

Selected references

Ashcroft D. M., Li Wan Po A., Williams H. C., Griffiths C. E. (2000) Combination regimens of topical calcipotriene in chronic plaque psoriasis: systematic review of efficacy and tolerability. *Arch Dermatol* **136**, 1536–1543.

Barker J. N., Ashton R. E., Marks R. *et al.* (1999) Topical maxacalcitol for the treatment of psoriasis vulgaris: a placebo-controlled, double-blind, dose-finding study with active comparator. *Br J Dermatol* **141**, 274–278.

Barna M., Bos J. D., Kapsenberg M. L., Snijdewint F. G. M. (1997) Effect of calcitriol on the production of T-cell-derived cytokines in psoriasis. *Br J Dermatol* **136**, 536–541.

Bleiker T. O., Bourke J. F., Mumford R., Hutchinson P. E. (1998) Long-term outcome of severe chronic plaque psoriasis following treatment with high-dose topical calcipotriol. *Br J Dermatol* **139**, 285–286.

Bourke J. F., Iqbal S. J., Hutchinson P. E. (1997) A randomized double-blind comparison of the effects on systemic calcium homeostasis of topical calcitriol (3 micrograms/g) in the treatment of chronic plaque psoriasis vulgaris. *Acta Derm Venereol* **77**, 228–230.

Bourke J. F., Iqbal S. J., Hutchinson P. E. (1996) Vitamin D analogues in psoriasis: effects on systemic calcium homeostasis. *Br J Dermatol* **135**, 347–354.

Bourke J. F., Mumford R., Whittaker P. *et al.* (1997) The effects of topical calcipotiol on systemic calcium homeostasis in patients with chronic plaque psoriasis. *J Am Acad Dermatol* **37**, 929–934.

Castelijns F. A. C. M., Gerritsen M. J. P., van Erp P. E. J., van de Kerkhoff P. C. M. (2000) Efficacy of calcipotriol ointment applied under hydrocolloid occlusion in psoriasis. *Dermatol* **200**, 25–30.

Dam T. N., Kang S., Nickoloff B. J., Voorhees J. J. (1999) 1-alpha, 25-dihydroxycholecalciferol and cyclosporine suppress induction and promote resolution of psoriasis in human skin grafts transplanted on to SCID mice. *J Invest Dermatol* **113**, 1082–1089.

Durakovic C., Malabanan A., Holick M. F. (2001) Rationale for use and clinical responsiveness of hexafluoro-1, 25-dihydroxyvitamin D_3 for the treatment of plaque psoriasis: a pilot study. *Br J Dermatol* **144**, 500–506.

Duweb G. A., Abuzariba O., Rahim M. *et al.* (2001) Occlusive versus nonocclusive calcipotriol ointment treatment for palmoplantar psoriasis. *Int J Tissue React* **23**, 59–62.

Green C., Ganpule M., Harris D. *et al.* (1994) Comparative effects of calcipotriol (MC903) solution and placebo (vehicle of MC903) in the treatment of psoriasis of the scalp. *Br J Dermatol* **130**, 483–487.

Inoue M., Matsui T., Nishibu A. *et al.* (1998) Regulatory effects of 1-alpha, 25-dihydroxyvitamin D_3 on inflammatory responses in psoriasis. *Eur J Dermatol* **8**, 16–26.

Jensen A. M., Llado M. B., Skov L. *et al.* (1998) Calcipotriol inhibits the proliferation of hyperproliferative CD29 positive keratinocytes in psoriatic epidermis in the absence of an effect on the function and number of antigen-presenting cells. *Br J Dermatol* **139**, 984–999.

Kang S., Yi S., Griffiths C. E. *et al.* (1998) Calcipotriene-induced improvement in psoriasis is associated with reduced interleukin-8 and increases interleukin-10 levels within lesions. *Br J Dermatol* **138**, 77–83.

Katayama I., Ohkawara A., Ohkido M. *et al.* (2002) High-concentration (20 μg/g) tacalcitol ointment therapy on refractory psoriasis vulgaris with low response to topical corticosteroids. *Eur J Dermatol* **12**, 553–557.

Kaufmann R., Bibby A. J., Bissonnette R. *et al.* (2002) A new calcipotriol/betamethasone dipropionate formulation (Daivobet) is an effective once-daily treatment for psoriasis vulgaris. *Dermatol* **205**, 389–393.

Klaber M. R., Hutchinson P. E., Pebvis-Leftick A. *et al.* (1994) Comparative effects of calcipotriol solution [50 micrograms/ml] and betamethasone 17-valerate solution [1 mg/ml] in the treatment of scalp psoriasis. *Br J Dermatol* **131**, 678–683.

Kondo S., Hozumi Y., Mitsuhashi Y. (2000) Comparative inhibitory effects of vitamin D_3 and an analogue on normal and psoriatic epidermis in organ culture. *Arch Derm Res* **292**, 550–555.

Kowalzick L. (2001) Clinical experience with topical calcitriol (1,25-dihydroxyvitamin D_3) in psoriasis. *Br J Dermatol* **144** (Suppl. 58), 21–25.

Kragballe K., Barnes L., Hamberg K. J. *et al.* (1998) Calcipotriol cream with or without concurrent topical corticosteroid in psoriasis: tolerability and efficacy. *Br J Dermatol* **139**, 649–654.

Langner A., Ashton P., van de Kerkhof P. C. M. *et al.* (1996) A long-term multicentre assessment, of the safety and tolerability of calcitriol ointment in the treatment of chronic plaque psoriasis. *Br J Dermatol* **135**, 385–389.

Lebwohl M. (2002) Vitamin D and topical therapy. *Cutis* **70**, 5–8.

Milde P., Hauser U., Simon T. *et al.* (1991) Expression of 1,25-dihidroxyvitamin D_3 receptors in normal and psoriatic skin. *J Invest Dermatol* **97**, 230–239.

Molin L., Cutler T. P., Helander I. *et al.* (1997) Comparative efficacy of calcipotriol (MC903) cream and betamethasone 17-valerate cream in the treatment of chronic plaque psoriasis. A randomized, double-blind, parallel group multicentre study. *Br J Dermatol* **136**, 89–93.

Papp K. A., Guenther L., Boyden B. *et al.* (2003) Early onset of action and efficacy of a combination of calcipotriene and betamethasone dipropionate in the treatment of psoriasis. *J Am Acad Dermatol* **48**, 48–54.

Pariser D. M., Pariser D. J., Breneman D. *et al.* (1996) Calcipotriene ointment applied once a day for psoriasis: a double-blind, multicenter, placebo-controlled study. *Arch Dermatol* **134**, 238–246.

Perez A., Chen J. C., Turner A. *et al.* (1996) Efficacy and safety of topical calcitriol (1,25-dihydroxy vitamin D₃) for the treatment of psoriasis. *Br J Dermatol* **134**, 238–246.

Perez A., Raab R., Chen T. C. *et al.* (1996) Safety and efficacy of oral calcitriol (1,25-dihydroxy vitamin D₃) for the treatment of psoriasis. *Br J Dermatol* **134**, 1070–1078.

Prystowsky J. H., Knobler E. H., Muzio P. J. (1996) Oral calcitriol does not augment UVB phototherapy for plaque psoriasis. *J Am Acad Dermatol* **35**, 272–274.

Queille-Roussel C., Duteil L., Parneix-Spake A. *et al.* (2001) The safety of calcitriol 3 microg/g ointment. Evaluation of cutaneous contact sensitization, cumulative irritancy, photoallergic contact sensitization and phototoxicity. *Eur J Dermatol* **11**, 219–224.

Reich K., Garbe C., Blaschke V. *et al.* (2001) Response of psoriasis to interleukin-10 is associated with suppression of cutaneous type 1 inflammation, downregulation of the epidermal interleukin-8/CXCR2 pathway and normalization of keratinocyte maturation. *J Invest Dermatol* **116**, 319–329.

Reichrath J., Muller S. M., Kerber A. *et al.* (1997) Biologic effects of topical calcipotriol (MC903) treatment in psoriatic skin. *J Am Acad Dermatol* **36**, 19–28.

Ring J., Kowalzick L., Christophers E. *et al.* (2001) Calcitriol 3 microg/g ointment in combination with ultraviolet B phototherapy for the treatment of plaque psoriasis: results of a comparative study. *Br J Dermatol* **144**, 495–499.

Ruzicka T., Lorenz B. (1998) Comparison of calcipotriol monotherapy and a combination of calcipotriol and betamethasone valerate after 2 weeks' treatment with calcipotriol in the topical therapy of psoriasis vulgaris: a multicentre, double-blind, randomized study. *Br J Dermatol* **138**, 254–258.

Scott L. J., Dunn C. J., Goa K. L. (2001) Calcipotriol ointment. A review of its use in the management of psoriasis. *Am J Clin Dermatol* **2**, 95–120.

Steinkjer B. (1994) Contact dermatitis from calcipotriol. *Contact Dermatitis* **31**, 122.

van de Kerkhof P. C., Berthe-Jones J., Griffiths C. E. *et al.* (2002) Long term efficacy and safety of tacalcitol ointment in patients with chronic plaque psoriasis. *Br J Dermatol* **146**, 414–422.

van de Kerkhof P. C., Franssen M., de la Brassine M., Kuipers M. (2001) Calcipotriol cream in the morning and ointment in the evening: a novel regimen to improve compliance. *J Dermatol Treat* **12**, 75–79.

van de Kerkhof P. C. M., Werfel T., Haustein U. F. *et al.* (1996) Tacalcitol ointment in the treatment of psoriasis vulgaris: a multicentre, placebo-controlled, double-blind study on efficacy and safety. *Br J Dermatol* **135**, 758–765.

Veien N. K., Bjerke J. R., Rossmann-Ringdahl I., Jackson H. B. (1997) Once daily treatment of psoriasis with tacalcitol compared with twice daily treatment with calcipotriol. A double-blind trial. *Br J Dermatol* **137**, 581–586.

19 Antimetabolites and sulfasalazine

Charles Camisa

Hydroxyurea

When the first therapeutic trial of hydroxyurea in patients with severe recalcitrant psoriasis was reported in 1970, an alternative to methotrexate was being sought. In a double-blind cross-over study, hydroxyurea at 500 mg twice a day clinically and histologically "improved" the psoriasis in nine of the 10 patients after 4 weeks of treatment. Further treatment cleared the psoriasis in six of the nine patients.

More than three decades later, the antimetabolite hydroxyurea has certainly not supplanted methotrexate, but it plays a minor role in the treatment of recalcitrant psoriasis. The drug is mainly used today by hematologists in the treatment of chronic myelogenous leukemia (CML), polycythemia rubra vera, essential thrombocythemia, and sickle cell anemia. Hydroxyurea inhibits cell proliferation by blocking DNA synthesis but does not impair RNA or protein synthesis.

Hydroxyurea is a simple compound with the empirical formula $CH_4N_2O_2$. It is well absorbed from the gastrointestinal tract and serum concentration peaks in about 2 hours. Excretion is primarily renal. The parent compound is probably the active drug.

Clinical studies

Layton *et al.* reported on the use of hydroxyurea for severe widespread chronic plaque psoriasis refractory to conventional topical therapy. Sixty percent (51/85) of patients achieved "complete to near complete clearing." The starting dose was usually 1.5 g daily, and the maintenance dose ranged from 0.5 to 1.5 g daily. In a prospective nonrandomized series, Kumar *et al.* treated 31 patients with extensive plaque psoriasis at a dose of 1–1.5 g/day for a median of 36 weeks. More than half of the patients achieved at least a 70% reduction of the PASI score.

Adverse effects

In the study of Layton *et al.*, adverse reactions occurred in 37 (43%) of 85 patients. The majority of the side-effects are hematologic: anemia, leukopenia, thrombocytopenia, pancytopenia, and macrocytosis. Treatment was discontinued because of adverse effects in 16 patients (18%). By contrast, in the study of Kumar *et al.* in Indian patients, the majority (58.6%) of the patients developed grayish-brown pigmentation of the nails, skin, or mucous membranes after a median of 4.3 weeks of the therapy. The adverse effects were considered mild and reversible, and no patient discontinued therapy because of them. Other, less common, adverse effects of hydroxyurea are xerosis, edema of the legs, oral ulcers, photosensitivity of psoriasis, diffuse alopecia, elevation of liver enzymes, and nausea. Recall erythema localized to previously x-irradiated areas and fixed drug reactions have been reported.

Two cutaneous reactions—leg ulcerations and a poikilodermatous rash of the backs of the hands with lichenoid papules—occur primarily in patients with blood dyscrasias, probably because they are more likely to be treated with long-term hydroxyurea. Both reactions occurred in an elderly woman treated for extensive psoriasis with hydroxyurea for 5 years. Hydroxyurea dermopathy, as it is called, is sometimes associated with low-titer antinuclear antibodies and may be confused with connective tissue diseases. It improves after cessation of the drug. Guidelines for the use of hydroxyurea are shown in Table 19.1.

Patient selection

All of the following treatments for chronic plaque-type psoriasis should be tried where appropriate before hydroxyurea is considered: conventional topical therapy, ultraviolet B (UVB) phototherapy, psoralen with ultraviolet A (PUVA) photochemotherapy, methotrexate, and acitretin. Cyclosporine, which is more toxic, and much more expensive, and the new biologic agents should take a second berth to hydroxyurea. In contrast to cyclosporine, hydroxyurea is not effective for pustular or erythrodermic psoriasis or psoriatic

Table 19.1 How to use hydroxyurea.

---

1 Complete blood cell count (CBC), chemistry profile, and urinalysis should be performed at baseline

2 Repeat CBC weekly for the first month and then every 2–4 weeks thereafter

3 Repeat liver profile and urinalysis monthly

4 Start therapy at 1 g daily. About half of the hematologic side-effects relating to myelosuppression and megaloblastic erythropoiesis can be avoided at this dose

5 Reduce the dosage if hemoglobin drops more than 2 g/dl, the white blood cell count decreases to <3500/µl, or the platelet count decreases to <100,000/µl

6 Improvement is usually evident at 6–8 weeks of therapy. If no improvement occurs by this time, and the hematologic parameters remain acceptable, increase the dose to 1.5 g daily and follow counts weekly

---

arthritis. The combination of low dose cyclosporine 2.5 mg/kg/day and hydroxyurea 500 mg/day was effective at clearing seven out of eight patients with severe psoriasis after 8 weeks. Hydroxyurea is contraindicated in pregnancy and lactation. Significant hepatic or renal disease are relative contraindications.

Maintenance

Since hydroxyurea is only mildly to moderately effective in most cases of extensive plaque-type psoriasis, it is a good choice for intermittent treatment when rotating systemic drugs which have different target organs of toxicity such as acitretin (skeleton, lipids); methotrexate (liver); and cyclosporine (kidneys).

Hydroxyurea has been effective as short-term continuous treatment for up to 36 weeks, and as intermittent treatment for up to 18 months. In general, an attempt should be made to decrease the dose or stop the drug after maximal improvement has been achieved.

Thiopurine antimetabolites

The thiopurine antimetabolites including azathioprine (AZA), 6-mercaptopurine (6-MP), and 6-thioguanine (6-TG) are used as immunosuppressive and steroid-sparing agents for many diseases (Fig. 19.1).

AZA is metabolized to 6-MP which is then converted into 6-MP ribotide. This is the active agent that, because of its structural

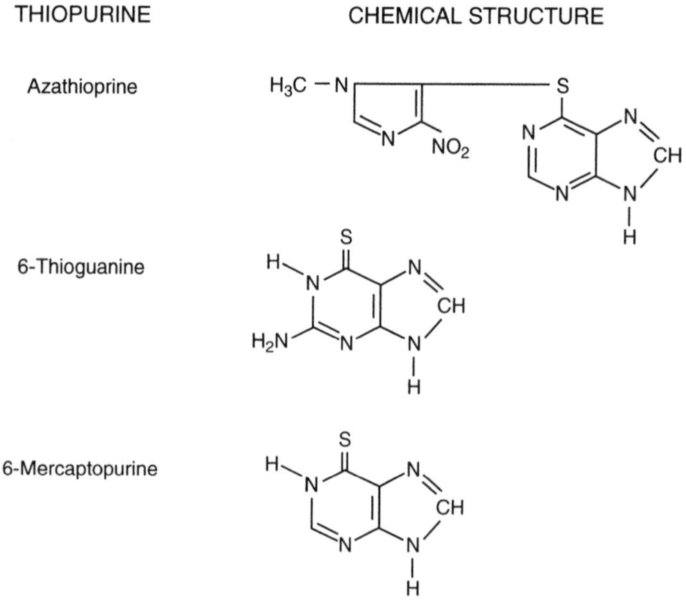

THIOPURINE   CHEMICAL STRUCTURE

Azathioprine

6-Thioguanine

6-Mercaptopurine

Figure 19.1 Chemical structures of selected thiopurine antimetabolites.

similarity to inosinic acid, competes with enzymes involved in guanylic and adenylic acid synthesis, thereby inhibiting DNA synthesis.

AZA was used to treat 29 patients with severe plaque-type psoriasis as well as erythroderma and pustular variants. Nineteen (66%) of 29 patients benefited with 50–100% improvement on doses of 75–200 mg/day. The main side-effects are gastrointestinal and hematologic: macrocytic anemia, leukopenia, and thrombocytopenia.

In human cells, simple genetic polymorphism controls activity of the enzyme thiopurine methyltransferase (TPMT), which rapidly converts AZA to inactive metabolites. Since 90% of subjects have high levels of TPMT, they are susceptible to underdosing with AZA if it is administered at the lower end of the therapeutic range, 1–3 mg/kg/day. Heterozygous individuals have intermediate levels of TPMT which may place them at increased risk of myelosuppression, and 1/300 patients have almost no TPMT activity and are at risk from profound myelosuppression with any dose of AZA. The solution is to measure TPMT activity before AZA treatment is started

Table 19.2 How to use azathioprine.

1 Contraindications: pregnancy, severe liver dysfunction, concomitant administration of allopurinol
2 Complete blood cell count (CBC), chemistry profile and urinalysis at baseline
3 Repeat CBC and liver profile every 4 weeks while escalating dose; check amylase if liver enzymes are elevated
4 Unless TPMT level is known (see text), start azathioprine at 50 mg/day; increase by 50 mg/day every 4 weeks until satisfactory response or dose-limiting toxicity occurs
5 The average dose is 150–200 mg/day; the maximum dose is approximately 300 mg/day
6 When the dose has stabilized, monitor CBC and chemistry profile every 2–3 months

and to select a dosage appropriate to the individual. TPMT activity can be determined in red blood cell lysates, which correlates with activity in the liver, but the test is not readily available. Until the assays become more widely available, I suggest initiating treatment at 50 mg/day, and increasing by 50 mg each month to a maximum of 300 mg/day (Table 19.2) while monitoring for myelosuppression.

Gastrointestinal reactions—nausea, vomiting, diarrhea—are usually well tolerated especially when dosages are gradually escalated. The more serious complications—idiosyncratic hepatitis, hepatic veno-occlusive disease, pancreatitis, drug fever, myelosuppression—occur in 1% or fewer patients. The latter is much more likely to occur in patients who have low TPMT activity or who take concomitant allopurinol, a xanthine oxidase inhibitor. Thrombocytopenia is likely to be the first sign of bone marrow toxicity. The theoretical risks of increased infection and cancer have not been observed in the treatment of dermatologic disorders because of lower doses, shorter duration, and absence of concomitant immunosuppressive drugs (i.e. corticosteroids, cyclosporine, mycophenolate mofetil).

6-TG is an antimetabolite in purine synthesis that is structurally related to 6-MP and AZA. It also inhibits DNA synthesis. 6-TG is metabolized primarily by the liver, and it is used mainly to treat acute myelogenous leukemia. Its chief toxicity is myelosuppression.

Zackheim *et al.* treated 76 patients with recalcitrant plaque-type psoriasis with 6-TG at 80 mg/day or 120–160 mg twice weekly. About 50% of patients responded and were maintained for 33

Table 19.3 How to use 6-thioguanine.

1 Complete blood cell count (CBC), chemistry profile, and urinalysis should be performed at baseline
2 Repeat CBC weekly during dose escalation period and then every 2 weeks thereafter
3 Repeat liver and kidney profile monthly during dose escalation and at least every 3 months thereafter
4 Unless TPMT level is known (see text), start therapy at 20 mg/day. Increase by 20 mg every 2 weeks until satisfactory response is obtained or dose-limiting toxicity occurs
5 Reduce dose or discontinue if white blood cell count decreases to <4000/µl, platelet count decreases to <125,000/µl, or hemoglobin drops to 11 g/dl
6 After desired clearing is obtained, taper dose to twice-weekly or thrice-weekly administration if possible

months. Palmoplantar pustulosis and generalized pustular psoriasis may also respond very well to 6-TG. The response is usually evident within 2 months of starting therapy (Table 19.3). Using a pulse-dosing schedule of 120 mg twice weekly or 160 mg thrice weekly, Silvis and Levine achieved 75% improvement in 70% of patients. Further, 14 (78%) of 18 patients showed >90% improvement with escalating dosages of 6-TG varying from 20 mg twice weekly to 120 mg daily.

Myelosuppression is the most common side-effect (47%) that necessitates discontinuation of therapy. Thrombocytopenia may appear before leukopenia and anemia. Clinical improvement seems to correlate with some degree of myelosuppression. Two patients with dramatic clearing of psoriasis and profound myelosuppression, respectively, were determined to have intermediate levels of TPMT. Elevation of liver enzymes occurred in 25%. The second most common adverse effects are gastrointestinal complications: nausea, vomiting, diarrhea, reflux, and elevated liver enzymes. Hepatic veno-occlusive disease may be associated with higher initial doses of 6-TG (160 mg/day). Patients previously treated with long-term MTX may be more sensitive to the bone marrow and liver toxicity of 6-TG. It may be necessary to measure TPMT activity prior to initiating 6-TG therapy because homozygous individuals should not receive it. The current standard of empiric therapy is to use lower doses in elderly patients and those with a history of myelosuppression.

Mycophenolic acid

Mycophenolic acid (MPA) is a potent, selective, reversible inhibitor of inosine monophosphate dehydrogenase and therefore inhibits de novo synthesis of guanosine nucleotide. MPA does not interfere with the production of interleukin (IL)-1 and IL-2, but it does block the coupling of these events to DNA synthesis, thereby selectively suppressing proliferation of T- and B-lymphocytes. The prodrug of MPA, mycophenolate mofetil (MMF, CellCept), has greater bioavailability and was approved by the FDA in 1995 for the prevention of organ rejection in patients receiving allogeneic renal transplants at a dosage of 2–3 g/day. MPA, however, was first studied for psoriasis as early as 1971. Double-blind placebo-controlled trials confirmed the efficacy of MPA (68% decrease in mean severity scores) after 12 weeks, and patients were subsequently treated with 1.6–4.8 g/day for 2 years. The main side-effects related to the gastrointestinal tract (nausea, vomiting, diarrhea) and genitourinary tract (dysuria, urgency, frequency). The incidence of herpes zoster was 4%. The sponsor discontinued the national clinical trial in 1977, but 85 patients continued therapy on a compassionate-use basis for up to 13 years. At stable doses (3 g/day at 5 years), the severity scores remained consistently low. Some patients reported cessation of joint paint and effusions. The gastrointestinal and genitourinary complications decreased over time, but the overall incidence of herpes zoster increased to 11.6%. Leukopenia occurred early in several patients and was the dose-limiting side-effect in some. After MPA therapy for 1 year, almost one-third of patients reported no significant adverse effects. In patients with renal allografts (not psoriasis), MMF, compared to AZA, was associated with a slightly higher incidence of diarrhea, leukopenia, and cytomegalovirus infections. Anecdotally, MMF has been reported to be effective in the treatment of autoimmune diseases: bullous pemphigoid, pemphigus vulgaris, pyoderma gangrenosum, and systemic vasculitis associated with anti-neutrophil cytoplasmic antibodies. A randomized, controlled study of 1% MPA incorporated into an ointment base was ineffective when applied to psoriasis plaques under occlusion for 3 weeks.

The results of MMF in the treatment of psoriasis have not been as successful as for MPA, although the reports have been anecdotal or small open trials. For example, in a 6-week trial of MMF dosed at 2 g/day for 3 weeks, the mean PASI score was reduced from 30.5 to

Table 19.4 How to use mycophenolate mofetil.

---

1 Patient selection: recalcitrant psoriasis of all types

2 Contraindications: pregnancy, leukopenia, thrombocytopenia

3 Baseline laboratory: complete blood cell count (CBC), chemistry profile, urinalysis, pregnancy test (where appropriate)

4 Monitoring laboratory: CBC weekly for first month, CBC twice monthly for second and third month, CBC monthly thereafter for first year. Other tests every 3 months or as indicated by symptoms

5 Dosage: initiate mycophenolate mofetil at 1 g bid for 12 weeks. If the patient's response is unsatisfactory, increase by 250 mg each month to maximum 2 g bid

6 After 1 year on stable dose, taper mycophenolate mofetil by 250 mg each month until psoriasis begins to flare (usually one month after attaining ineffective dose level)

7 If gastrointestinal symptoms occur, try qid dosing of same total dosage before reducing dosage

---

16.1 (47%). The lower dose and the short duration of treatment were probably insufficient. However, a longer 10-week study of MMF monotherapy (2 g/day) showed that patients with moderate, but not severe, chronic plaque-type psoriasis, and refractory psoriatic arthritis, improved.

MMF is clearly not as effective as cyclosporine in controlling severe psoriasis. When eight patients were rotated to MMF after long-term treatment (mean of 7.6 years) with cyclosporine, the disease deteriorated significantly in five patients and slightly in three patients over a period of 2–32 weeks. MMF, however, did allow renal function to improve in all six patients with cyclosporine-induced nephrotoxicity. Moreover, MMF (up to 3 g/day) combined with low-dose cyclosporine (2.5 mg/kg/day) may yield moderate disease control while avoiding cyclosporine-induced nephrotoxicity.

Because MPA has been proven effective for psoriasis and can be tolerated for many years with sustained efficacy, MMF at dosages of 2–3 g/day should be considered as fourth-line innovative therapy after PUVA, MTX and retinoids, or in combination as a "cyclosporine-sparing" agent (Table 19.4).

Sulfasalazine

Sulfasalazine (salicylazosulfapyridine, Azulfidine) is used as a steroid-sparing agent for inflammatory bowel disease. It has also been shown to be effective as second-line disease-modifying therapy for rheumatoid arthritis and ankylosing spondylitis. It may have anti-inflammatory activity in these diseases and psoriasis by inhibiting 5-lipoxygenase.

After oral administration, one-third of sulfasalazine is absorbed in the small intestine and two-thirds pass to the colon where it is split by bacteria into its components, sulfapyridine (SP) and 5-aminosalicylic acid (5-ASA). Most of the SP and about one-third of 5-ASA is absorbed. Serum concentrations of SP and metabolites tend to be higher in patients with a slow acetylator phenotype. These patients are more likely to have adverse reactions to sulfasalazine.

Sulfasalazine has been evaluated as monotherapy in the treatment of psoriasis. In two open-label trials, 50% of patients completing 6–8 weeks of therapy with 3–4 g of sulfasalazine daily showed a marked to excellent response; the other half had minimal to modest improvement. In a double-blind analysis, 17/23 patients randomized to receive sulfasalazine completed 6 weeks of treatment, compared to 26/27 placebo-treated patients. Significant improvement in global severity, scale, erythema, thickness, and total body surface area involved was evident at 4 weeks and further improvement was noted at 8 weeks. In the placebo-treated patients, the psoriasis was unchanged or worse. Overall, of the 17 evaluable patients in the sulfasalazine-treated group, seven had a marked response (60–89%), seven had a moderate response (30–59%), and three had minimal response (0–29%).

Arachidonic acid and eicosanoids were measured in lesional plaques pretherapy and following 1 and 8 weeks of sulfasalazine treatment. There were no significant changes in the levels of arachidonic acid, LTB_4 12-HETE, and 15-HETE after 1 week. At 8 weeks, there was a trend toward arachidonic acid reduction and a significant decrease in LTB_4 only. Keratinocyte intercellular adhesion molecule-1 (ICAM-1) expression was unchanged at 1 week and significantly reduced at 8 weeks. All of these changes were detected after significant clinical improvement had occurred and do not help to elucidate the mechanism of action of sulfasalazine in psoriasis.

Side-effects of sulfasalazine occur frequently. While usually not severe, the most common side-effects, anorexia, nausea, vomiting, fatigue, headaches, and cutaneous eruptions, frequently lead to discontinuation of sulfasalazine before any therapeutic benefit can be expected. Enteric-coated tablets (Azulfidine EN-tabs) are indicated for patients who cannot take regular sulfasalazine tablets because of gastrointestinal side-effects (i.e. nausea and vomiting) after the first few doses. In the studies cited, the incidence of a drug-induced rash was 18%. The rash is the typical generalized erythematous maculopapular pruritic variety and is reversible. Photosensitivity can occur with sulfasalazine and concomitant UVL should be used with caution, if at all. Transient neutropenia and elevated liver enzymes have been reported. Mild hemolytic anemia with decreased hemoglobin or cyanosis may occur. Other adverse reactions occur rarely but are more likely with a daily dosage of 4 g or more, or in slow acetylators who have a total serum SP level above 50 μg/ml.

Some patients treated with sulfasalazine experienced improvement of their psoriatic arthritis. Several groups of investigators evaluated sulfasalazine in the treatment of ankylosing spondylitis and psoriatic arthritis. The results have been variable, but the data suggest that sulfasalazine is less effective for spinal disease than for peripheral joint involvement. A double-blind trial of sulfasalazine, 3 g/day, for 8 weeks in 24 patients with active psoriatic arthritis revealed significantly improved physician and patient global assessments and duration of morning stiffness. Efficacy was observed as early as the fourth week of treatment. Cutaneous improvement with regard to erythema, scale, induration, and total body surface area was also significant, but the decrease in the activity of arthritis did not necessarily correspond to skin improvement in individual patients. A lower dose of sulfasalazine than is needed for cutaneous psoriasis may be effective for arthropathy. Newman *et al.* treated 10 patients with polyarticular psoriatic arthritis with sulfasalazine, 2 g daily for 16 weeks. Joint count score, morning stiffness, and global assessment of disease activity were significantly improved. Two large multicenter double-blind studies of sulfasalazine at 2 g/day for psoriatic arthritis showed trends favoring a response to sulfasalazine, with decreased pain and decreased erythrocyte sedimentation rate.

Despite the relatively high dropout rate during 8 weeks of therapy (25%), Gupta and coworkers emphasize that an equal proportion of patients may experience efficacy of sulfasalazine comparable to PUVA, methotrexate, or retinoids. Therefore, a trial of sulfasalazine is justified for patients with moderate to severe psoriasis with or without arthropathy whose disease is no longer

Table 19.5 How to use sulfasalazine.

1 Obtain baseline complete blood cell count, urinalysis, liver function and renal function tests; repeat at 2 weeks, 1 month, then every 3 months thereafter
2 Instruct patient to take 500 mg tid for 3 days; if tolerated, increase to 1 g tid
3 If gastrointestinal symptoms occur, reduce the dose by 500 mg decrements until a tolerable dose is attained
4 If the patient cannot tolerate at least 1.5 g/day, switch to enteric-coated tablets
5 If a symptomatic drug rash or urticaria develop, discontinue sulfasalazine
6 Treat for at least 4–6 weeks before making final judgments about efficacy
7 Do not increase the dose to 4 g/day because toxicity is much more likely to supervene and improved efficacy has not been confirmed

controlled by topical or UVB phototherapy (Table 19.5). In the long-term, if effective, sulfasalazine at 3–4 g/day is less costly and less toxic than PUVA, methotrexate, acitretin, or cyclosporine.

Selected references

Azathioprine

duVivier A., Munro D. D., Verbov J. (1974) Treatment of psoriasis with azathioprine. *Br Med J* **1**, 49–51.
Snow J. L., Gibson L. E. (1995) A pharmacogenetic basis for safe and effective use of azathioprine and other thioprinine drugs in dermatologic patients. *J Am Acad Dermatol* **32**, 114–116.

Hydroxyurea

Boyd A. S., Neldner K. H. (1991) Hydroxyurea therapy. *J Am Acad Dermatol* **25**, 518–524.
Daoud M. S., Gibson L. E., Pittelkow M. R. (1997) Hydroxyurea dermopathy: A unique lichenoid eruption complicating long-term therapy with hydroxyurea. *J Am Acad Dermatol* **36**, 178–182.
Kirby B., Harrison P. V. (1999) Combination low-dose cyclosporine (Neoral) and hydroxyurea for severe recalcitrant psoriasis. (Letter to editor). *Br J Dermatol* **140**, 186–187.
Kumar B., Saraswat A., Kaur I. (2000) Mucocutaneous adverse effects of hydroxyurea: a prospective study of 30 psoriasis patients. *Clin Exp Dermatol* **27**, 8–13.
Kumar B., Saraswat A., Kaur I. (2001) Rediscovering hydroxyurea: its role in recalcitrant psoriasis. *Int J Dermatol* **40**, 530–534.

Layton A. M., Sheehan-Dare R. A., Goodfield M. J. D., Cotterill J. A. (1989) Hydroxyurea in the management of therapy resistant psoriasis. *Br J Dermatol* **121**, 647–653.

Leavell U. W., Yarbro J. W. (1970) Hydroxyurea: a new treatment for psoriasis. *Arch Dermatol* **102**, 144–150.

Varma S., Lanigan S. W. (1999) Dermatomyositis-like eruption and leg ulceration caused by hydroxyurea in a patient with psoriasis. *Clin Exp Dermatol* **24**, 164–166.

Mycophenolate mofetil

Ameen M., Smith H. R., Barker J. N. (2001) Combined mycophenolate mofetil and cyclosporine therapy for severe recalcitrant psoriasis. *Clin Exp Dermatol* **26**, 480–483.

Davison S. C., Morris-Jones R., Powles A. V., Fry L. (2000) Change of treatment from cyclosporine mycophenolate mofetil in severe psoriasis. *Br J Dermatol* **143**, 405–407.

Epinnette W. W., Parker C. M., Jones E. L., Greist M. C. (1987) Mycophenolic acid for psoriasis. A review of pharmacology, long-term efficacy, and safety. *J Am Acad Dermatol* **17**, 962–971.

Geilen C. C., Arnold M., Orfanos C. E. (2001) Mycophenolate mofetil as a systemic antipsoriatic agent: positive experience in 11 patients. *Br J Dermatol* **144**, 583–586.

Geilen C. C., Mrowietz U. (2000) Lack of efficacy of topical mycophenolic acid in psoriasis vulgaris. *J Am Acad Dermatol* **42**, 837–840.

Grundmann-Kollmann M., Mooser G., Schraeder P. *et al.* (2000) Treatment of chronic plaque-stage psoriasis and psoriatic arthritis with mycophenolate mofetil. *J Am Acad Dermatol* **42**, 835–837.

Kitchin J. E. S., Pomeranz K., Pak G. *et al.* (1997) Rediscovering mycophenolic acid: a review of its mechanism, side effects, and potential uses. *J Am Acad Dermatol* **37**, 445–449.

Sulfasalazine

Combe B., Gouipille P., Kuntz J. L. *et al.* (1996) Sulfasalazine in psoriatic arthritis: a randomized, multicentre, placebo-controlled study. *Br J Rheumatol* **35**, 664–668.

Clegg D. O., Reda D. J., Mejias E. *et al.* (1996) Comparison of sulfasalazine and placebo in the treatment of psoriatic arthritis. A Department of Veterans Affairs Cooperative Study. *Arthritis Rheum* **39**, 2013–2020.

Gupta A. K., Ellis C. N., Siegel M. T. *et al.* (1990) Sulfasalazine improves psoriasis. A double-blind analysis. *Arch Dermatol* **126**, 487–493.

Gupta A. K., Grober J. S., Hamilton T. A. *et al.* (1995) Sulfasalazine therapy for psoriatic arthritis: A double-blind, placebo controlled trial. *J Rheumatol* **22**, 894–898.

Newman E. D., Perruquet J. L., Harrington T. M. (1991) Sulfasalazine therapy in psoriatic arthritis: clinical and immunologic response. *J Rheumatol* **18**, 1379–1382.

Thioguanine

Mason C., Krueger G. G. (2001) Thioguanine for refractory psoriasis: A 4-year experience. *J Am Acad Dermatol* **44**, 67–72.

Romagosa R., Kerdel F., Shan N. (2002) Treatment of psoriasis with 6-thioguanine and hepatic venoocclusive disease. (Letter to editor). *J Am Acad Dermatol* **47**, 970–972.

Silvis N. G., Levine N. (1999) Pulse dosing of thioguanine in recalcitrant psoriasis. *Arch Dermatol* **135**, 433–437.

Zackheim H. S., Glogau R. G., Fisher D. A., Maibach H. I. (1994) 6-Thioguanine treatment of psoriasis: Experience in 81 patients. *J Am Acad Dermatol* **30**, 452–458.

20 Investigational treatments for psoriasis

Charles Camisa

Innovative therapies for psoriasis are constantly being developed. In this chapter, I discuss examples of novel medical and surgical psoriasis treatments.

Propylthiouracil

Propylthiouracil (PTU), 300 mg daily, an antithyroid drug, demonstrated clinical efficacy and decreased PASI scores in the treatment of psoriasis in an open study. Experimental evidence suggests that PTU is active in psoriasis because of antioxidant effects. After 8 weeks' treatment, TSH levels were elevated in all patients compared to baseline but within the normal range. PTU may be combined with thyroxine 0.025 mg/day to prevent hypothyroidism.

In a small double-blind trial, PTU 5% lotion applied three times daily improved clinical and histologic scores significantly more than did placebo after 4–8 weeks. There was no systemic benefit, and no patient developed hypothyroidism.

Fumaric acid esters

Systemic fumaric acid was introduced as a treatment for psoriasis in 1959. Efficacy was confirmed when the dimethyl, monoethyl, and monomethyl esters were combined. In a double-blind placebo-controlled trial, modest but significant improvement occurred in 70% of patients receiving 215–1240 mg/day orally after 16 weeks. Nail involvement and psoriatic arthritis also respond to fumaric acid esters (FAE) in some cases. FAE has gained acceptance as an antipsoriatic therapy in western Europe and is available as Fumaderm.

The mechanism of action of FAE is not fully understood; however, recent experimental data indicate that the drug skews the

Th1-dominant T-cell response in psoriasis toward a Th2-like pattern and inhibits proliferation of keratinocytes. In a cohort of 12 patients followed for 24 months during FAE therapy, significant reduction of interferon-gamma secretion by peripheral blood mononuclear cells was followed by downregulation of IL-4 but not IL-10. Hoxtermann *et al.* followed 10 patients treated with FAE for over 1 year. In all cases, marked improvement of the psoriasis was associated with leukopenia and lymphopenia. Flow cytometric analysis of lymphocyte subsets revealed a reduction of CD8+ T-cells.

The most common adverse effects are gastrointestinal complaints (diarrhea, nausea, abdominal cramps) and flushing which occur in 56% and 31% of cases, respectively, and may lead to withdrawal from the drug. They are usually mild and subside over time. Minor laboratory abnormalities of liver and kidney functions may develop as well as transient eosinophilia.

A study of the combination of FAE in escalating doses with calcipotriene or vehicle ointment demonstrated that the active combination was significantly more effective (PASI score reduction 76% vs. 52%), more rapidly than FAE plus placebo. Moreover, calcipotriene yielded a slight but significant FAE-sparing effect: the final dose of FAE was reduced by 156 mg/day compared to FAE plus vehicle ointment, thus improving the risk–benefit ratio.

Fish oil

The rationale for using fish oil dietary supplements as a therapeutic modality for psoriasis is sound. Arachidonic acid (AA) and its pro-inflammatory metabolites are markedly elevated in lesional skin. Marine fish oil contains omega-3 polyunsaturated fatty acids, which could theoretically compete with AA as substrate for lipoxygenase and cyclooxygenase. The less chemotactically active leukotriene B5 may be formed as well as the relatively noninflammatory prostaglandins of the 3-series (PGE_3, TXA_3, PGI_3).

Unfortunately, in open and controlled trials, fish oil showed only minimal to modest improvement of plaque-type psoriasis, when used as monotherapy in doses ranging from 1.8 to 13.5 g/day. In order to overcome the slow kinetics and limited bioavailability of dietary fatty acids, intravenous infusions of a fish-oil-derived lipid emulsion containing 4.2 g of both eicosapentaenoic acid (EPA) and docosahexaenoic acid (DHA) were compared to a conventional omega-6-lipid emulsion in the treatment of chronic plaque-type psoriasis. The reduction in the PASI score was greater in the omega-3-treated group. Within days of initiating the omega-3 lipid infusion, but not the omega-6-treated group, there was a manifold rise in neutrophil LTB5, and platelet TXA_3 formation, accompanied by an increase in the plasma-free EPA concentration. Thus was proved the concept that omega-3 fatty acid administration improves psoriasis by increasing plasma EPA levels that compete with liberated AA as substrates for inflammatory mediators.

Monoclonal antibodies

Infusion of chimerized murine anti-CD4 monoclonal antibody infusions improve severe psoriasis, but the side-effects (fever, chills, headache, lymphopenia), and a potential host immune response to the antibody limit the practicality of this treatment. A humanized anti-CD4 IgG4 monoclonal antibody (OCTcdr4a) was infused into patients with severe psoriasis in two courses of 750 mg each 6 weeks apart. The PASI score decreased from 17.4 at baseline to 7.7 at day 99. The infusions were well tolerated. Sustained saturation of CD4 receptors by the antibody was not mandatory for sustained clinical response. There were no significant reductions of CD4+ T-cell counts.

A fusion protein called denileukin difitox (Ontak), which incorporates the membrane translocating and cytoxic domains of diphtheria toxin coupled to human interleukin-2, was used to treat patients with extensive chronic plaque-type psoriasis in a pilot study. Denileukin difitox selectively destroys activated T-cells that bear high-affinity IL-2 receptors. Side-effects include flu-like syndrome, itching and transiently elevated transaminases.

A recent dose escalation trial demonstrated that the most effective dose, 5 µg/kg/day administered for 3 consecutive days every other week, achieved a 50% reduction in PASI score in about 50% of the patients. Alternative options for blocking the binding of IL-2 to IL-2 receptors and treating psoriasis include daclizumab (humanized antibody to alpha-subunit [CD25] of IL-2R).

Flashlamp pulsed dye laser

Several studies have evaluated the flashlamp-pumped tunable dye laser (585 nm) for selective photothermolysis of dermal vasculature in the treatment of stable psoriatic plaques usually every 2 weeks up to five times. Most patients obtained significant clinical improvement lasting up to 13 months. There was no difference between short and long pulse-width lasers. Lesions with vertically oriented vessels and few horizontal vessels had a better prognosis whereas those with numerous tortuous vessels at the base of dermal papillae were associated with a poor response to pulsed dye laser treatment. Patients developed crusting and erosion of the epidermis that was not completely healed by 2 weeks. Textural and pigmentary changes developed at the sites of laser-induced erosions, but the Koebner phenomenon did not occur. The practicality of this treatment is limited by the expense, small spot size, prolonged postoperative healing time, and patient acceptance.

Alternative laser treatments are low energy continuous emission with Nd:YAG laser below the pain threshold for four treatments over 2 weeks and ablation of the lesion by the Er:YAG laser. The latter treatment gave comparable results to dermatome shaving. Using either modality, the epidermis and the papillary dermis are removed.

Asawanonda *et al.* compared CO_2 laser resurfacing to electrodesiccation and curettage in the treatment of single plaques of psoriasis. Again, both modalities removed epidermis and papillary dermis and produced similar results. The CO_2 laser offered more precise depth control and better coagulation, but the operation with the Hyfrecator was executed much more quickly. All of the foregoing surgical methods carry a moderate risk of scarring and are not practical for extensive disease. They should be reserved for the short-term treatment of limited recalcitrant plaques.

Photodynamic therapy

The technique of photodynamic therapy (PDT) for malignant tumors has been evolving for 25 years. Originally, a photosensitizer such as hematoporphyrin derivative (HPD) was infused intravenously, followed 48 hours later by irradiation with red light from an argon laser (630 nm). Because of persistent photosensitivity of the skin for 4–6 weeks, this was impractical for treating psoriasis. Low doses (8 mg/m^2) of benzoporphyrin monoacid ring-A activated at 690 nm substantially improved psoriasis lesions compared to untreated control lesions after a single 3-hour exposure. Generalized photosensitivity lasts for about 1 week. A standardized regimen has not yet been promulgated.

Protoporphyrin IX (PpIX) is elevated in some psoriatic plaques as detected by in vivo fluorescence spectroscopy. An experiment to exploit elevated endogenous PpIX levels in plaques was made by repeatedly exposing them to blue light. Although complete photo-bleaching of PpIX occurred, there was no difference in the clinical score of treated plaques after 12 exposures compared to untreated control plaques. Topical 5-aminolevulinic acid (ALA) can be applied directly to psoriatic lesions or under occlusion, and is metabolized to the photosensitizer PpIX, which accumulates in the inflamed skin. It is more expensive but easier to use than systemic PDT. The lesions are then exposed to long wavelength visible light. The concentration of ALA used and the type of radiation (blue, red) determine the efficacy and toxicity (burning sensation). In one study of 19 treated sites, 10 (53%) responded after a range of 3–8 treatments. Biopsies confirmed that fluorescence was localized to the entire epidermis, but the level was inconsistent between different sections of the same biopsy. The authors (Robinson *et al.*) concluded that despite therapeutic efficacy for psoriasis, ALA-PDT may be impractical because of the need for repeated treatments, unpredictable response, and patient discomfort. The mechanism of action of PDT is un-known, but both PDT and PUVA had a similar effect—decreased secretion of cytokines—on psoriatic peripheral blood mononuclear cells irradiated in vitro. The theoretical advantages of PDT over PUVA are that porphyrins damage cell membranes or mitochondria rather than DNA, and the wavelength of visible light is less likely to be carcinogenic over time than ultraviolet light.

Retinoid inhibitor

Liarozole is an imidazole inhibitor of the metabolism of all-*trans*-retinoic acid. A double-blind placebo-controlled trial determined that 150 mg/day for 12 weeks produced marked improvement in 38% compared to 6% of the placebo-treated patients. Mucocutane-ous retinoid side-effects were infrequent and mild. The same dose of liarozole is also effective for palmoplantar pustulosis. Mild eleva-tions of triglycerides occurred. In males, the serum levels of testos-terone and leutinizing hormone rose significantly.

Mycobacterium vaccae immunotherapy

Another novel approach to the therapy of psoriasis is inoculation (two intradermal injections 3 weeks apart) with a heat-killed suspension of nonpathogenic *M. vaccae*. Several limited placebo-controlled and open trials demonstrated significant reduction in baseline PASI scores (>50%) in the majority of subjects, which lasted for at least 6 months.

Selected references

Propylthiouracil

Elias A. N., Dangaran K., Barr R. J., Rohan M. K., Goodman M. M. (1994) A controlled trial of topical propylthiouracil in the treatment of patients with psoriasis. *J Am Acad Dermatol* **31**, 455–458.

Utas S., Kose K., Yazici C. *et al.* (2002) Antioxidant potential of propyl-thiouracil in patients with psoriasis. *Clin Biochem* **35**, 241–246.

Fumaric acid esters

Altmeyer P. J., Matthes U., Pawlak F. (1994) Antipsoriatic effect of fumaric acid derivatives. Results of a multicenter double-blind study in 100 patients. *J Am Acad Dermatol* **30**, 977–981.

Gollnick H., Altmeyer P., Kaufmann R. *et al.* (2002) Topical calcipotriol plus oral fumaric acid is more effective and faster acting than oral fumaric acid monotherapy in the treatment of severe chronic plaque psoriasis vulgaris. *Dermatol* **205**, 46–53.

Hoxtermann D., Nuchel C., Altmeyer P. (1998) Fumaric acid esters suppress peripheral CD4- and CD8-positive lymphocytes in psoriasis. *Dermatol* **196**, 223–230.

Litjens N. H., Nibbering P. H., Barrois A. J. *et al.* (2003) Beneficial effects of fumarate therapy in psoriasis vulgaris patients coincide with down-regulation of type 1 cytokines. *Br J Dermatol* **148**, 444–451.

Mrowietz U., Christophers E., Altmeyer P. (1998) Treatment of psoriasis with fumaric acid esters: results of a prospective multicentre study. German Multicentre study. *Br J Dermatol* **138**, 456–460.

Mrowietz U., Christophers E., Altmeyer P. (1999) Treatment of psoriasis with fumaric acid esters: scientific background and guidelines for therapeutic use. The German Fumaric Acid Ester Consensus Conference. *Br J Dermatol* **141**, 424–429.

Fish oil

Camisa C. (1994) Miscellaneous treatments. In: Camisa C. (ed.) *Psoriasis.* Blackwell, Boston, 329–337.

Mayser P., Grimm H., Grimminger F. (2002) N-3 fatty acids in psoriasis. *Br J Nutr* **87** (Suppl. 1), 577–582.

Monoclonal antibodies

Gottlieb S. L. (1997) Response of psoriasis to a lymphocyte-selective toxin (DAB$_{389}$ IL-2): A phase I clinical study and histopathological assessment. *J Am Acad Dermatol* **36**, 272–273.

Krueger J. G., Walters I. B., Miyazawa M. *et al.* (2000) Successful in vivo blockade of CD25 (high-affinity interleukin 2 receptor) on T cells by administration of humanized anti-Tac antibody to patients with psoriasis. *J Am Acad Dermatol* **43**, 448–458.

Martin A., Gutierrez E., Muglia J. *et al.* (2001) A multicenter dose-escalation trial with denuleukin difitox (ONTAK, DAB (389)IL-2) in patients with severe psoriasis. *J Am Acad Dermatol* **45**, 871–881.

Lasers

Asawananda P., Anderson R. R., Taylor C. R. (2000) Pendulaser carbon-dioxide resurfacing laser versus electrodesiccation with curettage in the treatment of isolated, recalcitrant psoriatic plaques. *J Am Acad Dermatol* **42**, 660–666.

Boehncke W. H., Ochsendorf F., Wolter M., Kaufmann R. (1999) Ablative techniques in psoriasis vulgaris resistant to conventional therapies. *Dermatol Surg* **25**, 618–621.

Katugampola G. A., Rees A. M., Lanigan S. W. (1995) Laser treatment of psoriasis. *Br J Dermatol* **133**, 909–913.

Ruiz-Esparza J. (1999) Clinical response of psoriasis to low-energy irradiance with the Nd:YAG laser at 1320 nm report of an observation in three cases. *Dermatol Surg* **25**, 403–407.

Photodynamic therapy

Boehncke W. H., Elshorst-Schmidt T., Kaufmann R. (2000) Systemic photodynamic therapy is a safe and effective treatment for psoriasis. (Letter to Editor). *Arch Dermatol* **136**, 271–272.

Boehncke W. H., Konig K., Kaufmann R. *et al.* (1994) Photodynamic therapy in psoriasis: suppression of cytokine production in vitro and recording of fluorescence modification during treatment in vivo. *Arch Dermatol Res* **286**, 300–303.

Fergin P. (1996) Photodynamic therapy for psoriasis. *Australas J Dermatol* **37**, 87–88.

Lui H. (1996) Photodynamic therapy: when will the promise be kept? *Med Surg Dermatol* **3**, 137–139.

Maari C., Bissonnette R. (2002) Multiple exposures to blue light does not improve psoriasis in patients with elevated endogenous levels of photoporphyrin IX. *Photodermatol, Photoimmunol, Photomed* **18**, 104.

Robinson D. J., Collins P., Stringer M. R. *et al.* (1999) Improved response of plaque psoriasis after multiple treatments with topical 5-aminolaevulinic acid photodynamic therapy. *Acta Derm Venereol* **79**, 451–455.

Retinoid inhibitor

Berthe-Jones J., Todd G., Hutchinson P. E. *et al.* (2000) Treatment of psoriasis with oral liarozole: a dose-ranging study. *Br J Dermatol* **143**, 1170–1176.

Bhushan M., Burden A. D., McElhone K. *et al.* (2001) Oral liarozole in the treatment of palmo-plantar pustular psoriasis: a randomized double-blind placebo-controlled study. *Br J Dermatol* **145**, 546–553.

Mycobacterium vaccae immunotherapy

Balagon M. V., Tan P. L., Prestidge R. *et al.* (2001) Improvement in psoriasis after intradermal administration of delipidated, deglycolipidated Myobacterium vaccae (PVAC): results of an open-label trial. *Clin Exp Dermatol* **26**, 233–241.

Balagon M. V., Walsh D. S., Tan P. L. *et al.* (2000) Improvement in psoriasis after intradermal administration of heat-killed Myobacterium vaccae. *Int J Dermatol* **39**, 51–58.

21 Psoriatic arthritis

Thomas Osborn
William S. Wilke

Definition and pathogenesis

Inflammatory arthritis occurs in 6–10% of individuals with moderate to severe psoriasis. Approximately one-third of individuals with psoriasis complain of joint stiffness. Although the existence of psoriatic arthritis (PSA) as a specific clinical entity continues to be questioned, it clearly differs from rheumatoid arthritis (RA) in radiographic appearance, clinical presentation, and genetic predisposition. Although PSA and RA share some HLA allotypes, such as DR4, others, such as B27, BW38, DR7 and CW6, occur with significantly higher frequency in PSA. While HLA-Cw0602 has one of the strongest major histocompatibility complex (MHC) associations with psoriasis and psoriatic arthritis, it is found in only 17% of patients with psoriasis versus 9% of controls. Early work implicated genes in the Class I and Class II region of the MHC to be the important areas linked to the development of PSA. Recent work has associated mutations in the TNF-α gene within the Class III region of the MHC between HLA-B and HLA-DR with psoriasis and psoriatic arthritis.

While genetic factors certainly play a part in the development of PSA, the etiology of PSA is not entirely understood. The role of trauma, which might result in a deep Koebner phenomenon, has been considered. Patients frequently relate significant physical or emotional stress prior to or near the onset of their first arthritis flare. Psychological stress is a common risk factor for many of the inflammatory arthritides. Bacterial antigens, including those derived from *Mycobacterium tuberculosis*, heat shock proteins from *Escherichia coli* and various peptidoglycans derived from Gram-positive bacterial cell walls have also been shown to induce proliferation in PSA synovial fluid lymphocytes. In many cases, however, this response is nonspecific and has been demonstrated to occur in other forms of inflammatory arthritis, including RA. There is a clear association of HIV infection and severe PSA.

The pathogenic mechanisms thought to cause PSA include the participation of chemical mediators of inflammation, the humoral immune system, and the interaction of T-cells and dendritic macrophages. Cytokines, prostaglandins, leukotrienes and platelet-derived factors may act through modulation of interleukin 1 and/or stimulate keratinocyte growth. Serum levels of IgA-containing immune complexes correlate with disease activity. Suppressor/inducer CD4 subsets are reduced in synovial fluid in PSA as in RA. The synovium of active psoriatic arthritic joints contains high numbers of helper/inducer T-cells and few suppressor/inducer T-cells. In long-standing disease, there are few T- or B-lymphocytes in the synovium. The predominant cell appears to be a mononuclear phagocytic cell, the type I synoviocyte. Gamma/delta T-cells, a subset that preferentially proliferates in response to heat shock proteins and other bacterial antigens, have also been found increased in the synovial fluid in PSA. In addition, higher numbers of antigen-presenting dendritic macrophage cells are present in the synovial fluid in both PSA and RA. Exceptionally high levels of TNF-α and interleukin-1 (IL-1) have been found in the synovial fluid in joints with active PSA. All of these findings suggest that immune mechanisms are important to the pathophysiology of PSA.

Hyperplasia and hypertrophy of synovial lining cells occurs in PSA, but is not always as prominent as that seen in RA. Synovial blood vessels show capillary wall thickening, endothelial swelling and hypertrophy with polymorphonuclear infiltration of the wall. In early disease, T-lymphocytes are prominent as mentioned above. However, in established disease, inflammation is perpetuated by macrophage-derived synoviocytes, which generally express DR antigen on their surface. The level of this DR expression is at least in part hereditary and in part due to the individual's response to environmental stimuli.

Clinical manifestations

Arthritic patterns

Five classical patterns of peripheral and axial arthritis have been recognized. Once one of these patterns is established, it is unlikely to change.

1 **Symmetric polyarthritis.** This almost always involves the proximal joints of the fingers but may include any joint in the body. It looks and behaves exactly like rheumatoid arthritis. This is the most common form of PSA.

2 **Asymmetric oligoarticular arthritis.** This involves five or fewer joints. These often include a distal interphalangeal joint of a finger or toe resulting in a "sausage" digit. The "sausage" appearance of interphalangeal joints has recently been demonstrated to be due to flexor tendon swelling and inflammation. It is termed "dactylitis." Later onset oligoarticular arthritis of large joints has the best prognosis.

3 **Distal interphalangeal joint arthritis.** This is a "classic" presentation in which only the distal finger joints are involved. This occurs in only 5% of patients. It is almost always associated with nail changes.

4 **Proximal osteolysis of the small joints of the hands resulting in arthritis mutilans.** Fortunately this occurs in only 1–2% of patients with PSA. Arthritis mutilans is most often encountered in patients with early onset disease. It has the worst prognosis.

5 **Sacroiliac and spine pain.** This is often asymmetric. Radiographic changes are consistent with sacroiliitis and ankylosing spondylitis. Sacroiliitis tends to be unilateral. Symptoms may be absent despite radiographic findings. Radiographic sacroiliitis differentiates PSA from RA. Involvement of the spine occurs as frequently as sacroiliitis, but lumbosacral stiffness and loss of motion is less prominent than in ankylosing spondylitis.

Other features

New constitutional symptoms such as fever, fatigue and anorexia are rare, but occur most frequently at the outset of polyarticular diease and arthritis mutilans. Distal swelling with pitting edema may be the initial manifestation of peripheral arthritis in some patients.

Arthritis occurs after the onset of cutaneous involvement in approximately two-thirds of cases, is synchronous in approximately 15% and occurs before the onset of rash in approximately 15%. What this means from a practical standpoint is that one must do a thorough and repeated search in the later group of patients. A patient with a rheumatoid arthritis pattern of joint involvement but who remains seronegative should also be scrutinized carefully and repeatedly for a psoriatic lesion. However, 30% of patients with classic rheumatoid arthritis remain seronegative.

Extra-articular manifestations other than cutaneous involvement include nail pitting and/or dystrophy in at least 80% of patients with arthritis compared to only 20% of patients with psoriasis alone. Iritis and conjunctivitis may occur in up to 30% of patients with peripheral arthritis. Anterior uveitis is most common in patients with axial involvement. These may require aggressive local and systemic immunosuppressive therapy to control.

The joints involved do not relate to the location of the psoriatic skin lesions. The only exception to this is the close association between distal interphalangeal joint involvement and nail lesions.

Diagnosis

There is no specific diagnostic serologic test for PSA. Disease activity correlates with the degree of anemia, leukocytosis, thrombocytosis and elevation of acute phase reactants such as the Westergren sedimentation rate and C-reactive protein. Hyperuricemia, due to heightened cellular metabolism and turnover, occurs in 10–20% of patients and may result in acute gout. It is reasonable to examine these laboratory tests in the individual with new onset PSA.

The radiographic appearance of peripheral joint involvement demonstrates the enthesiopathic nature of PSA. Bony erosion begins at the joint margin but is most extensive at the proximal aspects of the small joints of the hands and feet. This same fluffy periosteal reaction can be seen at the Achilles insertion on the calcaneus. Bony proliferation at the distal portion of the joint completes the "pencil-in-cup" appearance of severe peripheral joint involvement. Such findings may help establish the diagnosis of PSA. Bony ankylosis with or without significant joint space narrowing represents the end-stage of peripheral joint inflammation. It is not uncommon to have the diagnosis of PSA made in a patient with seronegative rheumatoid arthritis after reviewing the x-rays.

Sacroiliac and spinal involvement tends to be less symmetric than in ankylosing spondylitis. In addition, nonmarginal syndesmophytes arise from spinal ligaments rather than from the vertebral margin as occurs in ankylosing spondylitis. Involvement of vertebral bodies tends to be random in PSA rather than ascending as in ankylosing spondylitis, which also differentiates the two diseases. Anterior ligamentous calcification is common in ankylosing spondylitis but uncommon in PSA. Newer information suggests that cervical spine involvement may occur more frequently than previously reported (up to 75%) and may include atlantoaxial subluxation which is usually not encountered in ankylosing spondylitis.

Treatment of mild PSA

1 *Patient education, joint protection, occupational therapy and physical therapy,* especially aerobic exercise, are as important for the treatment of PSA as they are for rheumatoid arthritis.

2 Although *nonsteroidal anti-inflammatory drugs (NSAIDs)* are often considered the primary treatment for mild PSA, very few comparative trials have been performed specifically for this type of arthritis. Alternatively, a large number of clinical trials using NSAIDs in patients with osteoarthritis and rheumatoid arthritis have demonstrated improvement of function and symptoms when compared to placebo. In general, NSAIDs control swelling, pain, morning stiffness and improve range of motion and activities of daily living versus placebo. Their effects on these symptoms are similar to aspirin. Newer NSAIDs, more specific for inhibiting cyclooxygenase-2 (Cox-2) have not been shown to be superior to older, less specific, NSAIDs in controlling arthritic symptoms. They do, however, appear to have less gastrointestinal toxicity. The NSAIDs have not been shown to alter the long-term course or prevent joint damage.

Potential side-effects that cause the most concern include NSAID allergy, gastritis, esophagitis, gastric or duodenal ulceration or bleed, peripheral edema, hypertension, salt retention, elevation of blood pressure, and hepatic toxicity. The most common and most serious adverse effect of NSAIDs is gastric mucosal damage resulting in erosions, bleeding and ulcerations. Prostaglandin E2, which is inhibited by NSAIDs, is responsible for maintaining the mucosal barrier. The resulting direct contact of gastric tissue with gastric acid allows ion trapping and injury to the mucosal epithelial cells.

The frequency of gastric erosion and ulceration is estimated to be 1.5–4% of all patients receiving NSAIDs. In addition, at least 60% of patients taking NSAIDs for 6 months or longer report gastrointestinal symptoms, especially dyspepsia. Unfortunately, endoscopically proven gastric or duodenal ulcerations may be asymptomatic. Therefore, relying on symptoms as a warning for ulceration is not appropriate. Patients taking NSAIDs over a long period should have their hemoglobin levels monitored and screened for occult blood in their stool every 6 months. The elderly, smokers, alcohol abusers, and patients with previous peptic ulcer disease are at greatest risk.

Although uncommon, four types of renal dysfunction have been reported with NSAIDs: (1) papillary necrosis; (2) interstitial nephritis; (3) acute oliguric renal failure; and, (4) interstitial nephritis with proteinuria. The greatest risk of renal dysfunction occurs in patients of advanced age, with evidence of renal-vascular disease and/or hypertension, and diabetes mellitus. Additional risk occurs in patients with atherosclerotic disease who use diuretic agents, and those with preexisting renal disease, congestive heart failure or known hepatic dysfunction.

Worsening or flares of psoriasis have been reported with indomethacin, meclofenamate, and phenylbutazone. In these patients, an increase in the number of new lesions, as well as an increase in size of the preexisting lesions, developed within 1–2 weeks of initiating the NSAID. The use of these agents may improve joint symptoms and at the same time make the skin worse. Generalized pustular psoriasis may be precipitated in susceptible individuals.

3 *Antimalarial drugs*, especially hydroxychloroquine given in a dose approaching 3.5 mg/lb/day, have been used to treat mild psoriatic arthritis. In one series, Kammer and associates reported 68% response among 32 patients treated with hydroxychloroquine 200–400 mg/day. Cutaneous adverse events occurred in 10 patients (20%) and led to drug discontinuation in six (12%). Other series have demonstrated a higher frequency of cutaneous adverse reactions with the use of chloroquine phosphate. The most common adverse effect of hydroxychloroquine is gastrointestinal disturbance, which includes nausea, vomiting, abdominal cramping and bloating but only occurs in 5% or fewer patients. The accumulation of drug in the melanin-containing tissues of the iris, choroid and retinal epithelium was at one time the main deterrent to rheumatologic use. If low dose hydroxychloroquine is employed (≤3.5 mg/lb/day), retinal deposition occurs in less than 5% of patients. For safety monitoring, patients should be examined by an ophthalmologist on a regular basis.

4 *Colchicine* at doses of 0.6 mg twice daily or 0.5 mg three times daily has been shown to be marginally effective in a small controlled trial. Acute lower abdominal toxicity consisting of cramping and diarrhea occurs in nearly half of patients treated with this dose.

5 *Low-dose corticosteroid* (5–10 mg of prednisone equivalent/day) has been used in patients with PSA and can provide sustained symptomatic relief. Corticosteroids might be chosen as "bridge therapy" while awaiting the onset of action of maintenance drugs for moderate or severe PSA. High dose, pulse corticosteroids (i.e. 200–1000 mg of IV methylprednisolone) have been associated with severe flares of psoriasis and are usually contraindicated. In our experience, and that of others, local intra-articular corticosteroid injection, especially of large joints for patients with oligoarticular disease, often provides significant benefit and rarely worsens skin disease.

Treatment of moderate-to-severe PSA

Many patients, especially those with polyarticular, small joint involvement that begins in young adulthood, do not respond adequately to NSAIDs, hydroxychloroquine, colchicine or low dose corticosteroids. Although there are no universal guidelines, most rheumatologists would employ other agents, either as monotherapy or combined, in an additive fashion for patients who continue to have swelling and pain on motion in their joints. This is particularly true if they have elevated acute phase reactants (ESR or CRP) or swollen joints after 3 months of conservative therapy.

1 *Methotrexate (MTX)* has been used extensively for the treatment of psoriasis and psoriatic arthritis. The usual starting dose is 7.5 mg once per week given as three tablets (2.5 mg each) all in one day. The dose may be increased up to 25 mg per week. This should be done gradually, assessing clinical response and toxicity on a monthly basis. Methotrexate should probably not be used in patients with preexisting liver problems, for example, hepatitis B or C virus infection, nonalcoholic steatohepatitis, or a current or a previous history of heavy alcohol consumption. If MTX therapy is added to other potentially hepatotoxic medical therapy, e.g. lipid lowering agents, the elevation of liver enzymes may require stopping more than one medication. Monitoring for mucosal lesions, hair loss, nausea, anorexia, along with laboratory tests for CBC, liver enzymes (AST, ALT), albumin, and creatinine are important. Minor toxicity including gastrointestinal symptoms, stomatitis and alopecia occur in 5–10% of MTX-treated patients. Hepatic enzyme elevations occur in up to 20% of patients. MTX should be held if liver enzymes elevate over twice the upper limit of normal. A liver biopsy after a cumulative dose of 4 g should be considered. By contrast, see the American Academy of Dermatology guidelines for liver biopsy in Chapter 16. Folate deficiency occurs with MTX therapy and is associated with liver toxicity. The simultaneous use of folic acid 1–2 mg/day, or folinic acid 5 mg two or three doses given at least 12 hours after MTX, reduce the incidence of elevated liver enzyme levels and the rate of discontinuation of MTX.

Severe pulmonary toxicity has been encountered in up to 6% of rheumatoid arthritis patients treated with MTX and may occur at any time during therapy. Discontinuation of MTX and bolus corticosteroid treatment usually prevents serious long-term sequelae. In rheumatoid arthritis patients, the degree of renal dysfunction is directly correlated with the frequency and severity of pulmonary toxicity. This is not surprising since MTX is renally excreted. Similar pulmonary toxicity has been reported to occur in PSA treated with MTX. The prevalence of pneumonitis in PSA has not been established, but it is considered to be very uncommon.

There are few placebo-controlled, double-blind studies for MTX in PSA. In most reports, a weekly dose of 0.1–0.2 mg/kg/week was given. Three controlled or comparative studies have been reported. In the first study, published in 1964, very large doses (up to 3 mg/kg/week) were employed, and although improvement was seen, serious hematological toxicity was encountered in 38% of patients. In another 12-week study, trends toward improvement in all efficacy measures were seen, but only physicians' assessment improved significantly. In a third study, MTX at a dose of 7.5–15 mg/week was compared to cyclosporine 3–5 mg/day in 35 patients followed for one year. Comparable improvements, which were statistically significant compared to baseline, were seen in most efficacy measures with both drugs. There was a trend toward increased withdrawal due to toxicity among cyclosporine treated patients. Despite demonstrated symptom control, MTX has not been shown to slow radiographic damage in PSA.

2 *The effectiveness of sulfasalazine* has been demonstrated in a total of 314 patients enrolled in four randomized, prospective, double-blind studies. Generally, at doses of 2–3 g/day, 40–50% improvement of active joint count, acute phase reactants, global assessment and function can be expected. Best results were seen when the dosage was quickly escalated over a few days to 3 g/day. Benefit generally occurred within 4–8 weeks. Toxicity, including gastrointestinal symptoms and rash, occur in 30–50% of treated patients. Thrombocytopenia may occur at any time during treatment in 5% or fewer patients. Monthly blood counts are recommended for safety monitoring. Sulfasalazine is often used in combination therapy but can be an effective monotherapy.

3 There is a rapidly emerging role for *the inhibition of tumor necrosis factor (TNF)* in the treatment of psoriatic arthritis and psoriatic skin lesions. Several therapeutic agents are currently available that specifically block TNF and more should be forthcoming. Several specific cytokines are known to play a central role in the development and continued stimulation of inflammation in PSA and psoriasis. These include TNF, IL-1, IL-6 and IL-8. The earliest and most pronounced is TNF.

Etanercept (Enbrel) and infliximab (Remicade) have both been shown to decrease psoriatic arthritis activity as well as improve psoriatic skin severity scores. Dosages range from 25 to 50 mg given subcutaneously twice weekly for etanercept and 3 mg/kg given by intravenous infusion every 8 weeks for infliximab. Pitfalls include risk of infection, high cost, and the paucity of studies and long-term experience with these agents. The risk of infection is of greatest concern because mycobacterial and deep fungal infections may be occult due to the anti-inflammatory nature of the treatment and begin insidiously. Moreover, the patients are often followed by a practitioner who may not be familiar with the diagnosis and treatment of such infections.

Etanercept, in Phase 2 and 3 trials, has been shown to be effective and safe in the treatment of PSA. Psoriatic Arthritis Response Criteria (PsARC) were used to follow these patients. There were relatively few adverse events. There have been a number of concerns, triggered by case reports, in using etanercept. Prior exposure to tuberculosis, multiple sclerosis and systemic lupus erythematosus are conditions that should be considered before this medication is prescribed. The use of both etanercept and infliximab has been associated with rising serum levels of antinuclear antibodies and anti-double-stranded DNA antibodies.

Two other agents may have a beneficial effect on PSA, adalimumab (Humira) and anakinra (Kineret). There have been no controlled studies published for the use of these medications in PSA. Adalimumab, a fully humanized monoclonal anti-TNF antibody, is given subcutaneously every 2 weeks. Anakinra, which blocks IL-1 receptors, is given subcutaneously daily.

4 *Leflunomide (Arava)*, a pyrimidine synthesis inhibitor, has been successfully used to treat patients with psoriatic arthritis. Individual case reports have shown that leflunomide decreases joint erosion caused by PSA. It can also induce reparative changes where joint erosions have occurred as a result of PSA. This has been shown more extensively in rheumatoid arthritis.

This drug is given at a single dose of 20 mg/day after an initial 3-day load of 100 mg/day. It is necessary to monitor the patient both clinically and by frequent laboratory testing. Particularly worrisome is the potential for liver toxicity with leflunomide, therefore the liver enzymes should be monitored monthly. Rash, hair loss, mucosal ulcers, nausea, abdominal pain, and diarrhea are the more common clinical side-effects. Caution should be exercised in using this medication in combination therapy.

5 *Azathioprine (Imuran)*, an immunosuppressive antimetabolite, given in a dose up to 3 mg/kg/day has been shown to reduce the mean active joint count by 50% in a small double-blind, placebo-controlled cross-over trial. Leukopenia can be expected in 10–20% of treated patients. This does not always require stopping therapy. Maintaining a WBC count between 3000 and 5000/mm^3 is often the goal for the best arthritic response. Compared to MTX, far fewer patients treated with azathioprine have been reported, and it is difficult to make firm recommendations about its use. It should not be used in combination therapy with other immunosuppressive drugs.

6 *Cyclosporine* in low doses (1.5–3 mg/kg/day) can be rapidly effective in treating PSA and psoriasis. Numerous studies have shown it to give clear improvement within 4 weeks. This may occur in patients with particularly resistant disease, and in some whose arthritis has failed to respond to MTX. An open trial treating 45 patients with PSA has been reported with cyclosporine, using dosages ranging from 3 to 6 mg/kg/day. Up to 70% of patients experienced a 50% or more reduction of active joint count, improved global assessment and reduced morning stiffness. Although serum creatinine rose in the majority, serious renal toxicity in short-term (3–12 month) studies has not been a problem. Other side-effects include hypertension, fluid retention, headaches, hypertrichosis and paresthesias. Occurrence of these should be considered a serious problem and lead to stopping or altering the dose of cyclosporine.

7 *Etretinate*, a synthetic retinoid, has been used alone in numerous open studies at a maintenance dose of 10–25 mg/day and may be useful in PSA. The only controlled study in PSA contained 20 patients. Etretinate showed no improvement compared to baseline in this study. Moreover, typical retinoid mucocutaneous toxicity caused withdrawal of one-third of patients. Retinoids may be most useful in combination with other treatments.

8 *Photochemotherapy with 8-methoxypsoralen (PUVA)* has been reported in an open study of 28 patients with PSA. Treatment was given two to three times each week and produced at least 30% improvement for patients with peripheral arthritis. Treatment was not as effective in axial arthritis.

The combination of retinoid therapy and PUVA (Re-PUVA) has been reported in 14 patients and resulted in modest improvement of PSA in approximately one-half of the cases.

Assessment and prognosis

Prognosis in PSA is different in each clinical subset. Oligoarticular and axial disease are less disabling than peripheral disease or classic ankylosing spondylitis. When severe disability occurs, it is usually in the subset of patients with severe peripheral arthritis, especially those with arthritis mutilans. Poor prognosis is associated with early onset of peripheral arthritis (before age 20), the severity of cutaneous psoriasis, a family history of arthritis, and an elevated Westergren erythrocyte sedimentation rate at the first visit.

One prospective longitudinal series of 40 psoriasis patients who were followed for a mean of 8 years suggested that aggressive treatment beyond nonsteroidal anti-inflammatory drugs initiated within the first 5 years was associated with improvement in functional class.

Clinical assessment of joint activity has been shown to be as reliable in PSA as it is in rheumatoid arthritis. This includes such simple measures as counting the number of joints that are painful, tender or swollen. There are, generally for research purposes, more complex disease activity scoring systems and radiographic scoring systems. Acute phase reactants including erythrocyte sedimentation rate and C-reactive protein may provide accurate measurement of disease activity in selected patients. More recently, the questions used in a version of the Stanford Health Assessment Questionnaire modified for PSA and the SF-36 have been shown to provide valid measurement of functional outcome in PSA but may not accurately correlate with the severity of cutaneous involvement.

Psoriatic arthritis, Reiter's syndrome and reactive arthritis associated with HIV infection

Human immunodeficiency virus (HIV) infection is sometimes complicated by rheumatic syndromes, which include arthralgia/arthritis. Debate remains concerning the link between HIV infection and joint disease. Initial studies of homosexual/bisexual men showed no difference in the frequency of psoriasis, psoriatic arthritis (PSA), Reiter's syndrome and reactive arthritis in HIV-infected compared to HIV-negative individuals. Other reports have demonstrated a prevalence of psoriatic skin as high as 20% in an HIV-positive cohort. Two other prospective comparative cohorts that compared HIV-positive to HIV-negative individuals with the same risk factors demonstrated a significantly higher frequency of arthralgias and Reiter's syndrome in the HIV-positive cohort. Clearly, joint symptoms, which include PSA, Reiter's syndrome, reactive arthritis, and miscellaneous arthralgias, are encountered at a frequency that is probably higher than in the general population in patients with HIV infection. These joint manifestations represent a significant source of morbidity to HIV patients and require early treatment.

1 Psoriasis occurs in approximately 2% of the general population and is at least as common in HIV-infected individuals. While psoriasis is complicated by inflammatory arthritis in approximately 6% of the uninfected population, the reported incidence of inflammatory arthritis in HIV-infected psoriatics is as high as 50%. Although HLA-B27 is not necessarily associated with a higher frequency of peripheral PSA in the non-HIV population, it is much more common in HIV-associated PSA, conferring a 12-fold higher risk of PSA in HIV-infected individuals.

The etiopathogenesis of psoriasis and associated arthritis is probably multifactorial and includes increased production of cytokines such as interferon gamma and interleukin-2, enhanced immune response to Gram-negative and Gram-positive bacterial antigens, and products of the HIV TAT gene that directly promote epidermal acanthosis and hyperkeratosis.

2 Classic Reiter's syndrome is comprised of the triad urethritis, conjunctivitis and oligoarticular inflammatory peripheral arthritis. In addition, characteristic skin and mucous membrane lesions are common. Asymmetric involvement of the sacroiliac joints and "skip-lesions" in the apophyseal and enthesis joints of the lumbosacral spine can also occur. For classification purposes, Reiter's syndrome

can also be considered to be a reactive arthritis because of its demonstrated association with infection by *Shigella flexneri, Campylobacter fetus, Yersinia enterocolitica* and *Chlamydia trachomatis*. In a review of 51 reported cases of HIV-infected patients with Reiter's syndrome, clinical features included urethritis (57%), conjunctivitis (45%), circinate balanitis (27%) and keratoderma blennorrhagicum (18%). As with PSA, the presence of HLA-B27 increases the likelihood of arthritis in these patients.

Some HIV patients present with features of several syndromes including PSA, nonspecific enthesitis and reactive arthritis, and do not fit any specific diagnostic category. Other patients experience self-limiting and nonprogressive arthralgias without associated swelling or radiographic destruction. This group includes patients with the "painful articular syndrome" which present with evanescent joint pain lasting for a few hours to a few days. Joint aspiration in these patients fails to demonstrate sodium urate or calcium pyrophosphate dihydrate crystals.

Treatment

The treatment of HIV-related psoriasis and PSA is complicated by the underlying immunodeficiency state and concern about worsening that state with anti-inflammatory/anti-immune agents. In the case of PSA, two strategies have been employed. Often improvement of skin lesions results in significant improvement of arthritis. In addition, medications directed specifically at joint inflammation are employed. In Reiter's syndrome and reactive arthritis, eradication of the underlying pathogen is also important.

1 Conservative therapy for arthritis includes nonsteroidal anti-inflammatory drugs, physical therapy, proper joint protection and analgesics. Systemic low dose corticosteroids (0.1–0.2 mg/kg prednisone-equivalent per day) can be helpful. Local intra-articular and intralesional corticosteroid injections have been recommended. Enthesial injection, at the tendon insertion, has also been helpful using a very limited amount of corticosteroid, i.e. 1–2 mg of triamcinolone acetonide.

2 Zidovudine, an inhibitor of HIV replication, has been demonstrated to be very effective for both HIV-related psoriasis and PSA. The usual dose is 1–1.2 g/day given in divided doses.

3 Retinoid therapy employing etretinate appears to be useful in HIV-related psoriasis, PSA and Reiter's syndrome. For instance,

etretinate at a dose of 0.75 mg/kg/day resulted in rapid clearing of skin lesions and improvement of arthritis in a 34-year-old male HIV-infected patient who had previously failed topical corticosteroids and oral methotrexate. This case report suggests that, if tolerated, etretinate might be the drug of choice for treatment of Reiter's syndrome associated with HIV.

4 Although PUVA is relatively contraindicated in HIV infection, it is uncertain whether it adversely affects the course of the disease. Therefore, the combination of retinoids and PUVA (Re-PUVA) may be used with caution for severe unresponsive PSA or Reiter's syndrome.

5 Hydroxychloroquine 200–400 mg/day improved arthritis and decreased the amount of recoverable HIV-1 RNA in plasma, and was not associated with worsening infection.

6 Sulfasalazine 2–3 g/day, was associated with improvement of the CD-4 count and symptoms of arthritis and arthralgia in HIV–Reiter's syndrome in four consecutive cases. Similar reports suggest that sulfasalazine may be useful and well tolerated in this clinical setting.

7 Initial reports using methotrexate for the treatment of HIV-related psoriasis, PSA or Reiter's syndrome demonstrated an increased frequency of opportunistic infection developing during treatment. More recent information suggests that methotrexate may be used if patients are treated with aggressive prophylaxis for opportunistic infections. Methotrexate should be used only after zidovudine, hydroxychloroquine, and sulfasalazine have proven to be ineffective or intolerable. An acceptable dose is 0.1–0.2 mg/kg per week given with folic acid supplementation.

8 Anecdotal reports have suggested that cyclosporine and auranofin may benefit HIV-related PSA without exacerbating immunodeficiency.

9 TNF inhibition is not currently recommended in HIV infected individuals. This is primarily due to the high risk of opportunistic infections and the reactivation of tuberculosis. The inhibition of IL-1 activity in patients with HIV infection remains unstudied.

Selected references

Abu-Shakra M., Gladman D. D., Thorne J. C. *et al.* (1995) Long-term methotrexate in psoriatic arthritis: clinical and radiological outcome. *J Rheumatol* **22**, 241–245.

Allen B. R. (1992) Use of cyclosporine for psoriasis in HIV-positive patients. (Letter). *Lancet* **339**, 686.

Belz J., Breneman D. L., Nordlund J. J. *et al.* (1989) Successful treatment of a patient with Reiter's syndrome and acquired immunodeficiency syndrome using etretinate. *J Am Acad Dermatol* **20**, 898–903.

Blackmore M. G., Gladman D. D., Husted J. *et al.* (1995) Measuring health status in psoriatic arthritis: the health assessment questionnaire and its modifications. *J Rheumatol* **22**, 886–893.

Blanche P., Saraux A., Taefann H. *et al.* (1992) Arthritis and HIV infection in Kigali, Rwanda. *Br J Rheumatol* **31** (Suppl.), 200.

Buskila D., Langevitz P., Gladman D. D. *et al.* (1992) Patients with rheumatoid arthritis are more tender than those with psoriatic arthritis. *J Rheumatol* **19**, 1115–1119.

Calabrese L. H. (1993) Human immunodeficiency virus (HIV) infection and arthritis. *Rheum Dis Clin North Am* **19**, 477–488.

Calabrese L. H., Kelley D. M., Meyers A. *et al.* (1991) Rheumatologic symptoms and human immunodeficiency virus infection: Influence of clinical and laboratory variables in a longitudinal cohort study. *Arthritis Rheum* **34**, 257–263.

Cantini F., Salvarani C., Olivieri I. *et al.* (2001) Distal extremity swelling with pitting edema in psoriatic arthritis: a case-control study. *Clin Exp Rheumatol* **19**, 291–296.

Cuchacovich M., Soto L. (2002) Leflunomide decreases joint erosions and induces reparative changes in a patient with psoriatic arthritis. *Ann Rheum Dis* **61**, 942–943.

Culy C. R., Keating G. M. (2002) Etanercept: an updated review of its use in rheumatoid arthritis, psoriatic arthritis and juvenile rheumatoid arthritis. *Drugs* **62**, 2495–2539.

Diez F., Del Hoyo M., Serrano S. (1990) Zidovudine treatment of psoriasis associated with acquired immunodeficiency syndrome. *J Am Acad Dermatol* **22**, 146–147.

Disla B., Rhim H. R., Reddy A., Taranta A. (1994) Improvement in CD4 lymphocyte counts in HIV-Reiter's syndrome after treatment with sulfasalazine. *J Rheumatol* **21**, 662–664.

Duvic M., Johnson T. M., Rapini R. P. *et al.* (1987) Acquired immunodeficiency syndrome associated psoriasis and Reiter's syndrome. *Arch Dermatol* **123**, 1622–1632.

Duvic M. (1990) Immunology of acquired immunodeficiency syndrome related to psoriasis. *J Invest Dermatol* **95**, S38–40.

Espinoza L. R., Cuellar M. L., Silveira L. H. (1992) Psoriatic arthritis. *Curr Opin Rheumatol* **4**, 470–478.

Espinoza L. R., Vasey F. B., Olt J. H. *et al.* (1978) Association between HLA-DW38 and peripheral psoriatic arthritis. *Arthritis Rheum* **21**, 72–75.

Farr M., Kitas G. D., Waterhouse L. *et al.* (1990) Sulfasalazine in psoriatic arthritis: a double-blind placebo-controlled study. *Br J Rheumatol* **29**, 46–49.

Feldges D. H., Barnes C. G. (1974) Treatment of psoriatic arthropathy with either azathioprine or methotrexate. *Rheumatol Rehab* **13**, 120–124.

Fraser S. M., Hopkins R., Hunter J. A. (1993) Sulfasalazine in the management of psoriatic arthritis. *Br J Rheumatol* **32**, 923–925.

Gaston L., Cromberz C., Lassonde M. *et al.* (1991) Psychological stress and psoriasis: experimental and prospective correlational studies. *ACTA Derm Venereol* **156** (Suppl.), 37–43.

Gladman D. D., Farewell V., Buskila D. *et al.* (1990) Reliability of measurements of active and damaged joints in psoriatic arthritis. *J Rheumatol* **17**, 62–64.

Gladman D. D., Farewell V. T. (1999) Progression in psoriatic arthritis: role of time varying clinical indicators. *J Rheumatol* **26**, 2409–2413.

Gladman D. D. (1992) Psoriatic arthritis: recent advances in pathogenesis and treatment. *Rheum Dis Clin North Am* **18**, 247–256.

Gladman D. D. (2002) Current concepts in psoriatic arthritis. *Curr Opin Rheumatol* **14**, 361–366.

Greaves M. W., Camp R. D. R. (1988) Prostaglandins, leukotrienes, phospholipase, platelet activating factor and cytokines: an integrated approach to inflammation of human skin. *Arch Dermatol Res* **280** (Suppl.), S33–S41.

Gupta A. K., Matteson E. L., Ellis C. N. *et al.* (1989) Cyclosporine in the treatment of psoriatic arthritis. *Arch Dermatol* **125**, 507–510.

Helliwell P., Marchesoni A., Peters M. *et al.* (1991) An evaluation of the osteoarticular manifestations of psoriasis. *Br J Rheumatol* **30**, 339–345.

Hochberg M. C., Fox R., Nelson K. E. *et al.* (1990) Human immunodeficiency virus infection is not associated with Reiter's syndrome. Data from Johns Hopkins Multicenter AIDS Cohort Study. *AIDS 1990* **4**, 1149–1151.

Hohler T., Kruger A., Schneider P. M. *et al.* (1997) A TNF-α promoter polymorphism is associated with juvenile onset psoriasis and psoriatic arthritis. **109**, 562–565.

Hopkins R., Bird H. A., Jones H. *et al.* (1995) A double-blind controlled trial of etretinate (Tigason) and ibuprofen in psoriatic arthritis. *Ann Rheum Dis* **44**, 189–193.

Husted J., Gladman D. D., Farewell B. T., Long J. A. (1996) Validation of the revised and expanded version of the arthritis impact measurement scales for patients of psoriatic arthritis. *J Rheumatol* **23**, 1015–1019.

Husted J. A., Gladman D. D., Farewell B. T. *et al.* (1997) Validating the SF-36 health survey questionnaire in patients with psoriatic arthritis. *J Rheumatol* **24**, 511–517.

Kammer G. M., Soter N. A., Gibson D. J., Shur P. H. (1979) Psoriatic arthritis: a clinical, immunologic and HLA study of 100 patients. *Semin Arthritis Rheum* **9**, 75–97.

Mease P. J., Goffe B. S., Metz J., Vanderstoep A., Finck B., Burge D. J. (2000) Etanercept in the treatment of psoriatic arthritis and psoriasis: randomized trial. *Lancet* **356**, 385–390.

Olivieri I., Barozzi L., Favaro L. *et al.* (1996) Dactylitis in patients with seronegative spondyloarthropathy. Assessment by ultrasonography and magnetic resonance imaging. *Arthritis Rheum* **39**, 1524–1528.

Pearlman S. G., Gerber L. H., Roberts R. M. *et al.* (1979) Photochemotherapy and psoriatic arthritis. A prospective study. *Ann Intern Med* **91**, 717–722.

Queiro R., Sarasqueta C., Belzunegui J. *et al.* (2002) Psoriatic spondyloarthropathy: a comparative study between HLA-B27 positive and HLA-B27 negative disease. *Semin Arthritis Rheum* **31**, 413–418.

Reveille J. D., Conant M. A., Duvic M. (1990) Human immunodeficiency virus-associated psoriasis, psoriatic arthritis and Reiter's syndrome: A disease continuum? *Arthritis Rheum* **33**, 1574–1578.

Roth S. H., Bennett R. E. (1987) Nonsteroidal antiinflammatory drug gastropathy. *Arch Int Med* **147**, 2093–2100.

Salaffi F., Manganelli P., Carotti M. *et al.* (1997) Methotrexate-induced pneumonitis in patients with rheumatoid arthritis and psoriatic arthritis: report of five cases and review of the literature. *Clin Rheumatol* **16**, 296–304.

Salvarani C., Cantini F., Olivieri I. (2002) Disease-modifying antirheumatic drug therapy for psoriatic arthritis. *Clin Exp Rheumatol* **20** (Suppl. 28), S71–S75.

Scander M. P., Ryan F. P. (1988) Nonsteroidal anti-inflammatory drugs and pain free peptic ulceration in the elderly. *Br Med J* **297**, 833–834.

Segal A. M., Wilke W. S. (1989) Toxicity of low-dose of methotrexate in rheumatoid arthritis. In: Wilke W. S. (ed.) *Methotrexate Therapy in Rheumatic Disease*. Marcel Dekker, New York, 147–178.

Seideman P., Fjellner P., Johannsson A. (1987) Psoriatic arthritis treated with oral colchicine. *J Rheumatol* **14**, 777–779.

Shakoor N., Michalska M., Harris C. A., Block J. A. (2002) Drug-induced systemic lupus erythematosus associated with etanercept therapy. *Lancet* **359**, 579–580.

Spadaro A., Riccieri B., Sili-Scadalli A. *et al.* (1995) Comparison of cyclosporine A and methotrexate in the treatment of psoriatic arthritis: a one-year prospective study. *Clin Exp Rheumatol* **13**, 589–593.

Steinsson K., Jonsdottir I., Valdimarsson H. (1990) Cyclosporine-A in psoriatic arthritis: an open study. *Ann Rheum Dis* **49**, 603–606.

Thivolet J., Robart S., Vignon E. (1981) Combined oral retinoid and PUVA therapy in the treatment of psoriasis and psoriatic arthritis. *Ann Dermatol Venereol* **108**, 131–137.

Torre Alonso J. C., Rodriguez Terez A., Arribas Castrillo J. M. *et al.* (1991) Psoriatic arthritis (PA): a clinical immunological and radiological study of 180 patients. *Br J Rheumatol* **30**, 245–250.

Van Ede E. A., Laan R. F. J. M., Rood M. J. *et al.* (2001) Effect of folic or folinic acid supplementation in the toxicity and efficacy of methotrexate in rheumatoid arthritis: a forty-eight-week, multicenter, randomized, double-blind, placebo-controlled study. *Arthritis Rheum* **44**, 1515–1524.

Wilfert H., Honigsmann H., Steiner G. *et al.* (1990) Treatment of psoriatic arthritis by extra corporeal photochemotherapy. *Br J Dermatol* **122**, 225–232.

Willkens R. F., Williams H. J., Ward J. R. *et al.* (1984) Randomized, double-blind, placebo-controlled trial of low-dose pulse methotrexate in psoriatic arthritis. *Arthritis Rheum* **27**, 376–381.

Wright V. (1956) Psoriasis and arthritis. *Ann Rheum Dis* **15**, 348–356.

Wright V. (1961) Psoriatic arthritis. A comparative radiographic study of rheumatoid arthritis and arthritis associated with psoriasis. *Ann Rheum Dis* **20**, 123–132.

Zboganova M., Trnavski K., Vicek F. (1974) Indomethacin in the treatment of psoriatic arthritis. *Czech Dermatol* **49**, 129–132.

22 Biologic immunotherapy of psoriasis

Kenneth Gordon

Over the past decade, advances in molecular biology have allowed for the development of new, targeted medications that can work to alter the course of many diseases. These new proteins can either mimic naturally occurring proteins, such as recombinant human insulin to treat deficiencies, or can interfere with ongoing patho-physiological processes by blocking the activity of a specific cell type or protein. As the mechanisms of disease are elucidated on the molecular level, these medications provide the hope that treatments can only target the processes central to the disease and leave normal systems and tissues intact. Thus, while these drugs may provide excellent efficacy, the central hope is that these medications can be given without significant multi-organ side-effects.

The advent of biologic medications for psoriasis is based on the observation that the most effective treatments for this disease modulate the immune response driving the keratinocyte reaction. Moreover, available therapies, including methotrexate, cyclosporine, and PUVA, are all limited by cumulative, dose-dependent side-effects on multiple organs. Thus, with the knowledge that psoriasis is a life-long disease, there is a need to find new, effective agents to treat the more severe forms of this condition with reduced risk of systemic toxicity. Biologic immunotherapies are being developed to fill this void for the benefit of patients with psoriasis.

Principles of biologic immunotherapy

Biologic agents are proteins that are designed through recombinant DNA technology to specifically interact with a cell surface protein or cytokine central to a disease process. In psoriasis, these drugs bind to specific markers on T-cells or on inflammatory cytokines that are central to the propagation of the disease. There are two methods to gaining the specificity required to make biologic medications that tightly interact with the target molecule but do not influence the function of normal tissues. The first is to make a monoclonal antibody. These antibodies are initially grown in animals, usually mice, to allow for the development of a specific binding site to a human protein. After the binding site is produced, the molecule is altered to make the remaining part of the monoclonal antibody as similar to human antibodies as possible. This "humanization" of the antibody makes it less likely a patient's own immune system will recognize the antibody as a foreign protein and develop a hypersensitivity response to the drug. The second method is to use the human body's own recognition tools to confer specificity. All target proteins for biologic medications also have their own receptor or group of receptors that are generally unique to that protein. Thus, using the binding site for this receptor with the addition of the Fc portion of human IgG to make the molecule last longer in the circulation, it is possible to make medications with the appropriate specificity. As this construct, termed a "fusion protein", is fully human, the likelihood of developing an immune response to the medication is reduced.

The target for these biologic medications is the immune response that drives the keratinocyte changes visible as a psoriatic plaque. As has been described elsewhere, psoriasis is a complex interaction between the innate and adaptive immune systems and keratinocytes. Effector T-cells must become activated and migrate to the skin, where they interact with the local innate immune cells including macrophages, dendritic cells, and natural killer T-cells, producing a series of cytokines, which alter the behavior of keratinocytes. There are multiple potential ways in which biologic areas can interact with, and inhibit this pathologic immune reaction. These include: (1) reducing the number of specific pathogenic T-cells; (2) blocking the ability of T-cells to become activated and migrate to the skin; (3) changing the pattern of cytokine secretion from a predominantly type 1 to type 2 response; or, (4) inactivating the post-secretory cytokines necessary for psoriatic changes. Each of these strategies has potential advantages and has been exploited during drug development.

Specific biologic medications for psoriasis

There are a number of medications in development for the treatment of psoriasis (Table 22.1). At the time of writing, there are three

Strategy 1	Strategy 3
Alefacept*	rhIL-4
Siplizumab	rhIL-10
	anti-IL-12

Strategy 2	Strategy 4
Efalizumab*	Etanercept**
CTLA-4Ig	Infliximab**
	Adalimumab**
	Anti-IFN-gamma

Table 22.1 Biologic medications being developed for psoriasis.

*FDA approved for psoriasis.
**FDA approved for indications other than psoriasis.

biologic medications approved by the United States Food and Drug Administration (FDA) for psoriasis-related indications: alefacept and efalizumab for psoriasis and etanercept for psoriatic arthritis. Infliximab has completed phase II studies in both psoriasis and psoriatic arthritis and is currently FDA approved for the treatment of Crohn's disease and rheumatoid arthritis. Though other biologics are in development programs, the discussion of specific agents will be limited to these four medications.

Alefacept

In February 2003, the FDA approved alefacept for the treatment of psoriasis, the first biologic medication approved for this indication. Alefacept is a fully human fusion protein consisting of two extracellular domains of leukocyte function-associated antigen type 3 (LFA-3) bound to the Fc portion of human IgG1. The LFA-3 binds to its natural ligand, CD2, expressed at high levels on CD45RO(+) T-cells, the effector T-cells that play the most significant role in the pathogenesis of psoriasis. While designed to block this important interaction for the activation of T-cells, the IgG portion can also bind to receptors on local macrophages and natural killer cells. These cells can, in turn, induce apoptosis in the effector T-cells. This second effect seems to account for a significant portion of the efficacy of the drug.

Alefacept can be given as either an intravenous (IV) push or intramuscular (IM) injection. In practice, more than 80% of U.S. dermatologists have preferred the IM route of administration. The injections are once a week for 12 consecutive weeks. While the FDA has approved alefacept for a single course, studies have used this medication in multiple courses after a 12-week period off-drug. Both of these methods have been demonstrated to be effective as monotherapy when compared to placebo in large, multi-center, placebo-controlled, phase III clinical trials (Table 22.2). In addition to the improvement in psoriatic plaques, alefacept seems to have the rather unique effect of inducing prolonged improvements in the overall disease, with the median length of clinically significant improvement of over 7 months for patients with excellent responses to the medication. Subsequent retreatment courses were well tolerated and as effective as the first course. For these reasons, the FDA has approved alefacept as a potential first line therapy for psoriasis in patients with moderate to severe disease who are candidates for any systemic therapy or phototherapy.

Safety has also been studied in detail with alefacept and the record in clinical trials is encouraging. Unlike traditional systemic treatments for psoriasis like cyclosporine, methotrexate, retinoids, and PUVA, there seems to be no toxicity to internal organs like the cardiovascular system, the kidneys, or the liver. Treatment of alefacept does lower the number of CD45RO(+) T-cells in the circulation, raising the possibility of a level of immunosuppression. However, in the clinical trials with this medication, there was no identifiable difference in the rate of infection in patients treated with alefacept when compared to placebo, and no opportunistic infections were seen. Moreover, there are data to suggest that novel immune responses to antigenic challenges in patients treated with alefacept remain intact. Nonetheless, the FDA recommends that patients' circulating CD4 counts be monitored and the drug held for counts less than $250/\mu l$. If counts drop below this level for four consecutive weeks, it is recommended that the medication be stopped. Care should be taken in using this medication, as with all potentially immunosuppressive drugs in patients who have ongoing infections or systemic cancer.

Table 22.2 Clinical efficacy of biologic immunotherapies for psoriasis.

Medication	Dose (duration)	PASI 50*	PASI 75*	Reference
Alefacept	15 mg IM/week	42% (week 14)	21% (week 14)	Ellis *et al.*
	7.5 mg IV/week	38% (week 14)	14% (week 14)	
Efalizumab	1 mg/kg/week SC (12 weeks)	57%	28%	Lebwohl *et al.*
	2 mg/kg/week SC (12 weeks)	55%	28%	Menter *et al.*
	1 mg/kg/week SC (24 weeks)	67%	44%	
Etanercept	25 mg SC b.i.w. (12 weeks)	58%	34%	Leonardi *et al.*
	50 mg SC b.i.w. (12 weeks)	74%	49%	Gottlieb, Leonardi, Zitnik
	25 mg SC b.i.w. (24 weeks)	70%	44%	
	50 mg SC b.i.w. (24 weeks)	77%	59%	
Infliximab	3 mg/kg IV infusion (week 0, 2, 6)		72% (week 10)	Gottlieb, Evans, Li *et al.* (2003)
	5 mg/kg IV infusion (week 0, 2, 6)		88% (week 10)	

*PASI refers to psoriasis area and severity index; 50 and 75 indicate ≥50% and ≥75% improvement in PASI score compared to baseline.
IM, intramuscular; IV, intravenous; SC, subcutaneous; b.i.w., twice weekly.

Etanercept

Etanercept is a fusion protein of the p75 receptor for tumor necrosis factor alpha (TNF) and the Fc portion of human IgG. This molecule binds and inactivates TNF in the target tissue and prevents its significant role in the development and propagation of the immune response in both psoriasis and psoriatic arthritis. It has been available for a number of years for the treatment of rheumatoid arthritis and in 2002 became the only medication approved by the FDA for the treatment of psoriatic arthritis. Etanercept has been clearly demonstrated to improve symptoms in patients with psoriatic arthritis. Even more importantly, however, etanercept seems to be a truly disease modifying medication as it prevents the progressive permanent bony degeneration seen in patients with psoriatic arthritis. Etanercept has also been shown to be effective as monotherapy for the treatment of psoriasis in large phase III randomized, placebo-controlled clinical trials. The recommended dose of etanercept for psoriatic arthritis is 25 mg, given subcutaneously twice a week. There is evidence in the phase III trials that a higher dose, 50 mg given subcutaneously twice a week, increases its efficacy for psoriasis (Table 22.2). A filing for approval for the treatment of psoriasis has been made with the FDA and approval is anticipated sometime in 2004.

Etanercept has been used to treat over 250,000 patients worldwide for rheumatoid arthritis and psoriatic arthritis. Thus, there is an extensive safety profile for this drug that is extremely good. As would be expected for a targeted biologic agent, there seem to be no significant multi-organ toxicities that require laboratory monitoring. The most common side-effect seen is a mild skin reaction at the injection site that occurs early in the course of therapy, is transient, and resolves with further dosing. There are, however, extremely rare side-effects that have been associated with treatment with etanercept for which a causal relationship is unclear. These include progression of demyelinating disease, possible drug-associated lupus erythematosus, worsening of congestive heart failure, and possible susceptibility to infections. TNF blockade in general has been associated with re-activation of preexisting tuberculosis, though there does not seem to be a causal relationship with etanercept. It should be remembered that all of these effects have not been definitively shown to be related to etanercept and should be viewed with caution when using this medication. To date, there are no limitations for the use of this medication in terms of total exposure or length of the course of therapy and many patients with rheumatoid arthritis remain on etanercept for multiple years.

Efalizumab

Efalizumab was approved by the FDA for the treatment of psoriasis in November 2003. Efalizumab is a humanized monoclonal antibody directed against leukocyte function-associated antigen type 1

(LFA-1), the primary ligand for intercellular adhesion molecule-I (ICAM-1). This interaction stabilizes the antigen presenting cell/ T-cell interaction, participates in co-stimulation, T-cell migration into the skin, and the ability of inflammatory cells to stay in activated plaques. Thus, efalizumab can block T-cell activation and migration into the skin. This medication is given as a subcutaneous injection once a week.

There has been an extensive phase III clinical trial program for efalizumab. Three multi-center, randomized, placebo-controlled trials of efalizumab have been performed with more than 2700 subjects. All of the trials demonstrate significant efficacy when compared to placebo at a dose of 1 or 2 mg/kg given once a week (Table 22.2). Importantly, ongoing long-term open label trials with efalizumab suggest that, during 21 months of efalizumab combined with UVB and topical anti-psoriasis therapy, patients continue to improve and retain their responsiveness to the medication. The drug is tolerated very well for extended periods of time with no increase in the incidence of adverse events. There are no multi-organ safety concerns identifiable in the clinical trials and there have been no significant drug-related laboratory abnormalities. The most significant side-effects are flu-like symptoms when the patient is given the first 2–3 doses, symptoms that resolve after the first few injections. Like most traditional treatments for psoriasis, the patient's disease tends to return quickly after discontinuation of the medication. It is likely that the medication's safety record, with no suggestion of cumulative multi-organ toxicity, will make efalizumab a continuous therapy to keep patients relatively disease-free.

Infliximab

Infliximab is a chimeric monoclonal antibody that, like etanercept, binds and inactivates TNF. Infliximab is approved for the treatment of Crohn's disease and rheumatoid arthritis and is in development for both psoriasis and psoriatic arthritis. Recent phase II results suggest that infliximab is extremely effective as monotherapy for psoriasis and with or without concomitant methotrexate in psoriatic arthritis. While long-term maintenance therapy with infliximab has been demonstrated to be effective in both of its indications, this has not yet been demonstrated in psoriatic disease, though this is being studied in the phase III trial program.

Infliximab is given as an IV infusion over 2 hours. The medication will likely be given with a loading regimen of 3–5 mg/kg given over 2 hours at weeks 0, 2, and 6 and an undetermined maintenance regimen.

The phase II safety profile of infliximab for psoriatic indications seems to be excellent (Table 22.2). Moreover, like etanercept, the safety profile of infliximab may be extrapolated from experience with more than 400,000 patients treated for nonpsoriatic indications. The most common side-effects of infliximab are infusion reactions occurring in some patients at the time the medication is given. The overwhelming majority of these reactions are mild and can be handled with pre-medication and slowing the rate of infusion. Fewer than 1% of infusions are associated with more severe reactions with nausea and hypotension. With infliximab, the association with reactivation with tuberculosis is more established and patients to be treated with this drug should have the appropriate tests for tuberculosis (purified protein derivative [PPD] and chest x-ray) prior to the initiation of therapy. The side-effects of the class of anti-TNF agents discussed with etanercept also apply to infliximab. While infliximab is earlier in development than the other agents discussed for psoriatic disease, this agent holds significant promise for the rapid treatment of patients for moderate to severe psoriasis.

Conclusion

Genetic engineering techniques have provided us with new medications that could offer significant improvements for acute and chronic care for patients with moderate to severe psoriasis. The specificity of these medications allows for effective treatment with fewer concerns for the multi-organ toxicities seen with more traditional therapies. With the recent approvals of alefacept and efalizumab for psoriasis and etanercept for psoriatic arthritis, and the continued development of infliximab, it is likely that practitioners and patients with psoriasis will have multiple new options of therapy for this disabling, chronic disease. See Table 22.3 for summary of how to use four new biologic immunotherapies for moderate to severe psoriasis.

Table 22.3 How to use biologic immunotherapy FDA-approved or likely to be approved for psoriasis.

Medication	Stage of development	Other indications	Prescribed or likely dose
Alefacept	FDA-approved	None	7.5 mg given as IV push or 15 mg IM given weekly for 12 weeks
Efalizumab	FDA-approved	None	0.7 mg/kg initial dose then 1.0 mg/kg given SC weekly
Etanercept	Completed Phase III	Psoriatic and rheumatoid arthritis	25 or 50 mg given SC twice a week
Infliximab	Completed Phase II	Rheumatoid arthritis and Crohn's disease	3, 5, or 10 mg/kg given as IV infusion weeks 0, 2, and 6 and then maintenance phase

Selected references

Asadullah K., Docke W. D., Ebeling M. *et al.* (1999) Interleukin 10 treatment of psoriasis: clinical results of a phase 2 trial. *Arch Dermatol* **135**, 187–192.

Baker B. S., Swain A. F., Valdimarsson H., Fry L. (1984) T-cell subpopulations in the blood and skin of patients with psoriasis. *Br J Dermatol* **110**, 37–44

Bos J. D., Hagenaars C., Das P. K. *et al.* (1989) Predominance of "memory" T cells (CD4+,CDw29+) over "naive" T cells (CD4+, CD45R+) in both normal and diseased human skin. *Arch Dermatol Res* **281**, 24–30.

Chaudhari U., Romano P., Mulcahy L. D. *et al.* (2001) Efficacy and safety of infliximab monotherapy for plaque-type psoriasis: a randomised trial. *Lancet* **357**, 1842–1847.

Ellis C. N., Krueger G. G. for the Alefacept Clinical Study Group (2001) Treatment of chronic plaque psoriasis by selective targeting of memory effector T lymphocytes. *N Engl J Med* **345**, 248–255.

Gottlieb A. B., Krueger J. G., Wittkowski K. *et al.* (2002) Psoriasis as a model for T-cell-mediated disease. Immunobiologic and clinical effects of treatment with multiple doses of efalizumab, an anti-CD11a antibody. *Arch Dermatol* **138**, 591–600.

Gottlieb A. B., Matheson R. T., Lowe N. J., Zitnik R. J. (2002) Efficacy of Enbrel in patients with psoriasis. *Presented at the 63rd Annual Meeting of the Society for Investigative Dermatology* **26** [abstract].

Gottlieb A. B., Evans R., Li S. *et al.* (2003) The efficacy and safety of infliximab induction treatment in subjects with severe plaque-type psoriasis. Presented at Summer Academy 2003 of the American Academy of Dermatology, July 25–29, Chicago, IL. Poster 49.

Gottlieb A. B., Leonardi C., Zitnik R. Efficacy and safety of etanercept in patients with psoriasis: results of a phase III study. Presented at Summer Academy 2003 of the American Academy of Dermatology, July 25–29, Chicago, IL. Poster 52.

Keane J., Gershon S., Wise R. P. *et al.* (2001) Tuberculosis associated with infliximab, a tumor necrosis factor alpha-neutralizing agent. *N Engl J Med* **345**, 1098–1104.

Krueger G. G., Papp K. A., Stough D. B. *et al.* (2002) A randomized, double-blind, placebo-controlled phase III study evaluating efficacy and tolerability of 2 courses of alefacept in patients with chronic plaque psoriasis. *J Am Acad Dermatol* **47**, 821–833.

Krueger J. G. (2002) The immunologic basis for the treatment of psoriasis with new biologic agents. *J Am Acad Dermatol* **46**, 1–23.

Lebwohl M., Papp K. A., Tyring S. *et al.* Continued treatment with subcutaneous efalizumab is safe: pooled results from two phase III trials. Presented at Summer Academy 2002 of the American Academy of Dermatology, July 31–4 Aug, New York, NY. Poster 47.

Leonardi C. L., Powers J. L., Matheson R. T. *et al.* (2003) Etanercept as monotherapy in patients with psoriasis. *N Engl J Med* **349**, 2014–2022.

Lowe N. J., Gonzalez J., Bagel J. *et al.* (2003) Repeat courses of intravenous alefacept in patients with chronic plaque psoriasis provide consistent safety and efficacy. *Int J Dermatol* **42**, 224–230.

Mease P. J., Goffe B. S., Metz J. *et al.* (2000) Etanercept in the treatment of psoriatic arthritis and psoriasis: a randomised trial. *Lancet* **356**, 385–390.

Mease P., Kivitz A., Burch F. *et al.* (2001) Improvement in disease activity in patients with psoriatic arthritis receiving etanercept (Enbrel): results of a phase 3 multicenter clinical trial. *Arthritis Rheum* **44**, S90.

Menter A., Toth D., Glazer S. *et al.* Efficacy and safety of 24-week continuous efalizumab therapy in patients with moderate to severe plaque psoriasis. Presented at Summer Academy 2003 of the American Academy of Dermatology, July 25–29, Chicago, IL. Poster 44.

Singri P., West D. P., Gordon K. B. (2002) Biologic therapy for psoriasis: the new therapeutic frontier. *Arch Dermatol* **138**, 657–663.

Index

Note: Page numbers followed by f indicate figures; those followed by t indicate tables.